CRITICAL
CARE
ASSESSMENT
HANDBOOK

CRITICAL CARE ASSESSMENT HANDBOOK

Sharron E. Murray, MS, RN

Former Faculty
California State University
Long Beach, California

Barbara S. White, DrPH, RN-Cs, ANP, GNP

Associate Professor
California State University
Long Beach, California

W.B. SAUNDERS COMPANY
A Division of Harcourt Brace & Company
Philadelphia   London   Toronto   Sydney   Montreal   Tokyo

W.B. SAUNDERS COMPANY

A Division of Harcourt Brace & Company

The Curtis Center
Independence Square West
Philadelphia, Pennsylvania 19106

Library of Congress Cataloging-in-Publication Data

Murray, Sharron E.
    Critical care assessment handbook / Sharron E. Murray, Barbara S.
White.
        p.   cm.
    Includes bibliographical references.
    ISBN 0-7216-6585-3
    1. Intensive care nursing Handbooks, manuals, etc.   2. Nursing
assessment Handbooks, manuals, etc.   I. White, Barbara S.
II. Title.
    [DNLM: 1. Critical Care—methods.   2. Nursing Assessment.
WY 154 M984c 1999]
RT120.I5M87   1999
610.73'61—dc21
DNLM/DLC
                                                                99-21517

CRITICAL CARE ASSESSMENT HANDBOOK   ISBN 0-7216-6585-3

Printed in the United States of America

Last digit is the print number: 9   8   7   6   5   4   3   2   1

To our patients who have taught us so much,
To the nurse at the bedside, the heartbeat of critical care nursing

And to our husbands, David and Dick,
who have become cooks and housekeepers on demand,
thank you for your unwavering support.

Sharron and Barbara

About the Authors

Sharron (Hayes) Murray, former faculty California State University Long Beach, has over 25 years of bedside, teaching, and consulting experience in critical care nursing and has taught courses in Canada and the United States in critical care nursing and physical assessment. She is a founding member of the British Columbia division of the Canadian Critical Care Nurses Association, a past CCRN, a member of the American Association of Critical Care Nursing, and a member of Sigma Theta Tau International Honor Society of Nursing. Previous publications include a variety of journal articles related to critical care nursing and physical assessment.

Barbara (Schwitz) White has been a nurse and educator for 30 years. Her clinical areas include medical-surgical nursing and coronary care. An adult/geriatric nurse practitioner since 1982 with experience both clinically and as an educator teaching physical assessment skills in a variety of acute and ambulatory settings, she currently practices in a geriatric clinic and teaches gerontological nursing to undergraduate and graduate nursing students.

Preface

The American Nurses Association Standards of Practice (ANA, 1991) emphasize that accurate and complete assessment of patients is essential to the diagnosis and treatment of human responses to actual or potential health problems. These beliefs are reflected in the American Association of Critical Care Nurses Process Standards (AACN, 1989), which specify that such data be collected on all critically ill adults.

Multiple nursing textbooks and handbooks address physical assessment techniques. Many of these references, however, do not discriminate between the full screening examination used for medical diagnosis and the physical assessment performed by the nurse at the bedside for evaluating the patient's response to actual or potential illness or treatment.

The *Critical Care Assessment Handbook* makes this distinction. The unique focus of the content is on how, when, and why to use these techniques in the care of the critically ill adult. Techniques that yield the most useful information are emphasized. Techniques that challenge the critically ill adult's ability to cooperate, as well as those that are difficult to perform, have been augmented with assessment tips to assist the practicing nurse and the nursing student achieve the best possible results in data collection. Because the focus of this comprehensive handbook is on assessment, discussion of interventions is minimal.

ORGANIZATION

The handbook is divided into three sections. Section I offers an overview of assessment techniques and introduces a framework for application of these techniques in the critical care setting. Because of the preponderance of elderly people in critical care areas, extensive geriatric considerations have been incorporated throughout the handbook and a separate chapter on the critically ill geriatric patient (Chapter 3) has been included. Section II offers a description of assessment techniques and applies these techniques to disorders frequently experienced in the critically ill adult. Section III incorporates a discussion of laboratory studies and bedside monitoring techniques commonly used to assist in the diagnosis of pathology in the critically ill adult.

Sections II and III are organized by body systems to facilitate retrieval of information and to correlate physical assessment findings with the pathophysiologic disorders, laboratory studies, and hemodynamic parameters. To foster an integrated approach to assessment of the critically ill adult, the Clinical Findings outlines in Section II, which apply assessment techniques to specific pathophysiologic disorders, are presented with laboratory and bedside monitoring findings inserted between history and physical assessment findings. In addition, because body systems do not function in isolation and pathology experienced in the critically ill adult often extends through one or more body systems, the reader is referred from section to section, chapter to chapter, and table to table for related information.

The *Critical Care Assessment Handbook* has been written to supplement the reader's current knowledge of anatomy, pathophysiology, and physical examination. Every effort has been made to keep explanations for normal findings and rationales for abnormal findings clear and concise yet comprehensive.

The range of normal values for laboratory studies and hemodynamic parameters is offered as a guideline. These values may vary slightly with different hospital laboratories and between the references cited. Numerous medications also may affect laboratory results, the scope of which is beyond this book. The reader is referred to drug and laboratory texts for more detailed discussions. In addition, because medication uses are continuously evolving, the reader is encouraged to review medication package inserts for specific information.

To keep the book a manageable size we have placed the reference list at the end of the text rather than at the end of each chapter. In addition to the reference list, a bibliography has been provided for the interested reader to explore.

Sharron Murray
Barbara White

Contents

Common Laboratory Studies and Bedside Monitoring Techniques, 613

I

Techniques and Types of Assessment

1

Techniques of Assessment

Physical assessment skills are a critical component of the nursing process. The data collected become the basis for nursing diagnoses and the planning, implementation, and evaluation of nursing care. Techniques used to collect data include the nursing history and the physical examination.

THE NURSING HISTORY

The nursing history is a detailed collection of subjective data focusing on the patient's physiological, psychological, and behavioral patterns. Often the critically ill adult is unable to participate in such an interview because of altered levels of consciousness, endotracheal tubes, tracheostomies, or the extent of the illness or injury. Interdisciplinary records, families, and significant others should be relied upon in such cases to provide the necessary information.

In the critical phase, only essential information should be collected (refer to Section II, "Focused Assessment: Techniques and System Disorders," Chapters 4 to 12, for essential data to be collected related to specific system disorders). General information that should be collected as the patient's condition and time permit is identified in the nursing history:

Table 1–1 *The Nursing History*

A. Identifying information
   1. Name
   2. Address and phone number

    3. Sex
    4. Birthdate, age
    5. Ethnic origin
    6. Marital status
    7. Religion
    8. Insurance
    9. Responsible party
  10. Advance directions for health care (living will, do not resuscitate, organ donation, etc.)

B. Chief complaint: A short description of the most important complaint, including duration.

C. History of present illness (HPI)
    1. Onset
      • Sudden or gradual
      • Mechanism of injury
      • Precipitating factors
    2. Characteristics of presenting symptom(s)
      • Location (exact and radiation)
      • Quality (crushing, burning, stabbing, aching, etc.)
      • Quantity or severity (must be measurable, i.e., pain scale, teaspoon, cup, etc.)
    3. Course
      • Timing (morning, evening, after meals, frequency, duration)
      • Factors that aggravate or relieve (rest, activity, medications, treatments)
      • Associated symptoms (cough, nausea, vomiting, etc.)
    4. Current medications (prescription and over-the-counter, including vitamins, minerals, herbs, and home remedies)
      • What medications are for
      • When last taken or omitted
    5. Impact of illness or injury on activities of daily living

D. Past medical history (PMH)
    1. Relevant childhood diseases
    2. Immunizations
    3. Allergies
    4. Addictions (smoking; medications, including analgesics, sedatives, alcohol, and recreational drugs)
    5. Major adult diseases
    6. Relevant hospitalizations, traumas, surgeries
    7. Environmental exposures

     8. Blood transfusions
     9. Foreign travel
   10. Sensory or motor limitations and prostheses

E. Family history
     1. Present state of health of relatives
     2. Presence of similar illness or symptoms in family members
     3. Chronic diseases
     4. Diseases with familial tendencies

F. Psychosocial, behavioral history
     1. Education
     2. Occupation
     3. Support systems (family, significant others), role relationships
     4. Spiritual, religious, and cultural practices; beliefs and values
     5. Personal habits and patterns (diet, food habits and preferences, elimination, activities, exercise, sleep, sexual and health practices)
     6. Self-concept (include mental and emotional status prior to hospitalization)
     7. Stress response (previous coping mechanisms)
     8. Communication needs or deficits

POINTS TO REMEMBER

▶ Use open-ended questions that will allow the person to explain the condition in his or her own words: This gives valuable clues to how the person perceives the condition.

▶ Ask questions that are critical to decision making first (HPI, PMH, drugs):
- Patients may not have energy for long discussions.
- When time is of the essence, patient history can be obtained simultaneously with the physical examination.

▶ If information is obtained from family members, it should be noted as such, because it may contain inaccuracies.

▶ Patients, families, and significant others should not be subjected to repeated questioning: To obtain information that is important but peripheral to an immediate situation, consider the following strategies:
- Conduct several short interviews.
- Use previously written records to fill in gaps (police and paramedic reports, physician notes).
- Be attentive to nonverbal clues such as body language in the patient, family, and significant others.

▶ Make every attempt to obtain an accurate translation for all non-English-speaking patients: The more accurate your history, the more you will be able to focus your physical examination.

Geriatric Considerations

- Make every attempt to obtain information directly from the elderly patient rather than from family members.
- The geriatric patient may appear confused or unresponsive due to alterations in vision or hearing that occur with aging. This can be corrected with strategies such as
  - Placing eye-glasses or hearing aid.
  - Facing the person when speaking.
  - Speaking with normal loudness and slightly lower pitch.
  - Decreasing distracting background noises.
- The geriatric patient often presents with one or several underlying chronic disease states that may affect treatment and response. Obtaining a complete and accurate past medical history is important.
- The geriatric patient may present with an extensive number of currently prescribed medications:
  - Retrieving information on all currently and recently prescribed medications and the history of their use is imperative (i.e., thyroid, digoxin, insulin, or oral hypoglycemics).
  - Look for indications of previous misuse (over- or under-medication); disuse (self-prescribed discontinuance); self-medication with borrowed, discontinued, expired, or over-the-counter drugs; and drug incompatibilities.

THE PHYSICAL EXAMINATION

The physical examination is a detailed collection of objective data using the techniques of inspection, palpation, percussion, and auscultation. These techniques are performed in sequence unless specified.

Inspection

Inspection involves the senses of sight, hearing, and smell:

- The eyes, ears, and nose are used to identify abnormalities that can be confirmed by other techniques of assessment.
- This may be described as "active looking."

Palpation

Palpation involves the sense of touch: The hands or fingertips are used to assess the size and shape of lesions and masses, texture and temperature of skin, character of pulsations and vibrations, symmetry of movement, and areas of tenderness.

Percussion

Percussion involves the use of the finger as a hammer to tap on the body surface to produce sound: In indirect percussion the finger strikes the examiner's stationary hand; in direct percussion the striking hand directly contacts the body surface.

The characteristic of a percussion tone is determined by the density of the medium through which the sound travels (the more dense the medium, the softer the tone):

- Air produces a loud sound referred to as resonance and hyper-resonance in the lung, and tympany in the abdomen.
- Fluid and organs produce a dull sound.
- Muscle and bone produce a flat sound.

Percussion is a useful tool to determine bladder fullness, as well as the abnormal presence of fluid or air in the abdomen or chest cavity.

Auscultation

Auscultation involves the use of a stethoscope to listen to sounds produced by the body:

- The diaphragm is used to auscultate high-pitched sounds such as the normal heart sounds (S_1 and S_2).
- The bell is used to auscultate low-pitched sounds such as extra heart sounds (S_3 and S_4).
- Major areas auscultated are the heart, the lungs, the abdomen, and the great vessels.

POINTS TO REMEMBER

▶ All of these techniques are not practiced all of the time on all critically ill patients. Rather, the nurse should be able to select the techniques that reveal the most appropriate and accurate information: How, when, and why to select the technique to fit the clinical situation are questions discussed in Section I, Chapter 2:

"Types of Assessment"; and in Section II, "Focused Assessment: Techniques and System Disorders," Chapters 4 to 12.

▶ Limit patient movement:
  • This is especially important for critically ill patients to conserve energy.
  • Limiting patient movement will also decrease oxygen demand.

▶ Tell the patient what you are doing and why, even when the patient is unconscious or sedated: Unexpected movements may stimulate the stress response, causing an increase in blood pressure, intracranial pressure, and oxygen demand.

▶ Maintain body alignment: Poor body alignment may cause a decrease in venous return and an increase in intracranial pressure. It may also be uncomfortable for the patient.

▶ Expose the area of the body being examined:
  • Inspection is not possible through bed linens.
  • Listening through bed linens distorts or obliterates sounds, giving inaccurate impressions that may lead to incorrect diagnoses.

▶ Use good lighting.

▶ Compare sides of the body: Look for *asymmetry* in appearance or response.

▶ Throughout the examination, maintain warmth and patient modesty:
  • Hypothermia may cause vasoconstriction, which in turn may decrease blood flow to the tissues.
  • Unnecessary exposure may cause anxiety, which in turn may stimulate the stress response, increase the metabolic rate, and increase oxygen demand.

2

Types of Assessment

Critically ill adults are found in a variety of settings in the hospital and the home. Many of these patients are elderly, debilitated, have major organ disease, or may have had surgical intervention. On the other hand, many of these patients are young, healthy adults with little or no history of previous illness who have become critically ill following severe trauma.

The type of assessment performed by the nurse varies with the needs of these specific populations of critically ill adults, and with the clinical situation. Four types of assessment facilitate efficient data collection to be used for clinical decision making: the initial or rapid assessment (Step 1), the baseline assessment (Step 2), the focused assessment (Step 3), and the ongoing assessment (Step 4).

INITIAL ASSESSMENT (STEP 1)

See Table 2–1.

The initial or rapid assessment (ABCDE) is completed in emergency situations or on first contact with the patient to identify life-threatening problems and facilitate immediate intervention.

ABC (Airway, Breathing, Circulation, and Consciousness)

The rapid assessment should begin with a careful observation of the PERSON in the bed, focusing on the ABCs.

D (Decision)

Life-Threatening Problem. If at any point during the ABC assessment a life-threatening problem is discovered, the appropriate

TABLE 2-1 Integration of Assessments of the Critically Ill Adult

Initial Assessment (Step 1)	Baseline Assessment (Step 2)	Focused Assessment (Step 3)

A. Airway Patency
1. Assess gas exchange:
  a. Look for chest expansion
  b. Listen with stethoscope for the presence of breath sounds
  c. Feel for the presence of expired air with a hand in front of mouth, nose, or artificial airway		

B. Breathing
1. Assess rate, depth, and regularity of respirations
	Respiratory System
	1. Inspect the chest for
	  a. Size
	  b. Shape
	  c. Symmetry of expansion
	2. Inspect the trachea for midline position
	3. Inspect respirations for
	  a. Rate
	  b. Depth
		Respiratory System
		1. Inspect nails for clubbing
		2. Palpate the chest for
		  a. Masses
		  b. Tenderness
		  c. Swelling
		  d. Crepitus
		  e. Fremitus
		3. Percuss the chest for
		  a. Resonance

b. Hyperresonance
c. Dullness

c. Breathing pattern
d. Use of accessory muscles
4. Auscultate breath sounds
   a. Normal
   b. Diminished or absent
   c. Adventitious
   d. Pleural friction rub
5. Note the presence of a cough; if productive, describe the amount, color, and consistency of sputum

C. Circulation
1. Assess quality, rate, and regularity of apical and carotid or radial pulses
2. Obtain blood pressure
3. Obtain body temperature reading

Cardiovascular System
1. Inspect color of skin and mucous membranes
2. Estimate capillary refill
3. Inspect jugular veins for distention
4. Inspect and palpate for edema: extremities, dependent areas
5. Palpate peripheral pulses and compare bilaterally
   a. Radial
   b. Femoral
   c. Pedal

Cardiovascular System
1. Inspect extremities and compare for
   a. Color
   b. Symmetry
   c. Hair growth
   d. Ulcerations
   e. Nail thickness
2. Palpate extremities for
   a. Temperature
   b. Pulses
      (1) Popliteal if pedal pulse(s) absent
      (2) Brachial if radial pulse(s) absent

Table continued on following page

TABLE 2–1 Integration of Assessments of the Critically Ill Adult *Continued*

Initial Assessment (Step 1)	Baseline Assessment (Step 2)	Focused Assessment (Step 3)

	6. Blood pressure
	7. Inspect the precordium for lifts, heaves, pulsations
	8. Auscultate the cardiac apex (mitral area) to evaluate heart sounds and heart rhythms
	  a. S_1 and S_2
	  b. Presence of extra heart sounds (S_3 and S_4)
	  c. Presence of murmurs
	  d. Presence of pericardial friction rub
	  e. Dysrhythmias
		3. Palpate the precordium for lifts, heaves, and thrills
		4. Evaluate the point of maximal impulse (PMI)
		5. Auscultate the neck for carotid bruits
		6. Auscultate the 5 cardiac areas to identify
		  a. Characteristics of S_1 and S_2
		  b. Characteristics of extra heart sounds
		  c. Characteristics of murmurs
		  d. Pericardial friction rub

C. Consciousness
1. Determine level of consciousness:
  a. Awareness and ease of arousal
  b. General response to verbal command
  c. General response to painful stimuli, if no verbal response
	Neuromuscular System
	1. Evaluate mental status:
	  a. *Conscious person*
	    (1) Level of orientation to time, place, person, and situation
	    (2) Memory for immediate, recent, and remote events
	    (3) Mood and behavior changes
		Neuromuscular System
		1. Assess sensory and motor function:
		  a. *Conscious person*
		    (1) Cranial nerves
		    (2) Muscle stretch and superficial reflexes
		    (3) Evaluation of muscle strength against resistance

(4) Level of physical and emotional comfort
b. *Altered consciousness:* Glasgow or other coma scale
2. Communication pattern *(conscious)*
   a. Ability to speak and any difficulties
   b. Method of communication, if unable to verbalize due to condition or equipment
3. Evaluate motor function and muscle strength
   a. *Conscious person*
      (1) Deformities
      (2) Range of motion
      (3) Voluntary and involuntary movement of extremities
      (4) Grip strength
      (5) Pedal pushes
   b. *Altered consciousness*
      (1) Cranial nerve tests that do not require consciousness, patient cooperation
      (2) Muscle stretch and superficial reflexes
      (3) Special reflex tests, as appropriate

Table continued on following page

13

TABLE 2–1 Integration of Assessments of the Critically Ill Adult *Continued*

Initial Assessment (Step 1)	Baseline Assessment (Step 2)	Focused Assessment (Step 3)
	b. *Altered consciousness* (1) Involuntary movements of extremities (2) Posturing	
D. Decision 1. Emergency intervention (hospital procedure and American Heart Association [AHA] cardiac care guidelines) 2. Position patient to minimize the work of breathing, maximize the outcome of respiratory effort, enhance tissue perfusion, and prevent complications		
E. Equipment *Airway/Breathing Support Equipment* 1. Note presence and type of artificial airway 2. Note presence and type of oxygen delivery system		

    a. Check for intactness and security of connections

    b. Ensure that prescribed flow rate is being delivered

3. Note presence of pulse oximeter and ensure oxygen saturation is within prescribed parameters

4. Note presence and type of mechanical ventilation

    a. Check for intactness and security of connections

    b. Ensure prescribed settings

    c. Verify that alarms are on

5. Note presence of a chest drainage system

    a. Check for intactness and security of connections and dressings

    b. Assess patency, water seal, pressure, bubbling, drainage

Table continued on following page

TABLE 2-1 Integration of Assessments of the Critically Ill Adult *Continued*

Initial Assessment (Step 1)	Baseline Assessment (Step 2)	Focused Assessment (Step 3)
Circulation Support Equipment		
1. Assess cardiac monitor equipment		
a. Check for intactness and security of connections		
b. Obtain rhythm strip		
2. Note presence and type of cardiac pacemaker		
a. Check for intactness and security of connections and dressings		
b. Ensure that method and mode of pacing are set as prescribed		

3. Evaluate central venous pressure, arterial and pulmonary artery catheters, and equipment
   a. Check for intactness and security of connections and dressings
   b. Calibrate equipment per hospital procedure and manufacturer's instructions
      (1) Obtain pressure readings
      (2) Obtain strips of waveforms
4. Evaluate other sources of life-support, such as intra-aortic balloon pumps and ventricular assist devices
   a. Check for intactness and security of connections and dressings
   b. Obtain pressure readings and strips of waveforms

Table continued on following page

TABLE 2–1 Integration of Assessments of the Critically Ill Adult *Continued*

Initial Assessment (Step 1)	Baseline Assessment (Step 2)	Focused Assessment (Step 3)

5. Assess peripheral and central lines for
   a. Medications, solution type, drip rate, and patency
   b. Assess infusion sites for swelling, heat, redness and other discoloration, and discharge
6. Note presence of urinary drainage systems
   a. Check for intactness and security of connections
   b. Assess for patency, color, and amount of urine.
7. Note presence and type of dialysis
   a. Check for intactness and security of connections and dressings
   b. Ensure patency
   c. Assess access sites for inflammation, discharge		

8. Assess wounds, dressings, drains, and orifices for bleeding or drainage and odor

Neurologic Support Equipment
1. Note presence of intracranial pressure catheter and equipment
   a. Check intactness and security of connections
   b. Calibrate per hospital procedure and manufacturer's instructions

Gastrointestinal System
1. Inspect the mouth and throat for secretions, obstructions, presence of dentures, loose teeth
2. Evaluate gag, cough, and swallow reflex
3. Inspect abdomen for contour, symmetry, pulsations, peristalsis, scars, lesions
4. Auscultate bowel sounds

Gastrointestinal System
1. Inspect the mouth and throat for masses, lesions
2. Inspect abdomen for distention, venous patterning
3. Measure abdominal girth in the presence of distention
4. Auscultate abdomen for bruits, venous hums

Table continued on following page

TABLE 2–1 Integration of Assessments of the Critically Ill Adult *Continued*

Initial Assessment (Step 1)	Baseline Assessment (Step 2)	Focused Assessment (Step 3)
		5. Percuss abdomen for tympany, dullness, shifting dullness
		6. Palpate abdomen for consistency, tenderness, masses
		7. Examine anus and rectum for impaction, stool color and consistency, masses
		8. Special tests
	Genitourinary System	**Genitourinary System**
	1. Urine	1. Evaluate urine specific gravity
	2. Inspect the suprapubic and perineal areas for distention, lesions, discharge	2. Percuss suprapubic area in the presence of distention
		3. Examination genitalia for
		a. Discharge
		b. Edema
		c. Lesions or masses
		d. Lymphadenopathy

Integumentary System

1. Inspect and palpate the skin for
   a. Color
   b. Temperature
   c. Moisture
   d. Turgor
2. Examine the skin for breaks in integrity
   a. Lesions
   b. Inflammation
   c. Pressure sores
   d. Invasive catheter sites
   e. Surgical incision sites
   f. Wounds

Integumentary System

1. Inspect and palpate lesions for
   a. Number
   b. Color
   c. Type
   d. Size
   e. Location
   f. Configuration
   g. Associated signs and symptoms (discharge, pruritus)

21

intervention is initiated per hospital procedure or emergency cardiac care guidelines (American Heart Association).

Positioning. The patient should be positioned to minimize the work of breathing, maximize the outcome of respiratory effort, enhance blood flow to the tissues, and prevent complications such as obstructed airway, aspiration of stomach contents, atelectasis, pneumonia, and increased intracranial pressure. General guidelines include

- The *unconscious patient* should be placed in a side-lying position to prevent airway obstruction and aspiration of stomach contents, and to facilitate the drainage of secretions, unless contraindicated by conditions such as physical injuries or surgical procedures.
- The *conscious patient* should be positioned with the head elevated 30 to 45 degrees to facilitate lung expansion and decrease workload on the heart, unless contraindicated by conditions such as spinal anesthesia or injury, surgical procedures, or hypotension.
- The *head-injured patient* should be positioned with the head elevated 30 degrees to decrease cerebral edema, unless otherwise indicated.
- Patients receiving *continuous feedings* through nasogastric tubes should be positioned with the head elevated at least 30 degrees to prevent aspiration, unless otherwise indicated.
- *Unstable critically ill patients,* conscious or unconscious, are usually intubated and mechanically ventilated and should be positioned with the head elevated 20 to 30 degrees to facilitate lung expansion and decrease workload on the heart where possible (sophisticated technology, hemodynamic instability, surgical procedures, spinal cord injury, and traumatic injuries may impose supine immobilization).
- *Patients with ventilation-perfusion mismatches* should be positioned to maximize gas exchange in the lungs (where possible, the good areas of the lung should be in the dependent position to match areas of ventilation with areas of blood flow).

E (Equipment)

The patient inspection is accompanied by an inspection of life-support equipment, bedside monitoring equipment, and patient equipment, including dressings, tubings, and drains. Providing a safe environment for the critically ill adult should be the priority:

- Oxygen or ventilatory support is established or maintained at the prescribed settings.
- Monitors, tubings, indwelling catheters, and drains are connected as ordered or assessed for intactness, security of connections, patency, and drainage.
- Central venous pressure, arterial, pulmonary artery, and intracranial catheters are connected and calibrated per hospital procedure, and baseline pressure readings and waveforms are obtained (see Chapter 14, "Hemodynamic Monitoring").
- Peripheral and central lines (including total parenteral nutrition) are assessed for intactness, security of connections, patency, drip rate, medications, and solutions.

POINTS TO REMEMBER

▶ Throughout the initial assessment, the nurse can decrease patient anxiety through verbal interactions, including simple explanations and reassurance where appropriate (this should be done for conscious and unconscious patients).

▶ Once the initial assessment is completed, a systematic assessment of the patient's major body systems should be performed (see Step 2, "Baseline Assessment").

BASELINE ASSESSMENT (STEP 2)

See Table 2–1.

In the critical illness setting, a complete data base related to specific pathology is collected by the physician(s) for the purpose of evaluating the etiology of the pathophysiological processes, and defining treatment. The nurse performs a systematic assessment of the patient's major body systems to establish a baseline of normals, so that response to treatment can be monitored and further problems may be anticipated and intervention initiated rapidly. This baseline assessment incorporates frequently performed skills and should be completed from head to toe to facilitate patient comfort, limit unnecessary movement, and conserve energy.

Respiratory System

In the baseline assessment, the priorities of respiratory assessment are airway patency and gas exchange. The baseline assessment includes an examination of the chest, trachea, respirations, breath sounds, and cough (see Table 4–1 for a detailed discussion of respiratory assessment techniques, and Chapters 13 and 14 for a discussion of the efficiency of gas exchange and respiratory monitoring).

Chest Size and Expansion. The chest should be inspected for size, shape, and symmetry of expansion:

- Increased anterior-posterior diameter (barrel chest) may be a sign of chronic obstructive lung disease or an indication of the normal aging process.
- Asymmetrical expansion may be related to conditions such as consolidation, pneumothorax, splinting at the site of injury or surgical incision, or a misplaced endotracheal tube.

POINT TO REMEMBER

▶ An increased thickness of the chest wall (barrel chest, obesity, muscular build) will diminish sound transmission during percussion and auscultation.

Trachea. The trachea should be inspected for midline position: Deviation from midline may be related to disorders such as tension pneumothorax.

Rate, Depth, and Pattern of Respiration and the Use of Accessory Muscles. Respirations should be assessed for the rate, depth, and pattern of respiration, and the use of accessory muscles:

- An increased respiratory rate may be seen in patients with conditions such as high anxiety levels, respiratory insufficiency, fever, shock, or brain-stem lesions.
- A decreased respiratory rate may be related to conditions such as the use of narcotics or sedatives, and neuromuscular disorders.
- Shallow respiration may be related to factors such as respiratory depression from drugs or alcohol, pain from injury or incisions, obesity, or tight dressings that restrict thoracic or abdominal movement.
- Rapid and deep respirations may be a sign of anxiety or metabolic or neuromuscular dysfunction.
- Cheyne-Stokes respirations may be seen in the elderly and the obese or associated with conditions such as central nervous system depression, cardiac and renal failure, and narcotic use.

- The use of neck and diaphragmatic muscles, intercostal retractions, bulging, tracheal deviation, and nasal flaring may indicate respiratory distress related to conditions such as airway obstruction, air trapping, and neuromuscular or respiratory disorders.

POINT TO REMEMBER

▶ In the adult patient the normal respiratory pattern varies with the gender:
  - The adult female usually demonstrates chest expansion with respiration while the adult male usually demonstrates abdominal expansion.
  - The geriatric patient, regardless of gender, demonstrates abdominal movement.

Auscultation of Breath Sounds. Anterior, lateral, and posterior lung fields should be auscultated to determine the presence of normal breath sounds, diminished or absent breath sounds, and adventitious sounds:

- Diminished or absent breath sounds on auscultation are abnormal findings that may indicate conditions such as pneumothorax, obstruction, atelectasis, fluid within the pleural space, or incorrect placement of an endotracheal tube.
- Adventitious sounds are abnormal sounds superimposed on normal breath sounds (crackles, sibilant wheezes, sonorous wheezes or rhonchi, and pleural friction rubs) and may indicate the presence of factors such as fluid overload, poor mobilization of secretions, obstruction to air flow, oscillation of upper airways, or inflammation of lung surfaces.

POINTS TO REMEMBER

▶ Auscultation of breath sounds may be difficult with the critically ill adult, because patients often cannot respond to the command to breathe deeper than normal through the mouth and are unable to sit forward.

▶ Position changes provide an invaluable opportunity to listen to posterior lung fields (see Table 4–1).

▶ An inspiratory wheeze may be heard over the trachea with upper airway obstruction and an expiratory wheeze may accompany lower airway obstruction.

▶ Secretions, particularly those associated with a cardiac cause, tend to pool in the dependent lung fields (pulmonary secretions may or may not be gravity dependent).

▶ Atelectatic crackles may be heard in the dependent portions of the lungs in the asleep and in the elderly population (atelectatic crackles will clear following a cough or a few deep breaths).

Cough
- A dry cough may indicate irritation or partial obstruction of the airways.
- A productive cough may be a sign of respiratory infection.

Cardiovascular System

In the baseline assessment, the priorities of cardiovascular assessment are the evaluation of cardiac output and blood flow to the tissues. The baseline assessment includes an examination of the skin and mucous membranes, nails, jugular veins, edema, peripheral pulses, blood pressure, precordium, and cardiac apex (see Table 5–1 for a detailed discussion of cardiovascular assessment techniques, and Chapter 14 for a discussion of oxygen delivery, oxygen consumption, and hemodynamic parameters).

Skin and Mucous Membranes
- The lips, ear lobes, and mucous membranes should be inspected for central cyanosis (a bluish discoloration resulting from a large amount of deoxygenated hemoglobin in the capillaries).
- The extremities should be inspected for peripheral cyanosis (a bluish discoloration resulting from diminished blood flow).

POINTS TO REMEMBER
▶ The anemic patient with hypoxia will be pale (not cyanotic) because of decreased hemoglobin.
▶ The polycythemic patient may be cyanotic when oxygenation is adequate.

Nails. The nail beds should be assessed for capillary refill:
- Blanching of the nail beds should produce a return of color in less than 2 seconds.
- Slow capillary refill time (greater than 2 seconds) may indicate decreased blood flow to the tissues.

Neck Veins. The neck veins should be assessed for flatness or distention:

- Flat veins with the patient in a horizontal position may indicate hypovolemia or massive vasodilation.
- Distended neck veins with the patient's head elevated 30 to 45 degrees may indicate conditions such as fluid overload, heart failure, cardiac tamponade, or tension pneumothorax.

Edema. The extremities and the periorbital, scrotal, and sacral areas should be inspected and palpated for edema:

- Unilateral edema may be related to a local or peripheral cause.
- Bilateral edema or generalized edema (anasarca) may be related to disorders such as right heart failure, kidney failure, distributive types of shock (neurogenic anaphylactic, septic), or multiple organ dysfunction.

Pulses. Bilateral peripheral pulses should be palpated and compared for rate, rhythm, and quality:

- Decreased or absent arterial pulses may result from decreased circulation to the extremities secondary to factors such as decreased cardiac output, obstruction to blood flow associated with peripheral vascular disease or invasive lines, and immobility.
- A decrease in the pulse on inspiration, pulsus paradoxus, may be a sign of pericardial tamponade.
- Pulsus alternans, alternating weak and stronger beats, is a sign of left ventricular failure.

Blood Pressure. Alterations in blood pressure readings are common in the critically ill adult. If possible, the patient's normal blood pressure should be ascertained for comparison.

- Hypotension may be associated with numerous factors, including hypovolemia, decreased cardiac output, peripheral pooling of blood, vasodilation, position changes, and medications.
- Hypertension may be associated with numerous factors, including anxiety, pain, hypovolemia, vascular disease, medications, and increased sympathetic activity in response to the stress of injury, illness, or hospitalization.

POINTS TO REMEMBER

► In the critically ill adult, blood pressure is usually monitored with an intra-arterial catheter (see Chapter 14, "Arterial Pressure").

► Mean arterial pressure is generally a more accurate reflection of blood flow in the hypotensive or vasoconstricted patient (cuff pressure may be unobtainable in the patient with shock).

Precordium. The precordium should be inspected in the supine position for visible heaves, lifts, and pulsations:

• Heaves or lifts may be associated with disorders such as heart failure.

• The point of maximum impulse (PMI) should be at the fifth intercostal space, midclavicular line (displacement may indicate disorders such as ventricular hypertrophy or thoracic masses).

POINT TO REMEMBER

► The PMI is often not visible in a large percentage of the population.

Heart Sounds. Heart sounds should be auscultated at the cardiac apex (mitral area):

• As the myocardium is depressed, heart sounds may decrease in quality and loudness.

• Muffled heart sounds may be an indication of disorders such as pericardial tamponade.

• Distant heart sounds may be the result of factors such as a thickened chest wall.

• Distant heart sounds are common in the elderly.

• Murmurs may be heard in association with disorders such as hypertension, valvular disease, and ventricular septal perforation; and in hyperdynamic states such as fever, anemia, or septic shock.

• An extra heart sound, such as S_3, may be heard in patients with conditions such as heart failure and fluid overload, or in the young adult.

• An extra heart sound, such as S_4, may be heard in patients with poorly compliant ventricles.

- An S_4 may be heard normally with aging.
- A pericardial friction rub may be heard with pericarditis.

POINTS TO REMEMBER

▶ For the beginning practitioner, many of these sounds are difficult to identify.

▶ Critical care and emergency areas are often noisy, making it difficult to isolate sounds.

▶ In the baseline assessment, the emphasis on assessing heart sounds should be on noting the clarity of S_1 and S_2, from whence changes can be identified.

Heart Rhythm. Alterations in heart rhythm are frequent in the critically ill adult (see Table 14–3 for a detailed discussion of dysrhythmias):

- Tachycardia may be associated with conditions such as fever, pain, anxiety, blood loss, hypoxemia, hypovolemia, shock, heart failure, an increased stress response, and metabolic problems.
- Bradycardia may be associated with conditions such as an increased vagal response, hypothermia, neurogenic shock, metabolic disorders, cardiac disease, and a physically conditioned adult.
- Ventricular and supraventricular ectopic beats may be associated with factors such as hypoxemia, electrolyte and acid-base imbalances, drug toxicities, and an increased stress response.

POINTS TO REMEMBER

▶ Tachycardia may be harmful to the critically ill adult, as it can decrease cardiac output and increase oxygen consumption.

▶ Bradycardia may be harmful to the critically ill adult, as it can decrease cardiac output and precipitate hypotension, chest pain, and dysrhythmias.

▶ Frequent ectopic beats may reduce cardiac output and become life-threatening.

Central Nervous and Musculoskeletal Systems

The central nervous system and musculoskeletal system are evaluated simultaneously. This simultaneous evaluation is referred to as the neuromuscular assessment. In the baseline assessment, the priorities of neuromuscular assessment include an examination of mental status, speech, motor function, and muscle strength (see Table 6–1 for a detailed discussion of neuromuscular assessment techniques, and Chapter 14 for a discussion of intracranial pressure monitoring).

Mental Status. Critically ill adults vary in levels of consciousness from fully awake to completely comatose.

Conscious Patient. The mental status evaluation includes an assessment of the level of orientation, memory, and behavior, as well as the level of physical and emotional comfort:

- Advancing age, unfamiliar environments, enforced isolation, and medications contribute to confusion, disorientation, and behavioral changes.
- Pain and anxiety are common in the critically ill adult.
- Feelings of helplessness and powerlessness may contribute to fear and anxiety and enhance the perception of pain.
- Clinical manifestations of pain and anxiety include increased blood pressure, tachycardia, increased respiratory rate, dilated pupils, increased muscle tension, cold and moist skin, and nausea.

POINT TO REMEMBER

▶ A thorough evaluation of all assessment parameters should be completed to identify the cause of behavioral deviations:
- In addition to pain, anxiety, and medications, restlessness, agitation, confusion, and disorientation may be related to cerebral hypoxia, bleeding, or increasing intracranial pressure.
- In the elderly, confusion may be the presenting sign of infection.

Patient with Altered Level of Consciousness. The mental status evaluation includes an assessment of spontaneous activity, response to verbal stimuli, and response to painful stimulation. In many critical care settings, the Glasgow coma scale (see Table 6–1) or some other coma scale is used to give an accurate reflection of the level of consciousness for patients with alterations:

- Assess for spontaneous activity before stimulating the patient.
- If there is no spontaneous activity, then proceed to verbal stimulation.
- If there is no motor response to a verbal command, proceed to painful stimulation:
  - The response to painful stimuli will vary with the degree of impairment of consciousness.
  - The patient may try to localize or push away from the stimulus, or as brain deterioration progresses, may exhibit abnormal reflex responses referred to as posturing.

POINTS TO REMEMBER

▶ Consciousness and voluntary movement are integrated and measured by the ability to obey a command.

▶ Often the critically ill adult is unable to respond to a command because of medication, traumatic injuries, paralysis, neuromuscular disorders, or lack of comprehension, *not because of loss of consciousness.*

▶ Every effort should be made to ascertain response, including examination of the eyes for tears, staring, and blinks, and assessment of the face for changes in expression.

Speech. Assessment of speech (coherency and appropriateness) may be difficult with the critically ill adult, as communication may be affected by artificial airways, altered levels of consciousness, and language barriers: Throughout the assessment, the nurse should be on the alert for patient attempts at nonverbal communication (groaning, grunting, and crying may be vocalizations of pain).

POINT TO REMEMBER

▶ Eye blinks and limited movement of the extremities, such as hand grips, may be the only method of communication for some critically ill adults.

Motor Function and Muscle Strength. In the conscious patient, motor function and muscle strength may be evaluated together: Extremities should be assessed for deformities, limitations in range of motion, voluntary and involuntary movement of extremities, weakness, and unequal hand grips or pedal pushes.

In the patient with an altered level of consciousness, spontaneous or involuntary movement of extremities may be present.

Gastrointestinal System

In the baseline assessment, the priorities of gastrointestinal assessment include an examination of the mouth and throat; evaluation of the gag, cough, and swallow reflex; inspection of the abdomen; and auscultation of bowel sounds (see Table 7–1 for a detailed discussion of gastrointestinal assessment techniques).

Mouth and Throat. The mouth and throat should be inspected for odor, swelling, lesions, blisters, hydration, intactness of teeth, dentures, and the presence of obstructive mucous or foreign objects:

- Odor, swelling, lesions, and blisters may be due to infection, trauma, immunologic or malignant disease.
- A dry mouth may be due to mouth breathing, a side effect of many drugs used by the elderly patient (for example: antihypertensives, anticholinergics, bronchodilators), or a sign of dehydration (oral mucous membranes will be dry, lips dry and cracked).
- Teeth, dentures, and mucous plugs may block the airway.

Gag, Cough, and Swallow Reflex. The presence of a gag, cough, and swallow reflex should be assessed: The gag reflex protects the airway and assists in the prevention of aspiration of stomach contents.

Abdomen. The abdomen should be inspected for distention, pulsations, and venous patterning:

- Distention may be related to disorders such as ascites, paralytic ileus, early intestinal obstruction, or obesity.
- Pulsations may be related to disorders such as hypertension and abdominal aortic aneurysm.
- Venous patterning may be related to disorders such as liver disease (cirrhosis or portal hypertension).

Bowel Sounds. Bowel sounds should be auscultated in all four quadrants:

- Hypoactive bowel sounds may be related to factors such as analgesics, late bowel obstruction, paralytic ileus following abdominal trauma or surgery, and shock (sluggish bowel sounds may be a sign of gastrointestinal shunting, see Chapter 14, Gastric Tonometry).
- Hyperactive bowel sounds may be related to early conditions such as bowel obstruction, diarrhea, and subsiding paralytic ileus.

Genitourinary System

In the baseline assessment, the priorities of genitourinary assessment include an evaluation of the urine and inspection of the suprapubic area and perineum (see Table 8–1 for a detailed discussion of genitourinary assessment).

Urine. The urine should be assessed for color, amount, and characteristics:

Color
- Colorless urine may be due to factors such as diuretics and overhydration, or disorders such as diabetes mellitus and diabetes insipidus.
- Cloudy, smoky, hazy urine may be due to infection (pyuria, bacteriuria).
- Red or pink urine may reflect hematuria due to trauma, infection, renal, or urinary tract disease.
- Dark yellow or orange urine may be due an increase in urine bilirubin related to liver disease.

Amount
- Decreased urine output may be due to conditions such as decreased cardiac output, hypovolemia, dehydration, or renal disease.
- As well, decreased urine output may be related to an inability to communicate the need to void, neurogenic bladder, and blockages in drainage systems.

Characteristics
- Urine may be concentrated with a high specific gravity due to factors such as an increase in the level of antidiuretic hormone

(ADH), dehydration, fever, proteinuria, glycosuria, adrenal insufficiency, or heart failure:

– An increase in the action or level of ADH may be related to conditions such as surgery, severe pain, increased stress response, syndrome of inappropriate ADH (SIADH), and to analgesics such as morphine or meperidine.

– Dehydration may be related to factors such as the decreased intake of fluid (for example, the elderly and unconscious patients are susceptible), or an increased fluid loss (for example, conditions such as severe diaphoresis, vomiting, diarrhea, and burns).

• Urine may be dilute with a low specific gravity related to conditions such as decreased levels of ADH (diabetes insipidus), diuretics, increased fluid intake, and renal disease.

POINT TO REMEMBER

▶ The ability of the kidneys to concentrate and excrete urine (specific gravity) decreases proportionately with age.

Suprapubic Area. The suprapubic area should be assessed for distention: In severe urinary retention a visible bulge may be seen in the suprapubic area (the area will be firm on palpation and dull to percussion).

Perineum. The perineal area should be inspected for lesions, swelling, discoloration, and discharge: Infection may be due to indwelling urinary catheters or vaginal or sexually transmitted diseases.

Integumentary System

In the baseline assessment, priorities of integumentary assessment include an evaluation of the color, temperature, moisture, turgor, and integrity of the skin (see Table 12–1 for a detailed assessment of the integumentary system).

Color. Alterations in color may be due to factors such as decreased blood flow to the tissues, hypoxemia, anemia, polycythemia, or local or generalized vasodilation or inflammation.

Temperature

- Generalized cold (hypothermia) skin may reflect a central circulatory disturbance related to disorders such as cardiogenic shock.
- Generalized warm (hyperthermia) skin may reflect an increased metabolic rate related to disorders such as fever (sepsis) or hyperthyroidism.

Moisture. Diaphoresis may reflect factors such as an increase in sympathetic nervous stimulation (anxiety, pain, stress response).

Turgor. Decreased turgor may be due to dehydration:

- Turgor should be analyzed with other indicators of hydration, because elasticity of the skin decreases with aging.
- Decreased turgor alone may not be a reliable finding.

Integrity. The integrity of the skin may be affected by factors such as decreased blood flow to the tissues, edema, immobility, surgical procedures, trauma, invasive catheters, and disease:

- The skin should be assessed for the presence of lesions and inflammation.
- Pressure sites should be evaluated for redness and breakdown (decubitus ulcers).
- Sites of invasive catheters should be evaluated for redness, heat, swelling, odor, tenderness, and drainage.
- Dressings, wounds, and exposed suture lines should be assessed for intactness and drainage:
  - Drainage should be described in terms of color, consistency, odor, and amount.
  - The amount of drainage should be quantified in measurable (objective) terms such as a $4'' \times 2''$, teaspoon, and cup (terms like *moderate* and *large* are subjective: the definition may change with the observer).

POINTS TO REMEMBER

▶ Throughout the baseline assessment, the nurse must be on the alert for abnormal clinical findings.

▶ Abnormalities may indicate the need for intervention or a more thorough assessment of the system or systems involved (see Step 3 and Section II, "Focused Assessment").

FOCUSED ASSESSMENT (STEP 3)

See Table 2–1 and Section II: Chapters 4 to 14.

The focused assessment is completed in addition to the initial and baseline assessments. The diversity and extent of the focused assessment is unique to the individual critically ill adult.

The focused assessment may incorporate less frequently performed skills in a more thorough examination of the system or systems involved with the primary disorder:

For example, a previously healthy, 19-year-old male presents with an acute head injury: The nurse may collect data in the initial assessment, the baseline assessment, and the focused neuromuscular assessment (see Tables 2–1 and 6–1 and Clinical Findings 6–1 to 6–4).

Many critically ill adults have multiple organ dysfunction. Focused assessments should be completed in addition to the baseline assessment for all the systems involved with the pathophysiological processes:

For example, a 65-year-old male presents with an extensive acute myocardial infarction and subsequently develops cardiogenic shock. Impaired contractility, reduced arterial blood flow, and vasoconstriction may lead to respiratory failure, cerebral ischemia, renal failure, and decreased peripheral blood flow: The nurse may collect data in the initial assessment, the baseline assessment, and the focused respiratory, cardiovascular, neuromuscular, gastrointestinal, and genitourinary assessments (see Tables 2–1, 4–1, 5–1, 6–1, 7–1, and 8–1, and Clinical Findings 4–1, 5–1 to 5–3, 8–1, and 12–3).

Geriatric patients often have multiple disease processes and are more easily compromised due to changes with aging. Focused assessments should be completed in addition to the baseline assessment for each underlying disease process:

For example, a 78-year-old woman with a history of heavy smoking, chronic obstructive lung disease, and heart failure is admitted with a cerebrovascular accident: The nurse may collect data in the initial assessment, the baseline assessment, and the focused respiratory, cardiovascular, and neu-romuscular assessments (see Tables 2–1, 4–1, 5–1, and 6–1 and Clinical Findings 4–8, 5–1, 5–2, and 6–5).

ONGOING ASSESSMENT (STEP 4)

The ongoing assessment is an evaluation of the critically ill adult's rapidly changing status:

- Selected skills may be used to evaluate isolated problems or the resolution of the problems: For example, breath sounds may be auscultated in bilateral lung fields before and after insertion of an endotracheal tube.
- A repertoire of skills may be used to continuously evaluate complex problems or the resolution of the problems: For example, breath sounds, heart sounds, blood pressure, and evaluation of the level of consciousness may be some of the skills used to evaluate blood flow to the tissues following cardiopulmonary arrest and successful resuscitation.

PUTTING IT ALL TOGETHER

The initial, baseline, and focused assessments should be completed in steps as the nurse makes the first contact with the patient (usually this occurs at the beginning of a shift, on admission to an emergency room or a nursing unit, or on initial contact during a home visit).

The assessment changes as the patient's condition improves or deteriorates (ongoing assessment):

- As the patient's condition deteriorates, the initial, baseline, and focused assessments may be repeated numerous times and not necessarily in sequence.
- As the patient's condition improves, more emphasis can be placed on psychosocial assessment and the health promotion needs of the patient and family.
- As the patient's condition becomes less critical, opportunity to focus attention on identification of pathologies that are not directly related to the acute problem but may affect patient outcomes and the quality of life may arise (e.g., breast mass or scrotal mass may be detected and reported to the physician).

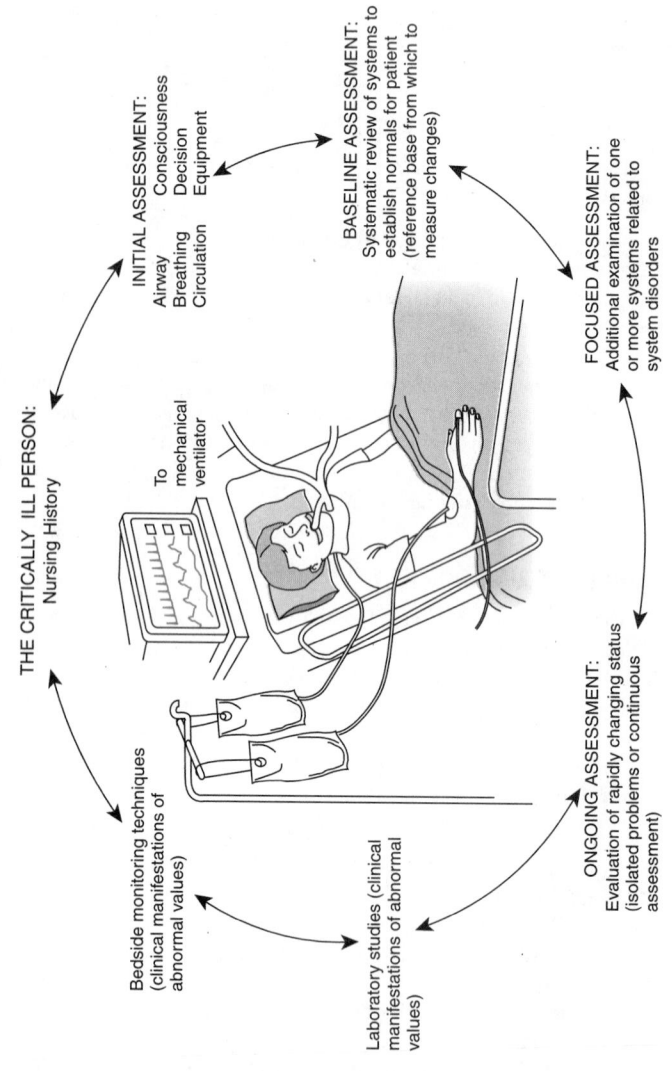

THE CRITICALLY ILL PERSON:
Nursing History

INITIAL ASSESSMENT:
Airway
Breathing
Circulation
Consciousness
Decision
Equipment

BASELINE ASSESSMENT:
Systematic review of systems to
establish normals for patient
(reference base from which to
measure changes)

To
mechanical
ventilator

FOCUSED ASSESSMENT:
Additional examination of one
or more systems related to
system disorders

Bedside monitoring techniques
(clinical manifestations of
abnormal values)

ONGOING ASSESSMENT:
Evaluation of rapidly changing status
(isolated problems or continuous
assessment)

Laboratory studies (clinical
manifestations of abnormal
values)

SUMMARY

In summary, collection of data in a logical and organized fashion assists the nurse in evaluating the response of the patient to actual problems, while anticipating and possibly preventing potential health problems. Throughout the assessment (initial, baseline, focused, or ongoing), the nurse is challenged to think critically:

- Is there a life-threatening problem requiring immediate intervention?
- Is there a problem requiring prompt intervention to prevent deterioration?
- Is there an abnormal finding requiring further investigation before any decisions can be made?

3

The Critically Ill Geriatric Patient

The high census of elderly in critical care areas will not only persist, but probably increase. It is estimated that beyond the year 2000 approximately 13% of the population of the United States will be 65 years of age or older. This percentage is expected to rise to almost 22% by the year 2030 when the "baby boomers" have all reached 65. Life expectancy is also increasing. Currently the fastest growing segment of the population is the age group that is 85 and older.

AGING AND DISEASE

It is not possible to make generalizations about the group of people who are 65 and older. Individual characteristics vary widely within this group. Age, by itself is not an adequate predictor of outcomes in the critically ill person, however, nurses must keep in mind trends that occur with aging when assessing the geriatric patient.

Study of human growth and development indicates that the response of older persons to illness events may not be exactly the same as that of younger adults. The nurse must, therefore, be attentive to possible variations in the expected physiologic and psychologic response to acute illness in the geriatric patient (see Table 3–1). These variations may be caused by the following:

- *Decreased immune response,* which may result in increased susceptibility to
  - Infection
  - Autoimmune response

TABLE 3–1 Factors Influencing Disease Development with Aging

Decreased immune response
Altered homeostatic mechanisms
Diminished functional reserve
Reaction to social losses
Alterations in physiologic and functional states with age
Multiple chronic disease states
Underreporting of symptoms
Atypical symptom expression
Altered physiologic response to therapy

  - Tissue rejection
  - Malignancy
- *Altered homeostatic mechanisms,* which may result in
  - Slower increase in heart rate in response to stress and slower return to baseline values
  - Less temperature elevation in response to infection
  - Glucose intolerance
  - Slowed response to changes in plasma volume
  - Altered response to drugs and less tolerance of multiple drug therapies
- *Diminished functional reserve* to deal with adverse events, which may result in
  - Atypical signs and symptoms of acute conditions
  - More rapid decompensation in the presence of physical and psychological stressors
  - Slower recovery from illness stressors
- *Social losses with aging,* which may affect response to illness and slow the pace of recovery
  - Death of family, friends
  - Economic losses
  - Role changes
  - Increased dependence on others

The critical care nurse is further challenged in assessing the geriatric patient due to possible changes in the response of the elderly person to treatment. The nurse must be aware of the following:

- *Underlying alterations in physiological and functional states,* including
  - Skin integrity
  - Sight, hearing, touch
  - Mobility
  - Nutrition
  - Continence
  - Sleep/wake cycle
  - Cognition/memory
- *Underlying multiple chronic disease states.* Some of the leading chronic conditions among the elderly living in the community may directly affect treatment in critical care areas:
  - Hypertension
  - Heart conditions
  - Diabetes mellitus
  - Arteriosclerosis
- *Effects of underlying chronic disease on a presenting illness*
  - Acute illness resulting from ineffective treatment of a chronic disease
  - Patient misuse of prescribed drugs
  - Polypharmacy: physician- or patient-induced
- *Underreporting of symptoms* possibly motivated by
  - Denial
  - Fear of dependence
  - Depression
  - Feeling that nothing can be done about the problem
  - Attributing symptoms to normal aging
- *Atypical symptoms of disease*
  - No symptoms
    ○ Sepsis without fever
    ○ Myocardial infarction without chest pain
  - Atypical symptoms
    ○ Pneumonia presenting as confusion without cough, dyspnea, fever
    ○ Urinary tract infection presenting as fatigue, loss of appetite, or confusion
    ○ Acute hyperthyroid state presenting as fatigue, malaise
- *Altered physiologic response to treatment*
  - Atypical or adverse drug reactions (see "Geropharmacology" below)

While disease cannot be equated with aging, it is estimated that most people over the age of 65 have at least one chronic disease. Critical illness in the older person may be caused by

- An exacerbation of a chronic disease
- An extension of a chronic disease to other body systems
- A condition that is not directly related to preexisting disease but that may affect or be affected by it

The nurse must be prepared to deal with multisystem disease and complications. Assessment of the geriatric patient must, therefore, be comprehensive of all major body systems, because each disease and its treatment affects the entire burden of disease. Frail elderly (those with multiple physiologic and functional limitations) respond poorly to the stressors of acute illness. They generally experience more prolonged hospitalization, more disease and treatment complications, and have a poorer prognosis for recovery. They present an additional challenge to health care providers and require added vigilance during assessment and treatment. For these reasons the nurse caring for critically ill elderly patients will be required to do the following:

- Distinguish symptoms, signs, and responses which are attributable to a previously compromised body system from those of the acute condition.
- Monitor treatment effects on multiple compromised systems simultaneously
- Maintain optimal functional ability during acute illness by
  - Maintaining mobility
  - Protecting skin integrity
  - Providing adequate nutrition
  - Providing frequent orientation to surroundings
  - Assuring sensory stimulation while preventing sensory overload
- Promote self-care and decision making to maintain the patient's independence
- Balance current treatment of the acute condition with realistic expectations for full recovery.
  - In the geriatric patient a full return to premorbid physiologic parameters may not be attainable.
  - The best predictors of long-term survival seem to be preadmission health and functional ability (Adelman, Berger, & Macina, 1994).

- Support family members through the critical care experience
  - Provide family members with frequent and simple explanations of patient condition and events. It may be helpful to identify one family member with whom to communicate.
  - Allow visitation to meet family needs.
  - Assess the family for stress and unresolved conflict, and make appropriate referrals.
- Support the patient and family through end-of-life decision making.

GEROPHARMACOLOGY

Drug therapy is a major contributor to morbidity and mortality in the older adult population. Hospitalization as a result of drug-induced illness is common in older adults. Elderly patients may also experience complications due to the multiple drug therapies prescribed during any hospitalization.

A major consideration in assessment and treatment of the critically ill geriatric patient is a potential alteration in response to drug therapy that may occur with aging and disease. The geriatric patient is more likely than a younger adult to have variable or unexpected responses to drugs, usually including the following:

- An increased drug sensitivity
- More frequent side effects or adverse drug reactions (ADRs).

This may be especially critical due to the frequent use of polypharmacy in treatment of the critically ill patient. Variability in response may be due to the following:

- Physiologic changes with aging
- Primary disease states affecting organs involved in drug processing
- Underlying disease states affecting organs involved in drug processing
- Previous misuse or abuse of prescribed or over-the-counter medications

Pharmacokinetics

The processes of drug absorption, distribution, metabolism or biotransformation, and excretion are collectively called pharmacokinetics.

These processes depend on the properties of specific drugs as well as on changes with aging and disease that may affect a drug's passage through the body. In the elderly these changes may include those described below.

Absorption

Decreased Gastric Acid, Mucosal Cells, Intestinal Blood Flow, and Altered Intestinal Motility. Any of these changes may affect the usually predictable rate and degree of absorption of drugs administered orally. Elevated gastric pH also occurs with antacid therapies. Changes in motility (hypo or hyper) may also be drug-induced.

Decreased Peripheral Blood Flow and Increased Connective Tissue. These changes may decrease drug permeability and the absorption rate of intramuscular injections.

Decreased Skin Hydration, Surface Lipids, Peripheral Blood Flow, Microcirculation, and Increased Tissue Keratinization. Such changes may decrease penetration and absorption of medications administered transdermally.

Distribution

Decreased Serum Albumin Concentration. Serum albumin is the principle plasma protein to which drugs are bound for distribution to specific target sites. Production of serum albumin can be altered by age, illness, or nutritional deficiencies. Lack of binding sites makes increased amounts of free, active drug available for distribution, pharmacological activity, metabolism, and elimination. Limited binding sites may also require several drugs to compete for available sites. This increases the possibility of overdose, adverse drug reactions, and toxicity.

Decreased Total Body Water. This is a normal change with aging and is exacerbated by dehydration states. This increases the concentration of water-soluble drugs in the body (decreased volume of distribution). Higher circulating drug levels may produce a therapeutic or toxic response at lower-than-expected doses. In the elderly this may require reduced loading doses of water-soluble drugs such as digoxin. If the critically ill person is in a state of fluid overload, however, this decreases the concentration of water-soluble drugs in the body (increased volume of distribution) and may require increased doses in order to produce a therapeutic effect.

Increased Body Fat. This is a normal change with aging occurring in both genders but with a somewhat greater increase in women. The condition is exacerbated by obese states. This allows fat-soluble drugs (e.g., diazepam) to accumulate (increased volume of distribution) and prolongs the duration of drug action.

Metabolism

Decreased Cardiac Output. This may delay transport of a drug to the liver for metabolism and to the kidney for elimination. It may also delay the drug effect at the target receptor site.

Decreased Hepatic Blood Flow, Liver Mass, and Changes in Liver Enzyme Activity. These are normal changes with aging, which can be exacerbated by diseases affecting blood flow to the liver (e.g., shock, congestive heart failure, primary liver disease). This may slow the rate of drug extraction and detoxification and produce side effects and toxicity at low doses. This may be especially critical for drugs that are usually metabolized during the first pass or oxidative phase of bio-transformation by the liver. Underlying nutritional deficiencies may also adversely affect liver enzyme activity, further contributing to slowed drug clearance and drug toxicity.

Elimination

Decreased Renal Blood Flow, Glomerular Filtration Rate (GFR), and Tubular Reabsorption or Excretion. This is a normal change with aging and can be exacerbated by diseases such as congestive heart failure, diabetes mellitus, dehydration, or nephrotic syndrome. This may reduce elimination of drugs commonly cleared by the kidneys, prolonging their effects in the body. Because of reduced lean body mass with aging, serum creatinine levels remain relatively stable in the healthy older person and cannot be used as an indication of decreased GFR and the ability of the body to clear drugs. A more direct measure of GFR is creatinine clearance. Drug doses for the geriatric patient should be calculated based on an equation that factors in age and gender for drugs excreted by the kidneys.

$$\text{Creatinine clearance}_{men} = \frac{(140 - \text{age}) \times \text{Body weight (in kg)}}{72 \times \text{Serum creatinine (in mg/dl)}}$$

$$\text{Creatinine clearance}_{women} = \text{Creatinine clearance}_{men} \times 0.85$$

Changes with aging and disease can also affect the half-life ($t_{1/2}$) of a drug, which is the time it takes to eliminate one-half of the amount of a drug remaining in the body. Theoretically it takes approximately seven half-lives to completely eliminate a drug from the body. It takes between four and five half-lives for a drug to reach a steady state in the body in which drug eliminated during a dosing interval equals the amount of drug administered. Half-life is directly affected by the volume of distribution of a drug and its clearance rate. Drugs, such as digoxin, with a narrow therapeutic index (the margin between therapeutic and toxic levels) can quickly produce toxicity if half-life is unexpectedly prolonged due to changes in distribution or clearance.

Pharmacodynamics

The action of a drug at a target site is called pharmacodynamics. It can be affected by age-related changes in target organ receptors or by altered homeostatic mechanisms. These may produce idiosyncratic responses such as

- Less reduction in cardiac output from β-blockers in proportion to the predrug value
- Increased susceptibility to hypotensive effects of vasodilators and calcium channel blockers
- Increased incidence of gastrointestinal bleeding and ototoxicity from aspirin
- Decreased response to central nervous system (CNS) stimulant drugs
- Enhanced response to CNS depressant drugs
- Stimulant response to certain depressant drugs (e.g., barbiturates)

The possibility of such adverse responses requires the nurse caring for an elderly patient to be especially vigilant in looking for therapeutic responses and drug side effects at unexpectedly low doses, as well as for atypical and adverse reactions.

POINTS TO REMEMBER

▶ Know the principle modes of action and major side effects and toxic effects of all drugs administered.

▶ Introduce drugs cautiously.
▶ Increase drug doses cautiously.
▶ Keep drug regimens as simple as possible.
▶ Routinely assess the elderly patient for adverse drug reactions, especially in the presence of acute, chronic, or developing disorders of the gastrointestinal/hepatic, circulatory, and renal systems.
  • Consider all changes in assessment as possibly drug-induced, and attempt to correlate such changes with drug introduction.
    – Look for favorable responses at lower doses.
    – Look for adverse responses at lower doses.
    – Look for slower-than-expected responses.
    – Look for cumulative responses.
  • If new drugs are added to a treatment regimen, look closely, in collaboration with the physician and pharmacist, at possibilities for discontinuing other drugs that might produce adverse effects in combination with those previously prescribed.

PAIN AND AGING

In addition to any pain associated with the primary cause(s) of critical illness, the geriatric patient may experience acute or chronic pain due to normal changes with aging (e.g., joint pain) or to preexisting or developing disease states. The nurse must be sensitive to the possibility of such discomfort, because unrelieved pain can increase anxiety and stress as well as slow recovery. The nurse should make every effort to assess for pain through both history and physical examination to discover its presence and its cause. The geriatric patient may underreport pain for a variety of reasons:

  • It is expected with aging
  • Fear of its meaning to illness prognosis
  • Not wanting to inconvenience or burden care providers
  • Cognitive impairment due to delirium, depression, or dementia

Even the elderly person with cognitive impairment can, with careful assessment, report pain accurately using a simple pain scale. Assessment must also occur after administration of pain therapies. In the elderly who have been administered analgesics, assessment must consider these factors:

- Altered pharmacokinetic effects with age
- Sedative effects
- Cumulative effects
- Drug interactions
- Other side effects (especially anticholinergic effects such as constipation).

Because of the complications that may accompany drug therapy in the elderly, independent nursing interventions (positioning, splinting) and complimentary therapies (music, guided imagery, etc.) for pain relief should be encouraged and their effects evaluated for effectiveness.

CONFUSION IN THE GERIATRIC PATIENT

The geriatric patient in critical care often appears confused. Aging is not, however, synonymous with cognitive impairment. Indicators of cognitive impairment should not be taken for granted, overlooked, or regarded as benign. Careful initial evaluation and continued monitoring of cognitive function in the elderly patient is an important assessment parameter. It is important to identify subtle as well as overt changes in cognition and awareness. Such changes may indicate

- Adverse physiological responses to drugs
- Disease state
  - Extension of presenting disease
  - Development of a new disease
  - Previously missed underlying disease
- Response to the critical care environment
  - Reaction to overstimulation (sensory overload)
  - Reaction to understimulation (sensory deprivation)
  - Unrecognized surroundings and people
  - Altered routines and schedules
- Psychological stress response
- Sensory changes with aging that reveal themselves as an elderly patient becomes increasingly aware of and responsive to the critical care environment
  - Hearing impairment
  - Vision impairment

- Normal changes in cognitive function with aging
  - Slowed processing of information
  - Slowed reaction and response time
  - Some loss of short-term memory
- Underlying alterations in mental status
  - Alzheimer's disease
  - Dementia-like symptoms related to severe depression or anxiety states
  - Dementia related to multiple brain infarcts or Parkinson's disease
  - Preexisting schizophrenia or manic-depressive disorder

The nurse caring for the critically ill geriatric patient must carefully evaluate the possible causes of confusion in the elderly person. This includes collecting information concerning the premorbid state of the individual, as a baseline, to evaluate current changes in mentation. The nurse should consider any acute change in cognition as a possible indication of delirium or reversible dementia. Such changes may be caused by

- Drugs
- Emotional disorders
- Metabolic and endocrine disorders
- Eye and ear disorders
- Nutritional deficiencies
- Trauma or tumor
- Infection
- Arteriosclerosis

The critical care nurse should also be alert to prevent the downward spiral of events that may follow from symptoms of confusion in the geriatric patient. With all good intentions on the part of health care providers, the treatment of geriatric confusion can inadvertently lead to disease complications, prolonged hospitalization, and a permanent decline in function and quality of life. This downward spiral is illustrated in Figure 3–1.

POINTS TO REMEMBER

▶ Assessment of the older adult presents the nurse with a challenge in the acute and critical care settings. In performing the initial, baseline, focused, and ongoing assessments of the geri-

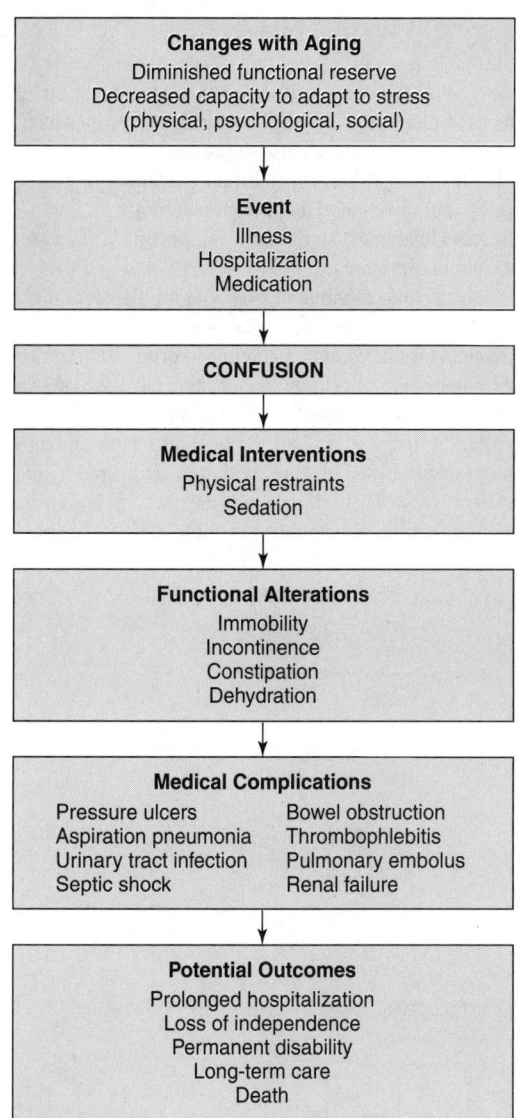

Changes with Aging
Diminished functional reserve
Decreased capacity to adapt to stress
(physical, psychological, social)

Event
Illness
Hospitalization
Medication

CONFUSION

Medical Interventions
Physical restraints
Sedation

Functional Alterations
Immobility
Incontinence
Constipation
Dehydration

Medical Complications

Pressure ulcers	Bowel obstruction
Aspiration pneumonia	Thrombophlebitis
Urinary tract infection	Pulmonary embolus
Septic shock	Renal failure

Potential Outcomes
Prolonged hospitalization
Loss of independence
Permanent disability
Long-term care
Death

FIGURE 3–1
Downward spiral of events that may follow confusion in the geriatric patient.

atric patient, the nurse must be attentive to conditions that may affect the older person's ability to maintain homeostasis during acute illness. The nurse must be prepared to

- Identify normal physiologic and psychologic changes with aging and distinguish them from pathology
- Be alert to atypical signs and symptoms of acute, chronic, and developing diseases
- Be attentive to possible or probable multisystem involvement in a disease process
- Be alert for unexpected responses to drug treatment caused by the interaction of normal age changes, disease processes, decreased immune response, and diminished functional reserve

▶ Finally, the nurse must find the human person among the presenting diseases and changes with age, and provide assessment and care that reflects dignity and respect for geriatric patients and their families during the vulnerable period of critical illness.

II

Focused Assessment: Techniques and System Disorders

4

Respiratory Assessment

FUNCTION OF THE RESPIRATORY SYSTEM

The principal function of the respiratory system is **gas exchange.** It delivers atmospheric oxygen to the blood stream and to hemoglobin molecules for use in metabolic activity at the cellular level. It eliminates carbon dioxide, a principle waste product of cellular metabolism. This is accomplished by **pulmonary ventilation,** which moves air to the lung alveoli during inhalation and to the atmosphere during exhalation, and by **alveolar ventilation,** in which gases diffuse between alveoli and pulmonary capillaries in response to concentration and pressure gradients. Alveolar ventilation requires

- Delivery of an adequate **volume of air** to alveoli
- Sufficient **alveolar surface** area for gas exchange
- Adequate **perfusion,** or pulmonary blood flow
- Alveolar and capillary membranes and interstitium that allow **diffusion** of gases to occur

In the healthy lung there is a match between ventilation and perfusion. Alveolar ventilation ($\dot{V}A$) is approximately 4 L/min. Pulmonary blood flow ($\dot{Q}$) approximates cardiac output at 5 L/min. Alveolar ventilation is enhanced by surfactant produced by specialized alveolar cells that decreases surface tension and prevents alveolar collapse. It is affected by gravity, lung volumes, respiratory rate, physiologic dead space, or by alterations in the supply or composition of inspired air. The pattern of pulmonary blood flow brings blood from the right ventricle through the pulmonary artery, into pulmonary arterial capillaries, and to the lungs, where it is oxygenated and relieved of its carbon dioxide.

Blood returns via pulmonary venous capillaries to the pulmonary vein and to the left atrium. Pulmonary blood flow is affected by gravity, right-to-left shunting, vasoconstriction, vascular occlusion, or cardiac failure.

Inhalation is normally regulated by the respiratory center in the pons and medulla in response to an increase in the partial pressure of carbon dioxide ($PaCO_2$) or a decrease in pH. Inhalation is primarily accomplished by nervous system innervation of (1) the diaphragm via the phrenic nerve, which arises from the cervical spine at C3–5, and (2) the external intercostal muscles via spinal motor nerves arising from the thoracic spine. Exhalation is largely a passive process of elastic recoil of respiratory tissue. Accessory muscles that may aid in inhalation include the ali nasi in the nose and the sternomastoid and scalene muscles of the neck. Accessory muscles that may assist in exhalation include the internal intercostals and the abdominal muscles. Lung volumes and capacities in the healthy individual are predictable and can be measured with pulmonary function tests.

The respiratory system has several other important functions:

- It helps to maintain **acid-base balance** through regulation of carbon dioxide tension and hydrogen ion concentration.
- It provides for **insensible water loss** of approximately 1 pint per day. This rate may be increased with fever and elevated respiratory rate.
- It contributes to the body's **immune response.** Mucus secretions in the respiratory system are rich in macrophages, polymorphonuclear leukocytes (PMNs), immunoglobulins, interferon, and antibodies that defend against foreign particles and organisms in inspired air and in blood. Ciliary action in the respiratory tree further assists in removal of foreign particles, as do the swallow, gag, and cough reflexes.
- It **converts angiotensin I to angiotensin II** a vasopressor that stimulates the secretion of aldosterone by the adrenal cortex.

The respiratory tree is situated in the mediastinum, which is enclosed by the rib cage, spine, diaphragm, and neck musculature. It shares space with the heart and great vessels, the thymus gland, and portions of the lymphatic system that drain the area. There are three lobes in the right lung and two in the left. The lungs are covered with

a two-layered pleura: the inner, or visceral, pleura covers the lung surfaces; the outer, or parietal, pleura is attached to the chest wall. The
pleurae are separated by a thin film of serous fluid that decreases friction during lung and chest wall movement. The functional units of the
lungs are the approximately 300 million small air sacs or alveoli
where gas exchange occurs. Large airways, including the nasal pas-
sages, mouth, pharynx, larynx, trachea, bronchi, and bronchioles,
transport air to alveoli through anatomic dead space in which no gas
exchange occurs. These structures, however, are lined with mucous
membranes that warm, humidify, and filter inspired air. The bronchi
and bronchioles are banded with smooth muscle which can affect airway resistance by dilating or contracting in response to autonomic
nervous system stimulation. The right mainstem bronchus is wider
and shorter than the left and branches from the trachea at the carina
at about a 10-degree angle. The left mainstem bronchus has a more
acute angle. Normal respiration requires both chest wall and lung
compliance or the ability of tissues to expand. Lung and chest wall
tissue must also have elastic recoil sufficient to expel air on exhalation. The bronchial arteries branch from the aorta to meet the nutritional needs of the lungs themselves. The bronchial veins empty into
the pulmonary veins or the vena cava.

Functioning of the respiratory system can be compromised by alterations in nervous system innervation, by ventilation, perfusion, or
diffusion defects, by cardiac failure, or by musculoskeletal injuries or
deformities. Respiratory symptoms may also occur secondary to medications, pain, or anxiety.

Changes with Aging

Lung volumes and capacities may be affected by chest wall
stiffness (decreased chest compliance), deconditioning and atrophy
of the primary muscles of respiration (diaphragm and intercostals), and loss of elastic recoil of lung tissue (increased lung
compliance).

There is an increased ventilation/perfusion ($\dot{V}A/\dot{Q}$) mismatch, especially in the supine position and with low volumes of air. This is due
to (1) increased physiologic dead space; (2) alveolar enlargement, thinning, and loss of septal surface area for gas diffusion; (3) early small
airway closure (increased closing lung volume) on exhalation; (4)
fewer alveolar capillaries; and (5) thickening of the alveolar-capillary

membrane. Along with some reduction in hemoglobin with age, this results in an expected decrease in PaO_2 of approximately 4 mm Hg per decade (PaO_2 mm Hg = $100.1 - 0.325 \times$ age). No significant changes in PCO_2 or pH are expected.

The aging person may have a diminished respiratory response to elevated levels of CO_2 (hypercapnia) and low levels of O_2 (hypoxemia). Return to normal concentrations can also be slower than in younger adults.

Decreased stimulation and force of the cough reflex, decreased respiratory macrophages and mucociliary action, and diminished antibody response to certain antigens compromise the immune response in the elderly. The elderly are more easily susceptible, therefore, to naturally occurring and nosocomial infections of the respiratory system. Diminished cough, swallow, and gag reflexes and supine position may also potentiate aspiration of gastrointestinal contents into the respiratory tree. Because of alterations in immunity, symptoms of respiratory compromise may be atypical, subtle, or nonexistent. Skin testing may result, at least initially, in an anergic response.

Prolonged exposure to environmental toxins, a history of smoking, sedentary lifestyle, obesity, central nervous system and respiratory depressant medications, circulatory disorders, and multiple chronic diseases contribute further to respiratory compromise. There is limited functional reserve capacity to deal with the respiratory demands of an acute/critical illness. The nurse must anticipate respiratory compromise through aggressive and careful initial, baseline, focused, and ongoing assessment. The nurse must also be prepared for the possibility that therapeutic responses involving the respiratory system may be slower or less dramatic than in the younger patient because of changes with aging and disease.

TABLE 4-1 Respiratory Assessment Techniques, Tips, Geriatric Considerations

Technique	Performance Tips	Description/Rationale	Geriatric Considerations
Pertinent History			
1. Related medical history	Review the patient's known medical history for **actual or potential disease states** that can affect respiratory function	Respiratory function may be affected by diseases that affect • Respiratory organs • Vascular supply to the respiratory system • Neurologic innervation of respiratory organs Respiratory function may also be affected by • Electrolyte, acid-base disorders • Immunocompromise • Chest or abdominal surgery • Chest trauma • Multisystem trauma • Recent anesthesia, analgesia, altered consciousness	In the elderly common conditions that affect the respiratory system include • COPD • Cardiovascular disease • Cerebral vascular disease • Pneumonia • Multiple disease states • Inactivity, immobility • Limited functional reserve capacity in acute illness • Altered inflammatory and immune responses

Table continued on following page

TABLE 4–1 Respiratory Assessment Techniques, Tips, Geriatric Considerations *Continued*

Technique	Performance Tips	Description/Rationale	Geriatric Considerations
		• Pain, immobility • Lifestyle behaviors: smoking, inhaling tobacco or drugs, obesity, exposure to environmental toxins • Recent cardiopulmonary resuscitation • Airway obstructions • Artificial airways, ventilators, chest tubes • Inappropriate oxygen therapy • Gastrointestinal tubes: aspiration • Central lines, hemodynamic lines	
2. Related drug history	Review the patient's recent past and current **drug therapy** for medications that may • Increase respiratory signs and symptoms • Mask respiratory signs and symptoms	Drugs taken prior to admission or administered in the critical care setting may affect respiratory function in a variety of ways. Such drugs include • Central nervous system stimulants or depressants	Because of altered pharmacokinetics and pharmacodynamics with aging • Unexpected drug responses may occur at usual doses • Drugs may have a cumulative effect

		• Drugs may cause an unexpected response (see Chapter 3) Polypharmacy may produce adverse side effects affecting respiratory function
	ASSESSMENT TIPS 1. Attempt to correlate a new symptom with a recently administered drug or with a recently discontinued drug or changed dose 2. Attempt to correlate improvement of a symptom with a recently administered drug or with a recently discontinued drug or changed dose	– Anesthetics – Analgesics • Respiratory stimulants or depressants • Anticholinergics • Sympathomimetics
3. Common complaints or observations that indicate the need for a focused assessment of the respiratory system	The most common sign and symptom is **dyspnea**, i.e., difficult or painful breathing	Dyspnea suggests inadequate ventilation, perfusion, diffusion, or insufficient circulating oxygen Dyspnea may indicate a respiratory, cardiovascular, neurologic, musculoskeletal, endocrine, or renal problem

Table continued on following page

TABLE 4–1 Respiratory Assessment Techniques, Tips, Geriatric Considerations *Continued*

Technique	Performance Tips	Description/Rationale	Geriatric Considerations

	ASSESSMENT TIPS
	1. Interview the alert patient about the exact nature of any discomfort
	2. Use the following mnemonic to assure that all major aspects and characteristics of the dyspnea have been evaluated
	P Precipitating factors, prodrome
	Q Quality, quantity
	R Region, radiation
	S Associated symptoms, setting
	T Timing, treatment effects
		Pertinent information should include
		• When the dyspnea occurred
		  – With rest, with activity (exertional dyspnea)
		  – During the day, at night
		  – Body position: lying, sitting, standing, always
		  – On inspiration, expiration, both
		  – Associated with any event, activity
		• Any treatment and effects
		• Associated symptoms
		  – Pain: location, duration
		  – Fatigue
		  – Cough, sputum	

Physical Examination: Inspection
1. General observations

• Mental status	*Look for*	These may be early indications of hypoxic changes that may result from
	• Restlessness, agitation, anxiety	• Changing physical condition
	• Confusion	• Adverse drug response
	• Apprehension, panic	
	• Feelings of impending doom	Changes in level of consciousness and mentation are often the *only* indications of changes in condition; classic symptoms may be absent (see Chapter 3)
	• Drowsiness, fatigue	
	• Breathlessness with speaking	
	• Feelings of suffocation	
• Integument	*Look at*	**Cyanosis** (bluish, dusky color) may be caused by
– Skin color	• General color	• Central cyanosis: increased concentrations of unsaturated hemoglobin (hypoxemia) in the arterial circulation (e.g., heart failure, pulmonary edema, right-to-left shunting)
	• Local variations	
	– Circumoral area	
	– Periorbital areas	
	• Vascular areas: lips, tongue, etc	• Peripheral cyanosis: increased venous desaturation (low cardiac
	ASSESSMENT TIPS	Epidermal thinning and decreased vascularity are normal changes with aging, and may give Caucasian skin a pale, transparent appearance accented by prominent blue veins
	1. Perform the examination in good light with minimal glare	

Table continued on following page

TABLE 4–1 Respiratory Assessment Techniques, Tips, Geriatric Considerations *Continued*

Technique	Performance Tips	Description/Rationale	Geriatric Considerations
	2. Use natural light, if possible; incandescent and fluorescent lighting may alter skin colors 3. Generalized changes in skin color, such as cyanosis or pallor, may be seen on the eyelids, nose tip, lips, tongue, buccal mucosa, ears, cheeks, fingertips, and nailbeds 4. Eyelid conjunctivae, lips, buccal mucosa, or palmar surfaces of the hands and feet will usually be better indicators of general color in dark-skinned patients	output, local vasoconstriction, venous stasis, hypothermia) **Pallor** (white, ashen-gray color) may be caused by anemia, blood loss, decreased tissue perfusion (local, systemic), vasoconstriction (local, systemic; e.g. hypothermia) **Erythema** (red, reddish-blue) may result from the following: • Increased blood flow, vasodilation (local or systemic inflammation, infection), fever • Increased RBCs (polycythemia) seen in severe pulmonary disease • Palmar erythema may be present in chronic liver disease	

5. Erythema in the dark-skinned person may present as an area of darker pigmentation
6. Inspection can be enhanced by simultaneous palpation

- Dependent rubor of the lower extremities is seen in chronic arterial insufficiency

– Skin temperature
– Skin moisture

ASSESSMENT TIPS
1. Look both for generalized and localized changes in skin temperature
2. Look for both generalized and localized changes in skin moisture
3. Use the back of the fingers or hand to assess skin temperature

General

Cool, moist, or dry skin may be due to hypoxemia, vasoconstriction, decreased perfusion, diaphoresis, decreased metabolic rate, sympathetic response to anxiety or stress, exposure to decreased environmental temperature

Warm, moist or dry skin may be due to fever, vasodilation, diaphoresis, inflammatory response, increased metabolic rate, exposure to increased environmental temperature

Decreased vascularity and altered immune response may limit temperature elevation in response to infection. In the elderly an oral temperature of 37.2° C (99° F) or 37.5° C (99.5° F) rectally on repeated measures should raise suspicion of infection

Decreased activity of sweat glands may minimize skin moisture in response to illness events

Table continued on following page

TABLE 4–1 Respiratory Assessment Techniques, Tips, Geriatric Considerations *Continued*

Technique	Performance Tips	Description/Rationale	Geriatric Considerations

— Mucous membranes
  ○ Buccal (oral)
  ○ Conjunctival
	ASSESSMENT TIPS
	1. Perform the examination in good light with minimal glare
	2. Use natural light, if possible; incandescent and fluorescent lighting may alter skin colors
	3. Pull down gently on the skin below each lower eyelid to expose the conjunctiva lining the lower lid
	4. Expose the lower lid enough to observe the en-
		Local
		Cool: arterial occlusion
		Warm: inflammation
		These are reliable places to evaluate true color with less pigment interference
			Mucous membranes may be dry in the elderly because of age-related decrease in salivary secretion, drug-induced dry mouth, or dehydration

tire lid since the outer canthus may normally be darker in color 5. Evaluate both conjunctivae to rule out local inflammation as a cause of membrane color		
– Nails ○ Plate	Thickened nails may indicate chronic peripheral vascular insufficiency or local trauma if isolated to one or several nails	Nail plates may become thickened, yellowed, less transparent, making assessment of the nail bed more difficult, especially on the lower extremities Thickened toenails may be a normal change with aging if not accompanied by other signs of peripheral vascular insufficiency (see below) Vertical ridges down all nails may be a normal finding with age
	Beau's lines: transverse ridges across all nails indicate a recent severe systemic disease that disrupted nail growth (see Fig. 4–1)	

Table continued on following page

TABLE 4–1 Respiratory Assessment Techniques, Tips, Geriatric Considerations *Continued*

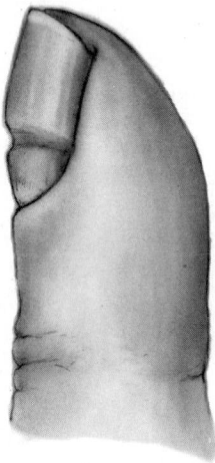

FIGURE 4–1

Beau's line. (From Jarvis, C. [1996]. *Physical examination and health assessment* [3rd ed., p. 264]. Philadelphia: W. B. Saunders.)

○ Beds: capillary refill

Nail beds are normally pink-tinged; after they are blanched, color should return in ≤2 seconds; slow or no color return may indicate hypoxemia or decreased tissue perfusion

Blanching effect may take 3 seconds in the frail elderly

ASSESSMENT TIPS
1. If nails are opaque because of polish or changes with aging, capillary refill can be assessed by compressing and releasing the finger or toe pads, ear lobes, or the tip of the nose
2. If capillary refill techniques are being used to assess general state of perfusion, confirm that the extremity being evaluated does not have compromised circulation

Table continued on following page

TABLE 4-1 Respiratory Assessment Techniques, Tips, Geriatric Considerations *Continued*

Technique	Performance Tips	Description/Rationale	Geriatric Considerations
○ Clubbing	*ASSESSMENT TIPS* 1. True clubbing must be distinguished from broad fingertips; this is done by assessing the nail angle 2. The angle formed by the nail plate and base is normally < 180 degrees. An angle ≥180 degrees indicates clubbing (Fig. 4-2) 3. Clubbing may be accompanied by a broadening of the nail plate 4. True clubbing is seen in all fingers	Clubbing is a physiologic adaptation to chronically decreased oxygen due to respiratory or cardiovascular disease; it may also be seen in colitis, cirrhosis, and thyroid disease	
○ Periungual area		Nicotine staining on the index finger and nail is an indication of smoking history and a risk for cardiorespiratory problems and vasoconstriction	

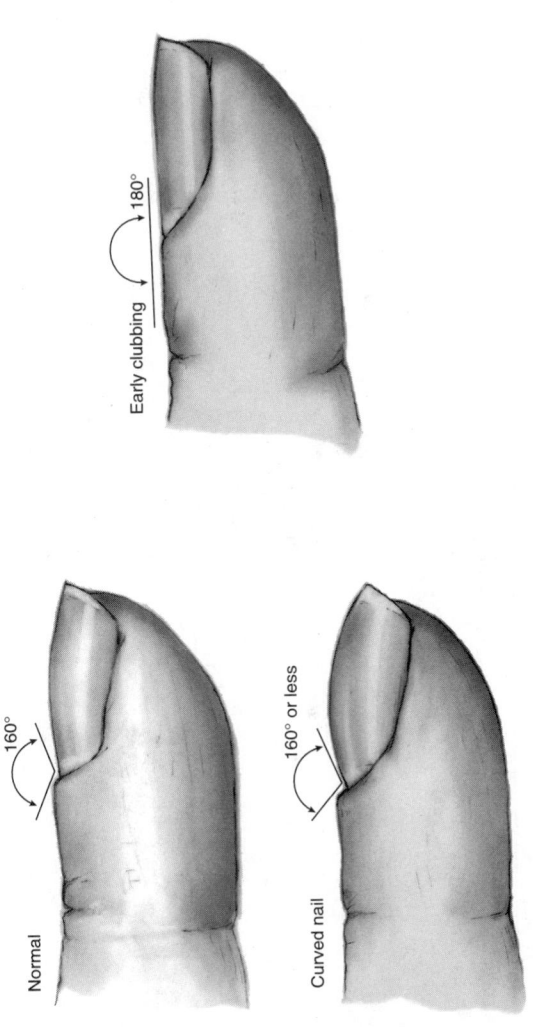

FIGURE 4-2

Assessment of nails for clubbing. (From Jarvis, C. [1996]. *Physical examination and health assessment* [3rd ed., p. 232]. Philadelphia: W. B. Saunders.)

Table continued on following page

TABLE 4-1 Respiratory Assessment Techniques, Tips, Geriatric Considerations *Continued*

Technique	Performance Tips	Description/Rationale	Geriatric Considerations
2. Physical obstruction of upper airways • Nasal airway obstruction	*Look for* • Nasal flaring • Mouth breathing	Upper airway obstruction may be caused by • Obstructive tubing (e.g., nasogastric, O_2 cannula) • Crusted drainage at nares • Nasopharyngeal edema, trauma	Mouth breathing is common in the geriatric patient
• Oral airway obstruction	*Look at* • Mouth • Throat • Neck	Oral airway obstruction may be caused by • Tongue (edema, displacement) • Secretions (copious, thick, crusted) • Injury, edema (pharynx, larynx) • Teeth (loose or dislodged, dentures) • Other foreign bodies • Tumor • Impairment of cranial nerves IX, X, or XI	Look for loose teeth in any patient with poor oral hygiene and in those with a history of limited dental care Ill-fitting dentures are common in geriatric patients who have experienced weight loss and those with a history of limited dental care Weakened cough, swallow, or gag reflex with aging or disease may increase the risk of oral obstruction
	ASSESSMENT TIPS 1. A mouth examination should always include inspection using a • **Pair of gloves** • **Tongue blade** (padded, if necessary)		

- **Light source** that allows clear visualization of mouth and pharyngeal structures
- **Gauze pad** to aggressively move the tongue from side to side and provide a clear view of structures

2. Examiner should always wear disposable gloves as a protection against contaminated oral secretions

3. Unresponsive and noncommunicating patients should have a mouth examination at least every shift; accumulation of thick secretions and other sources of obstruction can seriously

Table continued on following page

TABLE 4-1 Respiratory Assessment Techniques, Tips, Geriatric Considerations *Continued*

Technique	Performance Tips	Description/Rationale	Geriatric Considerations
	affect respiratory function and ability to speak 4. Carefully document loose, missing teeth, bridges, dentures		
• Tracheal obstruction	*Look for* • Crowing respirations (stridor) • Audible snoring, rattling, wheezes • Enlarged thyroid • Tracheal deviation from the midline • Tracheal tug (pulls out of midline with respiration) • Jugular venous distention (JVD)	Tracheal obstruction may be caused by direct, local obstruction: • Laryngeal, tracheal edema • Accumulated secretions • Foreign bodies, respiratory tumors • Following prolonged tracheostomy or intubation May also be caused by indirect, local obstruction: • Enlarged thyroid, glands, lymph nodes • Throat, neck tumors • Nasogastric intubation	Weakened cough, gag, and swallow reflexes may increase the risk of oral obstruction in the geriatric patient; this may be due to diseases associated with muscle weakness, immobility, prolonged inactivity, frailty There is a high incidence of mouth and throat cancer in patients with a history of smoking and alcohol use, especially males

3. Respiratory pattern

May also be caused by chest pathology:
- Mediastinal mass
- Pneumothorax, hemothorax

Rate, rhythm, and depth can be affected by
- **Disease or injury** that directly or indirectly affects respiratory function
  - Respiratory
  - Circulatory
  - Neurological
  - Endocrine
  - Kidney
- **Drugs** that directly or indirectly affect respiratory function
- **Metabolic reactions**
  - Acidosis
  - Alkalosis
  - Other electrolyte imbalances

Tracheal deviation in the elderly may be due to thoracic kyphosis due to osteoporosis or to scoliosis

The elderly may become dyspneic with mild exertion due to
- Diminished functional reserve capacity with aging
- Increased lung compliance
- Decreased thoracic compliance
- Respiratory muscle degeneration
- Supine position
- Diminished response to hypercapnia, hypoxemia

Lung volumes and capacities change with age (see Chapter 13)

ASSESSMENT TIPS

1. Respiratory pattern can be evaluated unobtrusively during assessment of radial or apical pulses; this allows the nurse to both see and feel respiratory movements, enhancing accuracy
2. While taking a radial pulse, place the patient's hand on his or her chest to evaluate respiratory rate, rhythm, depth, and effort
3. While performing cardiac auscultation, also evalu-

Table continued on following page

TABLE 4–1 Respiratory Assessment Techniques, Tips, Geriatric Considerations *Continued*

Technique	Performance Tips	Description/Rationale	Geriatric Considerations
	ate the patient's respiratory pattern as you observe the chest	• **Stress response** with concomitant release of catecholamines	
• Rate	*Look for* • Rates <10 or >25–30/min • Changes in rate from baseline		
• Rhythm (evenness)		(see Fig. 4–3) The normal ratio of duration of inhalation (I) to exhalation (E) = 1:2 or 2:3 (see Fig. 4–3)	
• Depth (tidal volume)			

• Effort	*Look for*
	 • Thoracic movement
	 • Use of accessory muscles
	   – Use of neck muscles
	   – Abdominal movement
	 • Position of comfort for breathing
		Usual Effort Patterns
		 Thoracic breathing: chest movement predominates on inhalation and exhalation; this is the usual finding in healthy adults, especially females
		 Abdominal breathing: abdominal movement predominates; this is the usual
			Abdominal breathing is a common pattern in aging, especially as the chest becomes stiffer and lungs more compliant with loss of elastic recoil; this pattern is seen more frequently in elderly males

FIGURE 4–3

Interpretation of respiratory rate, rhythm, and depth patterns.

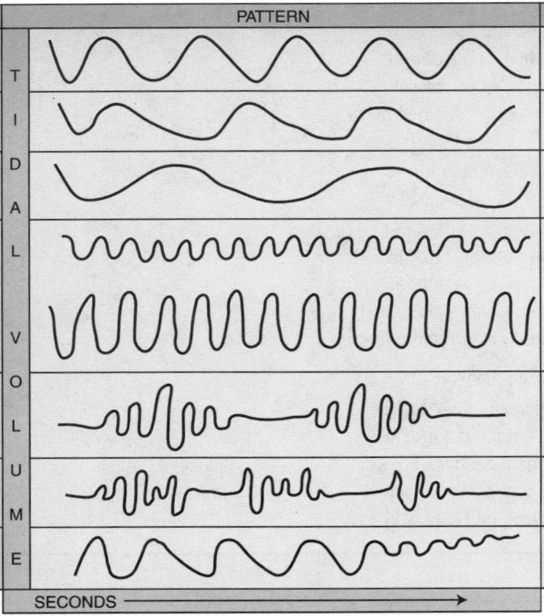

CHARACTERISTIC		PATTERN	POSSIBLE CAUSES
REGULAR RHYTHM: 1. Normal respiration	T		
2. Prolonged exhalation	I		Air trapping (e.g., emphysema)
3. Bradypnea	D		Metabolic alkalosis, CNS lesions, CNS depression (e.g., drug overdose)
	A		
4. Tachypnea (rapid, shallow)	L		Respiratory failure, pulmonary embolus, hypoxia, fever
Hyperventilation (rapid, deep)	V		Anxiety, pain, CNS lesions
Kussmaul (rapid, deep)			Metabolic acidosis
IRREGULAR RHYTHM: 5. Cheyne-Stokes	O		CHF, drug overdose, increased ICP, meningitis, advanced age, sleep pattern
	L		
6. Biot's respiration	U		Head trauma, brain infection or inflammation, spinal meningitis
	M		
7. Obstructive breathing	E		Chronic obstructive pulmonary disease
		SECONDS	

Table continued on following page

TABLE 4-1 Respiratory Assessment Techniques, Tips, Geriatric Considerations *Continued*

Technique	Performance Tips	Description/Rationale	Geriatric Considerations
	– Orthopnea – Upright position – Forward leaning	finding in infants; it may be usual in adult males and with rapid rates Occasional deep breaths (sighs) are part of the normal pattern of breathing; such periodic deep breaths aerate dependent lung areas ***Abnormal Effort Patterns*** Use of neck musculature to assist in inspiratory effort (e.g., airway obstruction, severe atelectasis, overexertion) • Scalene • Sternomastoid • Trapezius Use of rectus abdominis and intercostal muscles on expiration to push out air trapped in lungs; commonly seen in emphysema; may be accompanied by pursed-lip breathing	Use of abdominal muscles to assist in exhalation is often seen in persons with COPD and may be accompanied by pursed-lip breathing Abnormal patterns may be seen in otherwise healthy elderly in situations of exertion or stress due to changes in chest and lung compliance and decreased respiratory muscle strength with aging

Diminished or increased effort may also be due to

- Lung obstruction
- Lung collapse
- Chest injury
- Pleurisy
- Central nervous system injury
- Weakness, fatigue
- Pain
- Drug effects

Cranial nerves IX (glossopharyngeal) and X (vagus) innervate the posterior pharynx; function may be altered by central nervous system disease or by local irritation such as a nasogastric tube

Cough, swallow, and gag reflexes, and ciliary activity may be diminished with normal aging or due to neurological deficits affecting the cranial nerves or transmission of impulses; this increases susceptibility to aspiration

4. Cough and sputum
- Cough, swallow, and gag reflex

ASSESSMENT TIPS
1. Warn the alert patient before testing the gag reflex
2. Stimulate the back of the throat with a tongue blade
3. Observe how the person deals with accumulated saliva—is it swallowed or allowed to run from the mouth

Table continued on following page

TABLE 4-1 Respiratory Assessment Techniques, Tips, Geriatric Considerations *Continued*

Technique	Performance Tips	Description/Rationale	Geriatric Considerations
	4. Evaluate if swallowed secretions produce gagging or coughing		Continually evaluate the possibility of hypostatic pneumonia in the elderly patient due to persistent immobility and limited pulmonary hygiene through coughing and deep breathing
• Cough characteristics	*Look for* • Frequency • Voluntary or involuntary • Productive of mucus • Dry, hacking • Association with postural changes	May be an indication of • Acute changes • Chronic conditions • Local irritation, congestion	
• Sputum characteristics	*Look for* • Amount • Consistency • Appearance – Clear, mucoid: viral, asthma, irritation – Yellow: bacterial – Green: bacterial	Amount and consistency of sputum may be affected by drugs (e.g., sympathomimetics or anticholinergics, and by dehydration) It is important to distinguish between hemoptysis (coughing up blood) and hematemesis (bleeding from the gastrointestinal tract)	The incidence of human immunodeficiency virus (HIV) and pneumonia related to AIDS is increased in the elderly population and should not be disregarded as a possible etiology in the geriatric patient

- Gray: bacterial
- Rusty: pneumococcal, TB
- Currant jelly: *Klebsiella*
- Pink, blood-tinged: strepto-coccal or staphylococcal
- Pink, frothy: pulmonary edema
- Bloody, clotted: pulmonary emboli
- Fatty: fat emboli
- Foul-smelling: lung abscess

Characteristics of blood from the gastrointestinal tract include

- Red: active bleeding
- Brown, coffee ground: old blood

Common causes of hemoptysis include

- Irritated mucous membranes
  - Suctioning
  - Bronchiectasis
- Ruptured blood vessels
  - Tuberculosis
  - Pulmonary malignancy
  - Pulmonary emboli
- Blood from nasopharynx

Common causes of hematemesis include

- Esophageal irritation
- Esophageal varices (liver disease)
- Swallowed blood
- Gastric ulceration due to a **stress ulcer**
- Underlying gastric or colonic disease

Table continued on following page

TABLE 4-1 Respiratory Assessment Techniques, Tips, Geriatric Considerations *Continued*

Technique	Performance Tips	Description/Rationale	Geriatric Considerations

5. Respiratory excursion	***Paradoxical Chest Movements***
	Look for
	• Lag on inspiration
	• Guarding
	• Suprasternal retractions
	• Intercostal spaces, supraclavicular area
	  – Retraction of intercostal spaces on inhalation
	  – Bulging of intercostal spaces on exhalation
	• Ribs: pulling in on inspiration
	• Chest flailing: erratic, uncoordinated movements, unilateral or bilateral
	
	ASSESSMENT TIP
	Evaluation of chest movements may be enhanced
		Chest movements are usually full, equal, symmetrical.
		Lag may be due to severe obstruction of airflow (e.g., atelectasis, pneumothorax, hemothorax)
		Guarding may be due to pain
		Common causes of retraction include obstruction, atelectasis, tumor, COPD, pulmonary emboli
		Common causes of bulging include air-trapping (e.g., COPD), tension pneumothorax, massive pleural effusion)
		Common causes of rib and chest movement disorders are rib or sternal fractures or separation due to trauma or cardiopulmonary resuscitation efforts
			Respiratory excursion may be decreased with aging but should remain symmetrical
			Osteoporotic changes or history of falling put the geriatric patient at high risk for rib or vertebral fractures

6. Chest, back	by using both inspection *and* palpation (see below)	Barrel chest is common with chronic trapping of air in alveoli, as in chronic emphysema	Some barreling of the chest is a normal change with advancing age due to
• Chest diameters	**Chest**		• Kyphosis
	Look at		• Calcification of costal cartilages
	• Anteroposterior (AP) diameter		• Decreased elastic recoil of lungs with resultant increase in residual volume
	• Lateral diameter		Over time, this results in flattening of the rib angle and shortening of the thoracic cavity
	ASSESSMENT TIPS		Mild to moderate thoracic kyphosis is common with aging; severe kyphosis may suggest osteoporosis, especially in susceptible females, and less frequently in males
	1. Normal chest diameter can be estimated as anteroposterior diameter less than lateral diameter (AP < L)		
	2. Barrel shape is characterized by		
	• AP chest diameter approximately equal to the lateral chest diameter (see Fig. 4–4)		
	• Widening of the costal angle to ≥90 degrees		

Table continued on following page

TABLE 4–1 Respiratory Assessment Techniques, Tips, Geriatric Considerations *Continued*

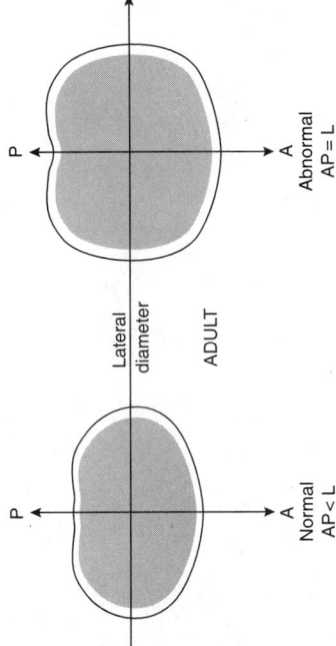

FIGURE 4–4

Normal and abnormal chest diameters (cross section). *A*, anterior; *P*, posterior. (Adapted from Jarvis, C. [1996]. *Physical examination and health assessment* [3rd ed., p. 487]. Philadelphia: W. B. Saunders.)

• Ribs and sternum	with flattening of the rib angle (see Fig. 4–5)	Osteoporosis can result in increased susceptibility to rib fracture
	Look for	
	• Injury	Ribs and sternum may be asymmetrical with fracture, separation, spinal deformity
• Spine	• Deformity	Rib, sternum, and spinal deformities may affect respiratory pattern
	– Kyphosis	
	– Scoliosis	
	– Lordosis	
7. Abdomen	**Discoloration**	
	Look for	
	• Ecchymoses	May indicate blunt trauma to the thorax
		Falls and elder abuse should be considered with any ecchymotic lesions
	• Petechiae	Petechiae may be visible with fat emboli
	• Spider nevi	Spider nevi may suggest liver disease
	Look for	
	• Distention	Abdominal distention or restriction may affect diaphragmatic movement, especially on inspiration, causing an increase in respiratory effort and a decrease in vital capacity
	• Recent abdominal surgery	
	• Restrictive dressings	Weakened diaphragmatic muscles with aging may severely compromise respiratory effort in the presence of increased intra-abdominal pressure

Table continued on following page

85

TABLE 4–1 Respiratory Assessment Techniques, Tips, Geriatric Considerations *Continued*

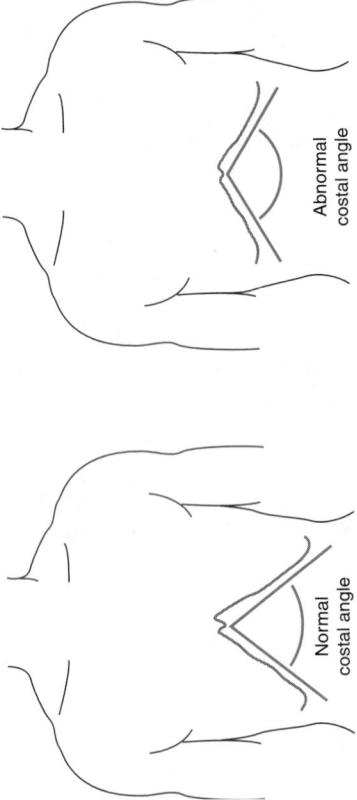

Normal costal angle

Abnormal costal angle

FIGURE 4–5
Alterations in costal angle with changes in lung and chest compliance.

Palpation

1. Respiratory excursion
(verification of inspection) (optional)

ASSESSMENT TIP
Place hands on lower rib cage with thumbs meeting in the vertical plane and pinching a fold of skin at midline:
- Skin fold disappears on deep inspiration.
- Movement should be symmetrical without lag or guarding.

(see Fig. 4–6)

This enhances inspection information about depth and symmetry of chest expansion with addition of the sense of touch

Abnormal findings may assist in identification of poor ventilation of a lung area due to
- Injury
- Displaced airway into the right mainstem bronchus in assisted ventilation
- Obstruction (e.g., severe atelectasis, pneumonia, pneumothorax, hemothorax)

Excursion may be diminished by
- Atrophy of accessory musculature
- Increased chest wall stiffness (decreased compliance) with aging

2. Tenderness, swelling

Palpate shoulder, clavicles, ribs, sternum, back, and spine for warmth, tenderness, and swelling

Pain in the thoracic area may lead to guarding and limit lung expansion

Tenderness or swelling may be due to injury, surgery, or increased sensitivity to touch

Table continued on following page

87

TABLE 4–1 Respiratory Assessment Techniques, Tips, Geriatric Considerations *Continued*

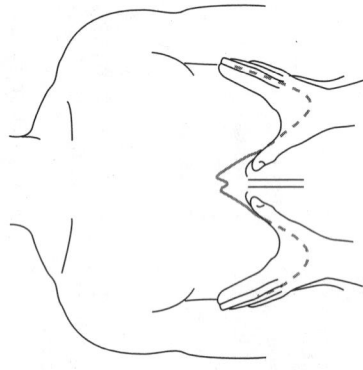

FIGURE 4–6
Assessing respiratory excursion on the anterior chest.

| 3. Crepitus | Examine the chest generally
Examine areas immediate to
• Trachea, tracheostomy (neck, face)
• Chest tube insertion site(s)
• Site of penetrating chest injury | A popping, crackling sensation on compressing the skin
Produced by air trapped in subcutaneous tissue; will resorb with time or with correction of the underlying cause:
• Rupture of an alveolar bulla in emphysema
• Pneumothorax
• Mediastinal air
• Air escape into subcutaneous tissue with assisted ventilation, especially with positive pressure | Crepitus is *not* a normal finding with aging |

ASSESSMENT TIPS

1. Crepitus is best felt with the pads of the fingers; it feels like popping bubbles
2. Crepitus sounds like crinkling cellophane
3. Define and record borders of any crepitant area; this can be used to evaluate improvement or deterioration in the condition

Table continued on following page

89

TABLE 4-1 Respiratory Assessment Techniques, Tips, Geriatric Considerations *Continued*

Technique	Performance Tips	Description/Rationale	Geriatric Considerations
4. Fremitus (optional)	Fremitus can be assessed during general palpation of the thoracic area It is found in the lower, anterolateral rib cage where there is increased pleural movement with breathing *ASSESSMENT TIP* Fremitus is best felt with the pads of the fingers or the metacarpal pads on the palms	Pleural friction fremitus is a grating felt over inflamed pleurae; it is verified with auscultation of a pleural friction rub (see below)	
Percussion (optional: use only in selected situations to confirm or enhance data obtained by inspection, palpation, or auscultation)	**All lung fields** (survey) **Areas of suspected pathology**	Gives an indication of lung tissue composition to a depth of about 3 cm Chest percussion notes: **Resonance:** Healthy lung tissue	Chest deformity with aging can alter the expected percussion note, producing unexpected dullness or hyperresonance

Hyperresonance: Overinflated lung tissue (e.g., emphysema, tension pneumothorax)

Dullness: Consolidating lung tissue (e.g., large pneumonia, large pleural effusion, hemothorax); percussion over the heart or liver

Hypertympanism: Tension pneumothorax, gastric bubble (with upward displacement of abdominal contents into the thoracic area)

The elderly have an increased susceptibility to pneumonia, which may present as dullness to percussion

COPD should be considered when hyperresonance is percussed

ASSESSMENT TIPS

1. The *pad* of the middle finger on the chest should be firmly placed (pleximeter finger); the rest of the hand remains off the chest

2. The *tip* of the middle finger of the dominant hand should strike the pleximeter finger proximal to the nail plate twice, briskly and then move to the next site

3. Percuss from side to side, comparing contralateral results immediately

4. Quality of sounds may be diminished by
   - Thickened chest wall
   - Obesity

Table continued on following page

TABLE 4-1 Respiratory Assessment Techniques, Tips, Geriatric Considerations *Continued*

Technique	Performance Tips	Description/Rationale	Geriatric Considerations
	• Large breasts • Muscular build • Shallow respirations 5. Do not percuss dependent areas with the patient in the side-lying position; dependent tissue is compressed and will produce a dull, pathological note even in the absence of disease; wait to assess these areas until the patient is turned 6. Dullness to percussion will be normal within the cardiac borders (mid and left chest) and over the upper margin of the liver (right lower chest)		

Auscultation
1. Normal breath sounds

ASSESSMENT TIPS

1. *Never* auscultate through clothing; movement of fabric under the stethoscope produces a sound similar to crackles

2. Movement of chest hair under the stethoscope produces a sound similar to crackles; wetting hair or pressing more firmly with the stethoscope may help

3. Quality of sounds may be diminished by thickened chest wall (obesity, large breasts, muscular build) and by shallow respirations

Table continued on following page

TABLE 4–1 Respiratory Assessment Techniques, Tips, Geriatric Considerations *Continued*

Technique	Performance Tips	Description/Rationale	Geriatric Considerations
	4. Instruct a cooperative patient to breath a little deeper than normal, through the mouth		
	5. Watch for hyperventilation and syncope but remember that deep breathing is also therapeutic		
	6. Auscultate from side to side, comparing contralateral results immediately		
	7. Initial assessment should include anterior, posterior, and lateral areas		
	8. To avoid fatiguing a weak patient, begin at		

the bases, posteriorly, where pathology is first expected

9. Because lung tissue is compressed in the side-lying position, assure accurate assessment by auscultating right posterior lung field in left side-lying position and vice versa

10. Empty ventilator tubing of water accumulated in dependent areas prior to auscultation; water movement can transmit sounds that may mask true breath sounds or be erroneously interpreted as adventitious

Table continued on following page

TABLE 4-1 Respiratory Assessment Techniques, Tips, Geriatric Considerations *Continued*

Technique	Performance Tips	Description/Rationale	Geriatric Considerations
	11. If you are unable to hear lung sounds over the bubbling of a chest tube, check for an air leak or loose connection, or decrease suction; chest tube bubbling should always be gentle 12. Record findings in terms of lung fields where abnormals were assessed; for example, • By area: anterior, lateral, posterior, right or left side • By approximate lung field, such as upper		

	(apex), middle, lower (base) • *Do not* attempt to describe by lobes, as this is not accurate	
	Bronchial breath sounds over large airways	Inspiratory and expiratory sounds are of similar, prolonged duration (see Fig. 4–7)
		Bronchial and vesicular breath sounds should be similar in young and old adults
	Vesicular breath sounds over peripheral lung fields	Inspiratory sound is of longer duration than expiratory sound (see Fig. 4–7)
2. Abnormal breath sounds	**Diminished breath sounds** (note specific area or side) • Generalized • Localized	Diminished sounds may be caused by shallow breathing or thick chest wall if sounds are symmetrical throughout lung fields; they may also indicate poorly ventilated lung field	Because of weakened respiratory muscles, decreased chest and lung expansion, and debilitated condition, the elderly patient may need increased encouragement to breathe deeply enough for you to hear breath sounds

	Absent breath sounds (note specific area or side)	Absent sounds usually indicate
		• Lung pathology; for example,
		  – Atelectasis
		  – Consolidation
			Diminished breath sounds throughout lung fields may be due to thickened chest wall and barrel chest

Table continued on following page

97

TABLE 4-1 Respiratory Assessment Techniques, Tips, Geriatric Considerations *Continued*

LOCATION OF STETHOSCOPE	TYPE OF BREATH SOUND	DURATION OF SOUND DURING AUSCULTATION OF THE LUNGS
Over trachea	Bronchial	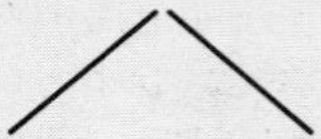
Over bronchi, large bronchioles	Bronchial	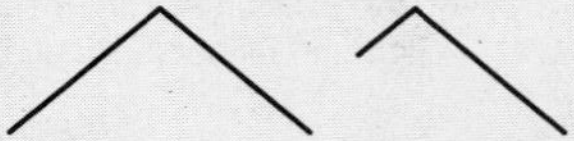
Over small airways	Vesicular	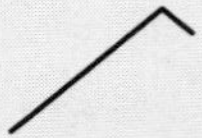

FIGURE 4-7
Duration of breath sounds during auscultation of the lungs.

	– Tumor – Pneumo-, hemothorax • Endotracheal tube displacement • Faulty stethoscope (check to see that the diaphragm is turned on by tapping on it with the earpieces in place)	
Bronchial breath sounds in a peripheral lung area	Solid tissue conducts sound better than aerated tissue; misplaced bronchial sounds indicate an area of consolidation, such as in a developing pneumonia, or other tissue thickening	Pay particular attention to bronchial breath sounds in the elderly because of their increased susceptibility to pneumonia; displaced bronchial breath sounds may be the only presenting sign

Table continued on following page

TABLE 4–1 Respiratory Assessment Techniques, Tips, Geriatric Considerations *Continued*

Technique	Performance Tips	Description/Rationale	Geriatric Considerations
3. Added breath sounds (adventitious) (terminology may vary in different practice settings)	**Crackles** (formerly called rales) *ASSESSMENT TIP* Estimate the pitch: • Fine (high-pitched, crackly, like strands of hair rolled between the fingers) • Coarse (low-pitched, bubbly) *ASSESSMENT TIP* Record where the sound is heard in the respiratory cycle: • Early, mid, or late inspiration • Expiration	A discontinuous, popping sound caused by equalization of gas pressures following late, forceful opening of airways against the resistance of fluid, mucus, or exudates (see Fig. 4–8) *Characteristics* Usually heard in early, mid, or late inspiration; rarer on expiration Usually will not clear with coughing Requires medical intervention *Causes* Early inspiratory crackles: obstructive disease	May be heard in dependent lung fields following prolonged periods of immobility, especially in the elderly; such crackles will usually clear with change of position, deep breathing, and coughing, as secretions are cleared

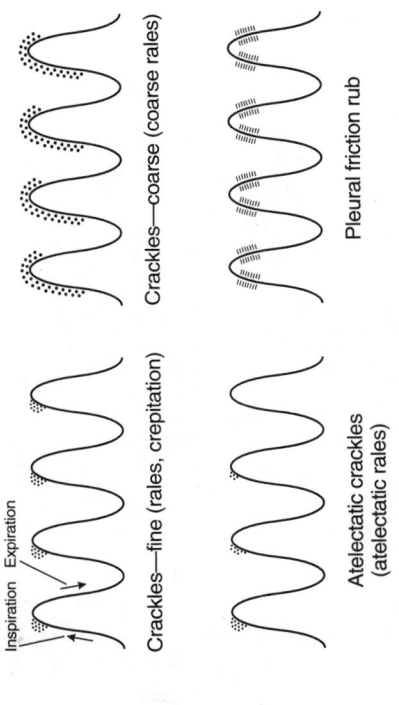

Inspiration Expiration

Crackles—fine (rales, crepitation)

Crackles—coarse (coarse rales)

Atelectatic crackles
(atelectatic rales)

Pleural friction rub

FIGURE 4-8

Discontinuous lung sounds. (Adapted from Jarvis, C. [1996]. *Physical examination and health assessment* [3rd ed., p. 502]. Philadelphia: W. B. Saunders.)

Table continued on following page

TABLE 4-1 Respiratory Assessment Techniques, Tips, Geriatric Considerations *Continued*

Technique	Performance Tips	Description/Rationale	Geriatric Considerations
		Late inspiratory crackles: restrictive disease	
		Fine, high-pitched crackles: pathology in lower, smaller airways	
		Coarse, low-pitched: pathology in higher, larger airways	
		Expiratory crackles: late airway opening	
Wheezes		A continuous musical sound caused by air moving through a narrowed opening such as edema, secretions, tumor, foreign body (see Fig. 4–9)	New onset asthma is rare in the geriatric patient
		Characteristics	Without a history of asthma, look for other possible causes of wheezing, such as
		May be heard on inspiration or expiration	• Cardiac disease resulting in left ventricular failure (cardiac asthma)
		Will often disappear or change with coughing and following inhaled bronchodilator therapy	• Aspiration
			• Pulmonary embolism
			• Tumor

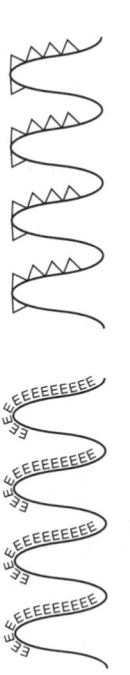

FIGURE 4–9

Continuous lung sounds. (Adapted from Jarvis, C. [1996]. *Physical examination and health assessment* [3rd ed., p. 503]. Philadelphia: W. B. Saunders.)

Wheeze—high-pitched (sibilant rhonchi)

Wheeze—low-pitched (sonorous rhonchi)

Table continued on following page

TABLE 4-1 Respiratory Assessment Techniques, Tips, Geriatric Considerations *Continued*

Technique	Performance Tips	Description/Rationale	Geriatric Considerations
	• Sibilant wheezes	Sibilant wheezes are high pitched and usually due to edema, spasm, tumor, or foreign body	With a history of asthma, look for triggers for an attack, such as respiratory inflammation or infection.
	ASSESSMENT TIP Sudden, unexplained disappearance may indicate complete obstruction of the involved airway		
	Sonorous wheezes (formerly called rhonchi)	Sonorous wheezes are low-pitched sounds like a vibrating reed; usually due to air colliding with secretions collected in large airways such as the trachea and bronchi	
	ASSESSMENT TIP These sounds indicate the need for position change, deep breathing, coughing, or tracheal suctioning		

Pleural Friction Rub

Low-pitched, grating sound like leather or ropes rubbing together; produced by inflamed pleurae rubbing together during breathing

Characteristics

May be heard on both inspiration (as inflamed plural surfaces contact each other) and during the initial period of expiration; the duration may be affected by the degree of inflammation

Does not clear with coughing

Pain may increase with coughing, deep breathing

Requires medical intervention

RESPIRATORY DISORDERS

Respiratory failure is defined as inadequate gas exchange to meet tissue metabolic needs. Causes of respiratory failure include any clinical situation where the body is unable to meet the tissue demands for oxygenation or for carbon dioxide removal. Blood gas diagnostic guidelines include an arterial partial pressure of oxygen (Pao_2) <50 to 60 mm Hg and a partial pressure of carbon dioxide (Pco_2) >50 mm Hg with a pH less than 7.30 for a patient breathing room air.

Types of respiratory disorders that may culminate in respiratory failure include (1) restrictive, (2) perfusion, and (3) obstructive lung disorders.

RESTRICTIVE LUNG DISORDERS

Restrictive lung disorders decrease lung expansion and therefore vital capacity and total lung capacity. Restrictive lung disorders, including adult respiratory distress syndrome, pulmonary edema, atelectasis, pneumonia, pleural effusion, and pneumothorax, generally cause acute respiratory failure.

Adult Respiratory Distress Syndrome (ARDS)

(high-permeability pulmonary edema, noncardiac pulmonary edema)

Pathophysiology

A number of cells and mediators have been identified as potential mechanisms of lung injury in ARDS. In particular, the overwhelming inflammatory response of alveolar macrophages, platelets, neutrophils, and endothelial cells is thought to be intensified by the activation of the complement system (C5a) and cytokines. Subsequently, toxic substances and degradative enzymes are generated and secreted. These substances, including toxic oxygen metabolites, proteases, arachidonic acid metabolites, and platelet-activating factor, can cause damage to the alveolocapillary membrane promoting pulmonary edema, changes in the small-caliber airways resulting in decreases in pulmonary compliance and bronchoconstriction, and disruption of pulmonary blood flow and coagulation resulting in pulmonary hypertension (see Fig. 4–10).

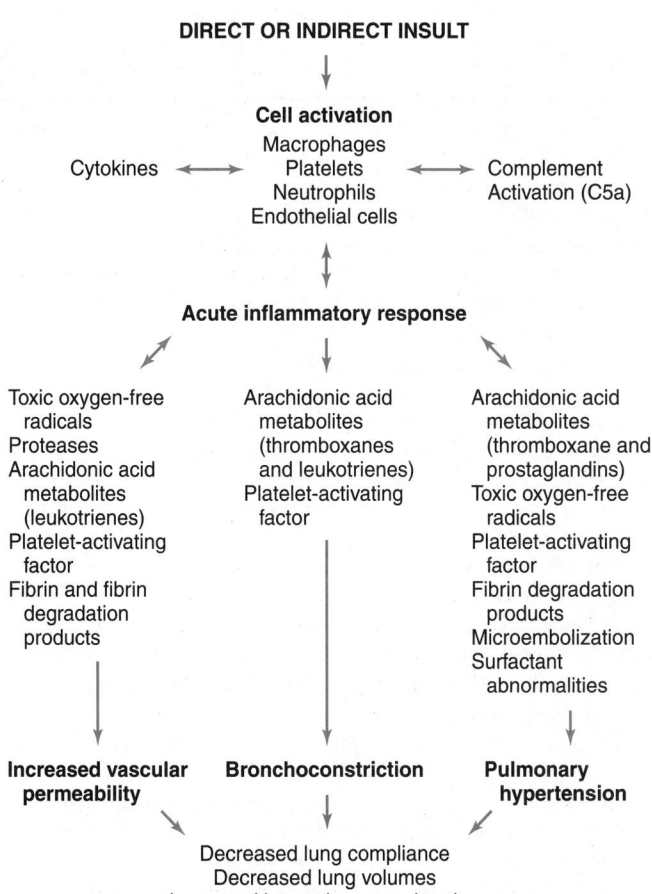

DIRECT OR INDIRECT INSULT

Cell activation
Macrophages
Platelets
Neutrophils
Endothelial cells

Cytokines ⟷ (cell activation) ⟷ Complement Activation (C5a)

Acute inflammatory response

Toxic oxygen-free radicals
Proteases
Arachidonic acid metabolites (leukotrienes)
Platelet-activating factor
Fibrin and fibrin degradation products

Arachidonic acid metabolites (thromboxanes and leukotrienes)
Platelet-activating factor

Arachidonic acid metabolites (thromboxane and prostaglandins)
Toxic oxygen-free radicals
Platelet-activating factor
Fibrin degradation products
Microembolization
Surfactant abnormalities

Increased vascular permeability   **Bronchoconstriction**   **Pulmonary hypertension**

Decreased lung compliance
Decreased lung volumes
Increased intrapulmonary shunting
Progressive arterial hypoxemia refractory to oxygen therapy

FIGURE 4–10

Cells and mediators that potentially intensify the pathologic disturbances in ARDS. (Adapted from Clochesy, J.M., Breu, C., Cardin, S., Whittaker, A.A., & Rudy, E.B. [Eds.]. [1996]. *Critical care nursing* [2nd ed., p. 662]. Philadelphia: W. B. Saunders.)

The chain of events is initiated by a catastrophic event that causes diffuse injury to the alveolar epithelium side (direct) or the pulmonary endothelium side (indirect) of the alveolocapillary exchanging membrane. The most common cause of direct injury is aspiration of stomach contents. The most common cause of indirect injury is septic shock.

Regardless of the initial insult, in the acute phase increased microvascular permeability allows large amounts of fluid, plasma, protein, and blood cells to leak into the pulmonary interstitial space, causing alveolar flooding. As the gas volume is replaced by fluid, the function of surfactant (reduction of surface tension) is thought to be inhibited by plasma proteins and inflammatory mediators. High surface tension causes collapse of alveoli, and surfactant is further inactivated secondary to atelectasis. The lungs become stiff, and compliance decreases.

Bronchoconstriction compounds the decrease in compliance, and the functional residual capacity is severely diminished. The work of breathing is dramatically increased.

Gas exchange is significantly compromised due to ventilation-perfusion mismatches and intrapulmonary shunting. Perfusion continues to flooded and underventilated alveoli, and ventilation may occur in the presence of pulmonary vasoconstriction. The alveolar-to-arterial difference in oxygen concentration widens, and hypoxemia resistant to oxygen therapy results.

Increased pulmonary vascular resistance contributes to increased pulmonary artery pressures and may lead to right heart failure. Decreased left ventricular filling pressures may decrease cardiac output.

Continued deterioration leads to the subacute or chronic phase of ARDS, which is characterized by the development of pulmonary fibrosis and the formation of hyaline membranes. Gas diffusion is severely compromised. Hypercapnia is reflective of severe membrane damage.

If the patient survives, changes in the injured lung parenchyma may be completely reversible. However, the mortality rate associated with ARDS remains high. Death may occur from prolonged respiratory failure or a complicating event.

Assessment

Initially, the predisposing factor dominates the clinical presentation. However, it is during this latent phase that changes in the alveolocapillary membrane begin to occur. At this time, respiratory assessment may reveal few or no abnormal pulmonary findings unless the precipitating event is respiratory in nature.

In the acute phase, breathing patterns, airway clearance, and gas exchange are compromised as protein-rich fluid moves into the pulmonary interstitium and then the alveoli. Clinical manifestations reveal abnormal pulmonary findings that indicate the disease has progressed beyond the early stages (see Clinical Findings 4–1).

POINTS TO REMEMBER

▶ Because the risk of developing ARDS increases significantly with the presence of more than one predisposing factor and the detection of ARDS in its early stages is very difficult, a thorough nursing history (see Tables 1–1 and 4–1 and Clinical Findings 4–1) is crucial to identify patients at risk (ARDS usually develops within 48 hours after the initial insult).

▶ Because the mortality rate of patients with ARDS increases with the severity and number of underlying disorders, in addition to the initial and baseline assessments (see Table 2–1), focused respiratory and cardiovascular assessments (see Tables 2–1, 4–1, and 5–1), as well as focused assessments of all systems involved in the underlying pathology, should be completed as often as the patient's condition dictates to detect or anticipate and prevent complications such as multiple organ dysfunction. (Tachycardia, dysrhythmias, decreased cardiac output, hypotension, decreased urine output, and alterations in the level of consciousness are warning signs of inadequate blood flow to the tissues.)

▶ Ongoing assessment incorporates (1) the evaluation of responses to diagnostic procedures and therapeutic interventions aimed at the recruitment of unstable alveoli and the improvement of gas exchange and (2) collaboration with other members of the health team to ensure optimal delivery of oxygen to the tissues and to prevent further injury.

Clinical Findings 4–1 *Adult Respiratory Distress Syndrome*

I. HISTORY

A. Predisposing factors

1. *Direct injury*
   - Aspiration of stomach contents
   - Inhalation of high concentrations of oxygen, smoke, or other chemicals

- Direct pulmonary trauma
- Viral, bacterial, or fungal pneumonia
- Near-drowning

2. *Indirect injury*
   - Septic syndrome
   - Shock of any kind
   - Multiple trauma
   - Pulmonary embolism (thrombotic, air, fat, or amniotic fluid)
   - Head injury (increased intracranial pressure)
   - Burns
   - Pancreatitis
   - Uremia
   - Cardiopulmonary bypass
   - Disseminated intravascular coagulation
   - Multiple blood transfusions
   - Drug overdose (heroin, methadone, barbiturates, propoxyphene [Darvon])

B. Subjective findings
1. Dyspnea related to increased physiological dead space and insufficient circulating oxygen
2. Fatigue related to increased work of breathing

II. LABORATORY AND BEDSIDE MONITORING FINDINGS

A. Pulmonary function studies (see Table 13–1 for related information on pulmonary function studies)
1. Increased minute ventilation related to increased physiologic dead space and the demand to maintain $PaCO_2$ at a tolerable level
2. Decreased functional residual capacity related to increased fluid in the air spaces and widespread atelectasis
3. Decrease in compliance (<50 mg/cm H_2O on mechanical ventilation) related to areas of consolidation and atelectasis
4. Increase in peak inspiratory pressure (>50 cm H_2O on mechanical ventilation) related to decreased compliance

B. Chest x-ray: Diffuse bilateral pulmonary parenchymal infiltrates

C. Arterial blood gas studies (see Chapter 13 for related information on arterial blood gas studies, efficiency of gas exchange, acid-base balance, and serum lactate levels. See Table 14–1 for related information on oxygen delivery and consumption parameters)
1. $PaCO_2$ may be decreased initially (<35 mm Hg) related to tachypnea and alveolar hyperventilation; it may be increased (>45 mm Hg) in later

stages related to decreased diffusion secondary to severe alveolocapillary membrane damage

2. Refractory hypoxemia (PaO_2 <55 mm Hg at a fraction of inspired oxygen [FiO_2] of 0.5 or higher) related to ventilation-perfusion mismatches
3. Increased shunt fraction ($\dot{Q}s/\dot{Q}t$) related to intrapulmonary shunting (right-to-left shunt)
4. Alveolar-arterial gradient (PAO_2-PaO_2) may be >20 mm Hg, reflective of intrapulmonary shunting (decreased gas exchange)
5. PaO_2/FiO_2 ratio may be <200, reflective of intrapulmonary shunting (inability of gas to diffuse into the blood)
6. pH may be >7.45 initially, related to hyperventilation (respiratory alkalosis); then it may be <7.35 in later stages, related to decreased blood flow to the tissues (metabolic acidosis) or hypercapnia (respiratory acidosis)
7. Plasma lactate may be increased (>2 mEq/L) if systemic oxygen delivery does not satisfy tissue oxygen requirements

D. Hemodynamic parameters (see Chapter 14, Table 14–2 and Fig. 14–2 for related information on hemodynamic parameters)

1. Pulmonary capillary wedge pressure (PCWP) is usually <18 mm Hg.
2. Pulmonary artery pressures are generally increased related to pulmonary hypertension (pulmonary artery diastolic pressure may be >5 mm Hg more than PCWP)
3. Cardiac output may be increased initially (compensatory mechanism to deliver the available but reduced amount of oxygen to the tissue); it may be decreased in later stages, related to decreased left ventricular filling pressures caused by pulmonary hypertension, right heart failure, or dysrhythmias

III. PHYSICAL ASSESSMENT FINDINGS

A. General observations (inspection)

1. *Mental status:* Restlessness, agitation, and confusion related to hypoxemia
2. *Skin*
   - Cyanosis may be present related to hypoxemia (late sign), peripheral vasoconstriction, or decreased blood flow to the tissues
   - Pallor may be present related to anemia secondary to initial insult or underlying disease process, or decreased blood flow to the tissues
3. *Nails:* Capillary refill may be >2 seconds because of decreased blood flow to the tissues
4. *Respiratory pattern:* Tachypnea or hyperventilation related to attempt by

lungs to move more oxygen and maintain $Paco_2$ levels
5. *Respiratory effort:* Use of accessory muscles and intercostal and supra-costal retraction related to the increased work of breathing (see Table 4–1)
6. *Cough and sputum*
   • Cough related to increased secretions in the lungs
   • Color of sputum will depend on the presence of infection or bleeding (see Table 4–1)
7. *Respiratory excursion:* Asymmetrical chest excursion related to altered air movement and atelectasis

B. Palpation
1. *Skin*
   • May be cool and moist because of decreased tissue perfusion (e.g., shock states)
   • May be warm and vasodilated because of hyperdynamic states (e.g., sepsis, fever)
2. *Chest wall and thorax:* Decreased or asymmetrical chest expansion related to altered air movement and atelectasis

C. Auscultation
1. *Abnormal breath sounds*
   • Diminished breath sounds related to decreased expansion secondary to decreased compliance
   • Bronchial breath sounds over areas of consolidation
2. *Adventitious breath sounds*
   • Crackles and sonorous wheezes (rhonchi) over fluid-filled airways
   • Sibilant wheezes may be present, related to bronchospasm

Pulmonary Edema

(low-permeability pulmonary edema, cardiac pulmonary edema)

Pathophysiology

An imbalance between hydrostatic pressure and osmotic pressure causes a fluid shift within the lungs that results in pulmonary edema. The permeability of the alveolocapillary membrane usually remains intact.

Hydrostatic pressure influences the outward movement of fluid. If hydrostatic pressure is higher in the capillary than in the interstitial space, fluid will move out of the capillary into the interstitium. If hydrostatic pressure is higher in the interstitium than in the capillary, fluid will move out of the interstitium into the capillary.

Osmotic pressure opposes hydrostatic pressure. Osmotic pressure is primarily generated by plasma proteins and molecules too big to cross the microvascular barrier. If osmotic pressure is higher in the capillary than in the interstitial space, fluid is pulled from the interstitium to the capillary. If osmotic pressure is higher in the interstitium than the capillary, fluid is pulled from the capillary to the interstitium.

Under normal conditions, both hydrostatic pressure and osmotic pressure are higher in the intravascular space than in the interstitial space. Consequently, there is a balance of forces moving fluid out of the capillary into the interstitium and pulling fluid out of the interstitium into the capillary. Excess protein and fluid that does not reenter the capillary is drained by the lymphatics.

A failing left ventricle (heart failure, cardiogenic shock), severe valvular disease, and excessive administration of intravenous fluids can cause a sustained increase in hydrostatic pressure. Fluid is forced from the capillaries (exceeding the capacity of the lymphatics) and moves into the interstitial and alveolar spaces, causing edema.

Assessment

Clinical manifestations of pulmonary edema vary with the severity of the edema and the underlying disorder (see Clinical Findings 4–2). The severity of edema can be estimated from the location of edema fluid. Initially, fluid accumulates in the dependent portions of the lungs (pulmonary blood flow is gravity dependent). As the fluid accumulation worsens, the edema moves up the lungs resulting in increased work of breathing, anxiety, and severely impaired gas exchange. An increased right-to-left shunt may result in hypoxemia.

POINTS TO REMEMBER

▶ Acute pulmonary edema is a life-threatening disorder that usually develops secondary to a cardiovascular disorder.

▶ The critically ill adult may present with acute pulmonary edema. As well, the critically ill adult is at risk for the development of acute pulmonary edema.

▶ A thorough nursing history (see Tables 1–1 and 4–1 and Clinical Findings 4-2) is crucial to identify the cause of pulmonary edema and to identify patients at risk for the development of pulmonary edema.

▶ In addition to the initial and baseline assessments (see Table 2–1), focused respiratory and cardiovascular assessments (see Tables 2–1, 4–1, and 5–1), as well as a focused assessment of the underlying or presenting pathology, should be completed as often as the patient's condition dictates to detect or anticipate and prevent complications such as acute respiratory failure, right heart failure, and decreased blood flow to the tissues.

▶ Ongoing assessment incorporates the evaluation of responses to diagnostic procedures and therapeutic interventions aimed at the reduction of fluid in the lungs, and involves collaboration with other members of the health team to support oxygenation and improve blood flow to the tissues.

Clinical Findings 4–2 *Pulmonary Edema*

I. HISTORY

A. Predisposing factors
1. Acute myocardial infarction
2. Left ventricular failure
3. Cardiogenic shock
4. Mitral or aortic valve disease
5. Excessive fluid replacement (the elderly are less tolerant of large increases in fluid volume)

B. Subjective findings
1. Dyspnea related to pulmonary congestion
2. Orthopnea and paroxysmal nocturnal dyspnea related to redistribution of blood flow in the supine position (failing heart is unable to pump extra blood, and pulmonary congestion is worsened).
3. Fatigue related to the increased work of breathing
4. Apprehension and panic related to feelings of suffocation

II. LABORATORY AND BEDSIDE MONITORING FINDINGS

A. Chest x-ray
1. Enlargement of the heart, pulmonary veins, capillaries, and lymphatics may be present, related to excessive blood volume
2. Aortic or mitral valve calcification may be present, related to valvular disease
3. Peripheral distribution of infiltrates

B. Arterial blood gases: PaO_2 may be >45 mm Hg, and $PaCO_2$ may be >40 mm Hg related to fluid-filled alveoli and decreased area for gas exchange

C. Serum enzymes (see Table 13–3 for related information on cardiac enzymes and Clinical Findings 5–3 for related information on acute myocardial infarction): Cardiac isoenzymes may be elevated because of acute myocardial infarction

D. ECG (see Table 14–3 for related information on dysrhythmias)

1. Tachycardia may be present, related to anxiety, hypoxemia, or decreased cardiac output
2. Dysrhythmias may be present because of myocardial hypoxia or underlying disorder
3. New Q waves may be present related to acute myocardial infarction
4. ST-T wave changes may be present, related to myocardial ischemia, injury
5. P wave changes may be present, related to mitral or left atrial disease (see Table 5–4 and Clinical Findings 5–1 to 5–3 for related information on cardiovascular disorders)

E. Hemodynamic parameters (see Chapter 14, Table 14–2, and Fig. 14–2 for related information on hemodynamic parameters)

1. Blood pressure (BP) may be normal or hypotensive related to decreased cardiac output
2. Increased left atrial pressure (25 to 30 mm Hg) related to excessive blood volume and the compensatory responses of atrial dilation and hypertrophy
3. PCWP >18 mm Hg related to excessive blood volume or impaired left ventricular contractility
4. Pulmonary artery diastolic pressure is usually ≤5 mm Hg more than PCWP (pulmonary hypertension, if present, is secondary to pulmonary venous congestion)
5. Cardiac output is usually decreased (<4 L/min) related to sluggish pumping of the left heart

III. PHYSICAL ASSESSMENT FINDINGS

A. General observations (inspection)

1. *Mental status:* Restlessness related to hypoxemia
2. *Skin:* Cyanosis may be present because of peripheral vasoconstriction (compensatory response secondary to decreased cardiac output), hypoxemia (late sign), or decreased blood flow to the tissues
3. *Nails*
   - Capillary refill may be >2 seconds, related to decreased blood flow to the tissues.
   - Clubbing may be present, related to chronic cardiovascular disease
4. *Respiratory pattern:* Tachypnea related to decreased area for gas exchange and need to move more oxygen and maintain acceptable CO_2 levels

5. *Respiratory effort:* In the conscious patient, the bolt upright position may be used to maximize respiratory effort
6. *Cough and sputum*
   - Productive cough related to bronchial irritation associated with congestion
   - Sputum blood-tinged, related to breakage of fragile capillaries, and frothy, related to fluid buildup in the alveoli
7. *Neck veins:* Jugular venous distention related to volume overload or venous congestion secondary to right heart failure (see Clinical Findings 5–2 for related information on right heart failure)

B. Palpation: *Skin*
   1. Cool, moist skin with decreased perfusion
   2. Peripheral edema related to right heart failure and venous congestion

C. Auscultation
   1. *Adventitious breath sounds:* Basilar to diffuse bubbly crackles related to the movement of air through partially fluid-filled alveoli (may begin in bilateral bases if in upright position and progress up to apices with severity of pulmonary edema)
   2. *Heart sounds*
      - S_3 related to ventricular failure
      - S_4 related to decreased ventricular compliance
      - Murmurs may be present related to valvular disorders, acute myocardial infarction, or heart failure. (see Clinical Findings 5–1 and 5–2 for related information on heart failure).

Atelectasis

Pathophysiology

Ineffective ventilation, decreased surfactant levels, or obstruction of conducting airways into the alveoli can cause collapse of lung tissue in the affected area. Atelectatic areas can potentiate ventilation-perfusion mismatches.

Constant shallow breathing at a reduced tidal volume can lead to the development of atelectasis. In normal respiration, some alveoli collapse at the end of expiration. A deep breath or sigh is sufficient to reexpand the atelectatic areas. With shallow breathing, the insufficient tidal volume is unable to reinflate collapsed alveoli and prevent the collapse of others.

Decreased production of surfactant may be attributed to a decrease in regional blood flow. As well, exposure to hypothermia, for example during cardiopulmonary bypass, may cause decreased production of surfactant.

Impaired cough mechanisms, damaged or inhibited cilia, increased viscosity of secretions, or prolonged immobility can lead to the accumulation of secretions in the dependent lung fields. Retained secretions or mucous plugs can block bronchioles. Lung gas distal to the blockages is absorbed, resulting in alveolar collapse.

Untreated or progressive atelectasis can lead to decreases in vital capacity, functional residual capacity, and compliance. Subsequently, the work of breathing is increased.

If perfusion continues to collapsed alveoli, a physiological shunt (right to left) occurs. Intrapulmonary shunting can lead to severe arterial hypoxemia.

Assessment

Nearly all critically ill adults are susceptible to the development of atelectasis. Patients at greatest risk are the immobile and those in whom ventilatory function is already impaired, mucous secretion is excessive or thicker than normal, or the cough reflex is suppressed (see Clinical Findings 4–3).

POINTS TO REMEMBER

▶ In addition to causing atelectasis, retained and pooled pulmonary secretions can act as a medium for the growth of bacteria and microorganisms and predispose the critically ill adult to the development of pneumonia (see Clinical Findings 4–4).

▶ A thorough nursing history (see Tables 1–1 and 4–1 and Clinical Findings 4–3) is crucial to identify patients at risk for the development of atelectasis.

▶ In addition to the initial and baseline assessments (see Table 2–1) and a focused assessment of the system involved with the original pathology, a focused respiratory assessment (see Tables 2-1 and 4-1) should be completed as often as the patient's condition dictates to detect or anticipate and prevent complications such as pneumonia.

▶ Ongoing assessment incorporates the evaluation of responses to diagnostic procedures and therapeutic interventions aimed at the facilitation of lung expansion and the elimination of secretions;

it includes collaboration with other members of the health team
to prevent hypoxemia and pneumonia.

Clinical Findings 4–3   *Atelectasis*

I. HISTORY

A. Predisposing factors
1. Thoracic or upper abdominal surgery or trauma
2. Pleural effusion
3. Splinting
4. Tight dressings or binders
5. Weakened thoracic muscles
6. Prolonged immobility (particularly the supine position)
7. Endotracheal intubation (bypasses normal host defenses and humidifying mechanisms of upper airway, can damage cilia, interfering with mucociliary clearance)
8. Thick, tenacious pulmonary secretions (dehydration, anticholinergic drugs)
9. Cardiopulmonary bypass
10. Altered levels of consciousness
11. Anesthetics, narcotics, or sedatives
12. Tumors
13. Aspiration of foreign objects

B. Subjective findings
1. Dyspnea related to restricted chest movement or increase in physiological dead space
2. Fatigue related to the increased work of breathing
3. Pain related to surgical incision or trauma

II. LABORATORY AND BEDSIDE MONITORING FINDINGS

A. Chest x-ray: Elevated diaphragm and patches of large areas of consolidation may be present
B. Arterial blood gases
1. PaO_2 may be decreased (<70 to 80 mm Hg) because of intrapulmonary shunting
2. $PaCO_2$ may be normal or decreased (<35 mm Hg) related to tachypnea

III. PHYSICAL ASSESSMENT FINDINGS

A. General observations (inspection)

1. *Mental status:* Restlessness related to hypoxemia (early sign)
2. *Skin*
   - Cyanosis may be present, related to peripheral vasoconstriction or hypoxemia (late sign)
   - Pallor may be present, related to anemia secondary to underlying disease or hypoxemia
3. *Respiratory pattern*
   - Shallow respiration may be present, associated with the reduction of diaphragmatic breathing related to pain, weakened respiratory muscles, restricted thoracic movement, drugs, or altered levels of consciousness
   - Tachypnea may be present, related to hypoxemia and the need to move more oxygen with severe atelectasis
4. *Respiratory effort:* Use of accessory muscles because of increased work of breathing with severe atelectasis (see Table 4–1)
5. *Respiratory excursion:* Asymmetrical chest expansion may be present, related to surgical incision, trauma, tight dressing or binder, or splinting secondary to pain

B. Palpation

1. *Skin:* Warm periphery with presence of fever
2. *Chest wall and thorax*
   - Tenderness may be present, related to surgical incision or trauma
   - Decreased chest expansion may be present, related to thoracic or upper abdominal surgery and trauma or weak thoracic muscles

C. Percussion: Dullness over collapsed or consolidated areas

D. Auscultation

1. *Abnormal breath sounds*
   - Diminished or absent breath sounds over large areas of collapse
   - Bronchial breath sounds over areas of consolidation
2. *Adventitious sounds:* Crackles may be heard in dependent lung fields over areas of retained secretions

Pneumonia

Pathophysiology

Acute pneumonia is an infective process that results in inflammation of the interstitial lung tissue, the alveoli, and often the bronchioles. The extent of pulmonary involvement depends on the defense mechanisms of the host and the characteristics of the invading organism.

Acute pneumonia may be caused by bacterial, viral, or mycoplasmal organisms, protozoan or fungal organisms, or chemical irritation. The infection may be community-acquired or hospital-acquired (nosocomial).

Bacterial pneumonia usually causes consolidation of lung tissue. Inflammatory exudate collects in the alveolar spaces and becomes difficult to expectorate. Ventilation-perfusion mismatches lead to impaired gas exchange. Causative organisms include gram-positive bacteria, such as *Staphylococcus aureus* (methicillin-resistant *Staphylococcus aureus*) and *Streptococcus pneumoniae (Pneumococcus),* and gram-negative bacteria such as *Klebsiella, Pseudomonas, Escherichia coli, Serratia, Haemophilus, Proteus, Legionella* species, and anaerobes: *Bacteroides* species, *Fusobacterium nucleatum.* Gram-negative bacteria are the most common cause of nosocomial pneumonia in the critically ill adult.

Viral pneumonia usually does not produce an exudate. Severe viral pneumonia causes the alveoli to fill with fluid, fibrin, red blood cells, and macrophages, producing refractory hypoxemia similar to ARDS (see Clinical Findings 4–1). Less severe viral pneumonia presents as patchy areas of infiltrate with a milder clinical presentation. The most common causative organisms include paramyxovirus, cytomegalovirus, measles, varicella viruses, and influenza viruses.

Mycoplasmal pneumonia is most common in young adults. It is often preceded by pneumonitis and bronchitis and may be associated with otitis media and myringitis.

Pneumocystis carinii pneumonia is an opportunistic infection caused by a protozoan. Patients whose immune systems have been compromised by chemotherapy or disease are susceptible. *Pneumocystis* pneumonia is the most common pulmonary infection in patients with AIDS (see Clinical Findings 11–1).

The incidence of fungal infection is increasing in the immunocompromised and critically ill populations. The most common causative organisms include *Candida, Cryptococcus, Aspergillus, Histoplasma, Coccidioides,* and *Blastomyces.*

Aspiration of stomach contents causes a chemical pneumonitis with a clinical presentation similar to ARDS (see Clinical Findings 4–1). Aspiration of oral bacteria (*Bacteroides* and *Fusobacterium*) may present as a lung abscess, necrotizing pneumonia, or empyema.

Assessment

Nearly all critically ill adults are susceptible to the acquisition of pneumonia. The patients most at risk are the immunocompromised and the elderly. The clinical presentation will vary with the patient's underlying disorder and the causative organism (see Clinical Findings 4–4).

POINTS TO REMEMBER

▶ The elderly are at risk for bacterial, viral, and aspiration pneumonias due to decreased inflation of basal alveoli, possible decreased cough and gag reflex, decreased ciliary action, and changes in the immune system with aging. In addition, the elderly patient's symptoms may be minimal or altered (see Chapter 3 for related information).

▶ Because nosocomial pneumonia is a contributing factor to mortality in ICU patients, a thorough nursing history (see Tables 1–1 and 4–1 and Clinical Findings 4–4) is crucial to identify patients at risk and facilitate preventative management.

▶ In addition to the initial and baseline assessments (see Table 2–1), a focused respiratory assessment (see Tables 2–1 and 4–1), as well as a focused assessment of the underlying disease process should be completed as often as the patient's condition indicates to detect or anticipate and prevent complications such as acute respiratory failure, refractory hypoxemia, ARDS (see Clinical Findings 4–1), atelectasis (see Clinical Findings 4–3), pleural effusion (see Clinical Findings 4–5), pleurisy (friction between layers of pleura), lung abscess, empyema, disseminated intravascular coagulation (see Clinical Findings 10–1), meningitis (see Clinical Findings 6–6), endocarditis (see Chapter 5, Valvular Disorders), or nephritis.

▶ Ongoing assessment incorporates the evaluation of responses to diagnostic procedures and therapeutic interventions aimed at the provision of airway clearance, oxygenation, and respiratory support; it includes collaboration with other members of the health team to prevent the spread of infection.

Clinical Findings 4–4   *Pneumonia*

I. HISTORY

A. Predisposing factors

1. *Compromised defense systems*
   • Elderly

- Immunocompromised
- AIDS
- Cancer
- Organ transplantation

2. *Chronic illness*
   - Chronic obstructive pulmonary disease (COPD)
   - Diabetes mellitus
   - Heart failure
   - Alcoholism

3. *Others*
   - Smoking
   - Malnutrition
   - Bronchitis, otitis media, myringitis *(Mycoplasma)*
   - Thoracic, upper abdominal surgery or trauma
   - Gastrointestinal surgery *(E. coli)*
   - Altered levels of consciousness
   - Inhibition of cough mechanism
   - Anesthetics, sedatives, narcotics
   - Anticholinergics
   - Histamine (H_2) antagonists and antacids (may allow gram-negative organisms to flourish)
   - Feeding tubes
   - Endotracheal intubation
   - Tracheostomy
   - Mechanical ventilation
   - Prolonged immobility (particularly the supine position)

B. Subjective findings
   1. Dyspnea related to decreased lung compliance and impaired gas exchange
   2. Fatigue related to increased work of breathing
   3. Headache, malaise, weakness, or myalgia related to infecting organism (bacterial, viral pneumonias)
   4. Chest pain related to inflammation of the parietal pleura (worse on inspiration and with coughing)
   5. Anxiety related to dyspnea and increased work of breathing

II. LABORATORY AND BEDSIDE MONITORING FINDINGS

A. Pulmonary function studies (see Table 13-1 for related information on pulmonary function studies): Decreased total lung capacity, decreased vital capacity, and decreased compliance associated with diffuse alveolar and interstitial disease such as *P. carinii* pneumonia

B. Chest x-ray

1. Dense infiltrates of one or more lobes or a patchy pattern with no consolidation with pneumococcal pneumonia
2. Unilateral or bilateral interstitial infiltrates progressing to consolidation with gram-negative bacterial pneumonia
3. Diffuse infiltrates involving one or more lobes (most commonly the lower lobes) with viral pneumonia
4. Segmental areas of consolidation (isolated in the lower lobes) with mycoplasmal pneumonia
5. Diffuse interstitial or alveolar infiltrates with *P. carinii* pneumonia
6. Infiltrates in dependent lung fields with aspiration pneumonia

C. Arterial blood gas studies (see Chapter 13 for related information on arterial blood gases and the efficiency of gas exchange)

1. May be normal
2. PaO_2 may be <60 mm Hg, and $PaCO_2$ may be <35 mm Hg with a pH >7.45, related to the extent of the pneumonia, intrapulmonary shunting, and tachypnea
3. May be increased PAO_2-PaO_2 gradient with severe intrapulmonary shunting

D. Other laboratory studies

1. Blood cultures may be positive in the presence of bacteremia
2. White blood cell (WBC) count may be elevated (12,000–30,000/ml) related to leukocytosis but may be normal in the debilitated and elderly patient (see Table 13–9 for related information on WBC)
3. Sodium and chloride may be elevated with dehydration (see Table 13–5 for related information on electrolyte imbalances)
4. Blood urea nitrogen (BUN) may be elevated related to catabolism, decreased glomerular filtration rate (see Table 13–6 for related information on BUN)
5. Sputum culture may or may not be diagnostic (Gram's stain may help to distinguish bacterial from viral infection, and gram-positive from gram-negative bacteria. Culture and sensitivity may help to define therapy)
6. Serological studies, bronchial washing, and lung biopsies may be required to identify many of the pathogens (*P. carinii*, mycoplasmas, anaerobic bacteria, fungi, legionellae)

E. ECG: May be tachycardic related to fever, hypoxemia

F. Hemodynamic parameters: May be hypotensive related to peripheral vasodilation or compromised cardiac function

III. PHYSICAL ASSESSMENT FINDINGS

A. General observations (inspection)

1. *Mental status:* Confusion related to dehydration or hypoxemia (common in the elderly)
2. *Fever:* Elevated temperature related to systemic response to infection (may be absent in the elderly)
3. *Chills:* Shaking related to body's attempt to increase heat production and raise metabolic rate
4. *Skin*
   - May be flushed, erythemic related to fever and increased metabolic rate
   - May be cyanotic with severe respiratory compromise
   - May have maculopapular rash with mycoplasmal pneumonia
5. *Nasal/oral airway*
   - Crusted drainage may be present at nares because of thick secretions (copious, thick secretions may block the oral airway)
   - Weakened cough, gag, and swallow reflexes may be a natural occurrence with aging, or related to altered levels of consciousness, or related to sedation, narcotics, or anesthetics (assessment of reflex essential to identify and protect patients at risk for aspiration of oral or gastric secretions; see Table 6–1)
6. *Tracheal obstruction:* Stridor, snoring, rattling, and wheezes may be present, related to accumulation of secretions (may increase the risk of oral airway obstruction and aspiration)
7. *Respiratory pattern:* May be tachypneic related to increased metabolic rate, hypoxemia
8. *Respiratory effort:* Use of neck and accessory muscles may be related to airway obstruction, atelectasis, increased work of breathing
9. *Cough and sputum*
   - Gram-positive bacterial pneumonias: cough may produce blood-tinged or rusty-colored sputum (relates to mix of red blood cells and inflammatory cells) or purulent yellow (pneumococcal or staphylococcal) sputum
   - Gram-negative bacterial pneumonias: cough may produce purulent yellow or green, often foul-smelling *(Pseudomonas)* or currant-jelly sputum *(Klebsiella)*
   - Nonproductive (dry) cough is usually associated with viral and *P. carinii* pneumonia
10. *Respiratory excursion:* May be asymmetrical related to unequal air movement secondary to atelectasis

B. Palpation
  1. *Skin:* Periphery may be warm and moist related to fever and diaphoresis or dry with poor turgor related to dehydration
  2. *Chest wall and thorax:* Chest expansion may be diminished, related to decreased compliance or atrophy of respiratory musculature
C. Percussion: Areas of consolidation will be dull to percussion
D. Auscultation
  1. *Abnormal breath sounds*
     - Breath sounds may be diminished or absent in atelectatic areas
     - Bronchial breath sounds may be present over consolidated areas
  2. *Adventitious sounds*
     - Crackles may be present over fluid-filled interstitial and alveolar areas
     - Wheezing may be present over inflamed and fluid-filled airways
     - Pleural friction rub may be present, related to inflamed pleurae

Pleural Effusion

Pathophysiology

A pleural effusion is associated with the accumulation of fluid in the pleural space in excess of the tiny amount normally present for lubrication. The accumulated fluid restricts lung expansion and can lead to compression of lung tissue and atelectasis.

Transudative infusions are associated with disorders that cause an increase in capillary hydrostatic pressure or a decrease in colloidal osmotic pressure. The accumulated fluid is watery and low in protein content.

Exudative infusions occur with disorders that damage the capillary membrane and allow leakage of fluid rich in plasma proteins, or with disorders that obstruct the lymphatic system and inhibit the drainage of protein. The accumulated fluid is generally high in protein and white blood cells.

An accumulation of pus (infection of protein-rich fluid) in the pleural space is referred to as an **empyema.** A collection of lymph fluid (chyle) in the pleural space is referred to as a chylous pleural effusion, or **chylothorax.** Blood in the pleural space is referred to as a **hemothorax.**

Assessment

Clinical presentation will vary with the size of the effusion and the underlying disorder (Clinical Findings 4–5). A small pleural effusion may cause little respiratory distress. A massive pleural effusion may cause a mediastinal shift (see Clinical Findings 4–6).

POINTS TO REMEMBER

▶ A pleural effusion is usually a sign of an underlying disorder, not a disease in itself.

▶ Because the critically ill adult may be susceptible to the development of a pleural effusion, a thorough nursing history (see Tables 1–1 and 4–1 and Clinical Findings 4–5) is crucial to identify patients at risk.

▶ In addition to the initial and baseline assessments (see Table 2–1), focused respiratory and cardiovascular assessments (see Tables 2–1, 4–1, and 5–1), as well as a focused assessment of the underlying disorder should be completed as often as the patient's condition dictates to detect or anticipate and prevent complications such as atelectasis (see Clinical Findings 4–3) and mediastinal shift (see Clinical Findings 4–6).

▶ Ongoing assessment incorporates the evaluation of responses to diagnostic procedures and therapeutic interventions aimed at elimination or reduction of the size of the pleural effusion; it includes collaboration with other members of the health team to support respiration and achieve an optimal level of lung expansion and ventilation.

Clinical Findings 4–5   *Pleural Effusion*

I. HISTORY

A. Predisposing factors

1. *Transudative infusions*
   - Congestive heart failure
   - Cirrhosis with ascites
   - Nephrotic syndrome
   - Peritoneal dialysis
   - Myxedema
   - Constrictive pericarditis
   - Superior vena cava obstruction
   - Pulmonary embolism

2. *Exudative infusions*
   - Pulmonary embolism (if embolism extends into pleural space)

- Malignancies
- Infections (viral, fungal, parasitic)
- Pancreatic disease
- Uremia
- Postmyocardial infarction syndrome
- Tuberculosis
- Chest trauma
- Chest surgery

B. Subjective findings

1. Dyspnea related to restricted lung expansion
2. Fatigue related to increased work of breathing
3. Pain related to inflammation of pleura
4. Apprehension or anxiety related to difficulty in breathing

II. LABORATORY AND BEDSIDE MONITORING FINDINGS

A. Chest x-ray

1. Large effusions may be seen as dense opacities
2. Trachea and mediastinal structures deviated from midline with massive effusion

B. Arterial blood gas studies

1. Hypoxemia (PaO_2 <60 to 70 mm Hg) may be present, related to atelectasis
2. $PaCO_2$ may be normal or decreased (<35 mm Hg) initially, related to tachypnea, and then increased (>45 mm Hg) if gas exchange is severely compromised, related to massive infusion and mediastinal shift
3. pH may be acidotic (<7.35) with severe hypoxemia or hypercapnia, related to massive infusion and mediastinal shift

C. Pleural fluid analysis

1. *Transudate fluid:* Low protein, low lactate dehydrogenase (LDH), increased glucose, and WBC count less than 1000/mm^3
2. *Exudate fluid*
   - Increased protein (pleural fluid to serum protein ratio >0.5)
   - Increased LDH (pleural fluid to serum LDH ratio >0.6)
   - Increased WBCs
3. *Pleural fluid (in general)*
   - pH <7.3 may indicate pleural effusion caused by cancer, pneumonia, empyema, rheumatoid arthritis, or tuberculosis
   - Hematocrit >50% of peripheral blood hematocrit may indicate hemothorax

D. ECG: Tachycardia may be present related to hypoxemia or decreased cardiac output secondary to massive infusion and mediastinal shift
E. Hemodynamic parameters (see Chapter 14, Table 14–2 and Fig. 14–2 for related information on hemodynamic parameters)
  1. Elevated central venous pressure (>6 mm Hg or 12 cm H_2O) related to venous congestion with massive effusion and mediastinal shift
  2. Hypotension related to decreased cardiac output with massive effusion and mediastinal shift

III. PHYSICAL ASSESSMENT FINDINGS
A. General observations (inspection)
  1. *Mental status:* Restlessness related to hypoxemia
  2. *Fever:* Elevated temperature related to infected pleural fluid or underlying disorder
  3. *Skin*
    • Flushed and erythemic related to fever
    • Cyanotic related to significant respiratory compromise or decreased peripheral blood flow associated with massive effusion and mediastinal shift
    • Pallor related to blood loss (anemia) or decreased blood flow to the tissues with massive effusion and mediastinal shift
  4. *Tracheal obstruction:* Tracheal deviation toward unaffected side related to massive effusion
  5. *Respiratory pattern:* Tachypnea related to hypoxemia
  6. *Cough and sputum:* Dry cough related to pulmonary infection or irritation
  7. *Respiratory excursion:* Asymmetrical related to restricted expansion of affected side
  8. *Neck veins:* Jugular venous distention related to pressure on great vessels and interference with venous return with massive effusion and mediastinal shift
B. Palpation
  1. *Skin*
    • Warm and moist periphery related to diaphoresis and fever
    • Cool and moist periphery related to decreased tissue perfusion with massive effusion and mediastinal shift
  2. *Chest wall and thorax:* Diminished chest expansion related to restricted movement of affected side
C. Percussion: Dullness over area of effusion

D. Auscultation
1. *Abnormal breath sounds:* Diminished or absent breath sounds over area of effusion
2. *Adventitious breath sounds:* Pleural friction rub related to inflamed pleura

Pneumothorax

Pathophysiology

A pneumothorax is associated with the accumulation of air in the pleural space. The increased pleural pressure can cause partial or total collapse of the lung.

A **spontaneous** (closed) pneumothorax occurs when air enters the pleural space from the rupture of a bleb within the lung. The rupture can occur spontaneously in young, healthy adults (tall, thin males between 20 and 40 years of age) or more commonly as a complication of blunt chest trauma, pulmonary disease, or mechanical ventilation.

A **tension** pneumothorax occurs when the air in the pleural space builds up under pressure. The lung tissue seals over on expiration, creating a one-way valve effect. Air continues to enter the pleural space on inspiration and is unable to escape on expiration.

An **open** pneumothorax occurs when atmospheric air enters the pleural space through an opening in the chest wall. Air is sucked in during inspiration. If the air is unable to escape during expiration, a tension pneumothorax may develop. An open pneumothorax occurs with penetrating chest trauma, thoracic surgery, or an unintentional puncture during invasive thoracic procedures.

Assessment

Clinical presentation depends on the size and type of pneumothorax (Clinical Findings 4–6). A small pneumothorax may result in a few symptoms, or it may cause severe distress in the presence of underlying disease.

POINTS TO REMEMBER

▶ Tension pneumothorax is a potentially fatal medical emergency. As the air accumulates in the pleural space, intrathoracic pressure increases, and the lung collapses. Pressure is exerted on the great vessels and the heart, causing a shift toward the unaffected side and leading to impaired venous return and decreased right ventricular filling. Decreased right ventricular output leads to decreased cardiac output, and ultimately, decreased blood flow to the tissues.

▶ The critically ill adult may present with a pneumothorax. As well, the critically ill adult may be susceptible to the development of a pneumothorax.

▶ A thorough nursing history (see Tables 1–1 and 4–1 and Clinical Findings 4–6) is crucial to identify the cause of a pneumothorax or to identify patients at risk for the development of a pneumothorax.

▶ In addition to the initial and baseline assessments (see Table 2–1), focused respiratory and cardiovascular assessments (see Tables 2–1, 4–1, and 5–1), as well as a focused assessment of the underlying or presenting disorder should be completed as often as the patient's condition dictates to detect or anticipate and prevent complications such as mediastinal shift and cardiovascular collapse.

▶ Ongoing assessment incorporates the evaluation of responses to diagnostic procedures and therapeutic interventions aimed at re-expansion of the involved lung; it includes collaboration with other members of the health team to promote ease of breathing, support ventilation, and facilitate gas exchange.

Clinical Findings 4–6   *Pneumothorax*

I. HISTORY

A. Predisposing factors
1. COPD
2. Lung cancer
3. Tuberculosis
4. Chest trauma
5. Chest surgery
6. Mechanical ventilation
7. Positive end-expiratory pressure (PEEP)
8. Thoracentesis
9. Central line insertion
10. Occlusion of chest tube

B. Subjective findings

1. Dyspnea related to lung collapse
2. Fatigue related to increased work of breathing
3. Sharp chest pain (may be unilateral or radiate to back, abdomen, shoulders and face) related to collapsed lung and pressure on parietal pleura
4. Agitation and or anxiety may be present, related to the increased work of breathing

II. Laboratory and Bedside Monitoring Findings

A. Pulmonary function studies (see Table 13–1 for related information on pulmonary function studies)

1. Decreased lung volumes and decreased compliance related to loss of lung function
2. Increased peak airway pressure related to partial or total collapse of lung

B. Chest x-ray

1. Air in pleural space
2. Contralateral shift of mediastinal structures, lowering of hemidiaphragm

C. Arterial blood gas studies

1. Hypoxemia related to increased pulmonary dead space (PaO_2 may be <60 to 70 mm Hg)
2. $PaCO_2$ may be decreased initially (<35 mm Hg), related to tachypnea and then increased (>45 mm Hg) with severe respiratory distress
3. pH may be acidotic (<7.35) with progressive hypoxemia and hypercapnia (mediastinal shift)

D. ECG: Tachycardia may be present, related to hypoxemia or reduced cardiac output associated with mediastinal shift

E. Hemodynamic parameters (see Chapter 14, Table 14–2 and Fig. 14–2, for related information on hemodynamic parameters)

1. Hypotension may be present, related to decreased cardiac output
2. CVP may be elevated (>6 mm Hg or 12 cm H_2O), related to venous congestion

III. Physical Assessment Findings

A. General observations (inspection)

1. *Mental status:* Restlessness related to hypoxemia
2. *Skin:* Cyanosis related to severe respiratory compromise and decreased blood flow to the tissues with tension pneumothorax and mediastinal shift
3. *Respiratory pattern:* Tachypnea related to hypoxemia

4. *Respiratory excursion:* Asymmetrical chest expansion related to collapse of the lung or trapped air
5. *Tracheal obstruction:* Tracheal deviation toward the unaffected side related to tension pneumothorax and mediastinal shift
6. *Neck veins:* Jugular venous distention related to venous congestion from pressure on the great vessels associated with tension pneumothorax and mediastinal shift (blood is unable to move forward from the right side of the heart to the left side of the heart as it should)

B. Palpation

1. *Skin:* Cool and moist periphery related to decreased peripheral blood flow with tension pneumothorax and mediastinal shift
2. *Chest wall and thorax*
   - Subcutaneous emphysema and crepitus in the chest and neck related to air escaping into the tissue
   - Abnormal chest wall movement related to collapsed lung or trapped air

C. Percussion: Hyperresonance on the affected side related to increased amount of air

D. Auscultation

1. *Abnormal breath sounds:* Decreased or absent breath sounds on affected side related to no air movement with respiration
2. *Heart sounds:* Distant or Hamman's sign (clicking or crunching sound correlated with heart sounds) related to air in the mediastinum

PERFUSION DISORDERS

Perfusion disorders affect blood flow in the lung. Perfusion disorders, including pulmonary embolism, generally cause acute respiratory failure.

Pulmonary Embolism

Pathophysiology

A pulmonary embolism is an occlusion of a pulmonary blood vessel by undissolved matter transported to the lungs by the venous system. Any substance can cause an embolism, including thrombi, air, fat, amniotic fluid, and foreign objects such as catheter tips.

The most common source of an embolism is a thrombus that has dislodged from the deep veins in the pelvis and legs (deep-vein thrombosis, or DVT). Factors that favor formation of DVT include venous stasis, hypercoagulability, and damage to the vessel wall.

Air can enter the venous system during procedures such as neurosurgery and central line cannulation. Air bubbles lodge in the small pulmonary vessels and cause obstruction.

Fat emboli can occur with major soft tissue injury or fractures of the pelvis and lower extremities (long bone fracture). The release of fatty acids causes destruction of the pulmonary endothelial tissue leading to pulmonary edema and a course similar to ARDS (see Clinical Findings 4–1).

Amniotic fluid embolism is a rare, often fatal, complication that can occur during pregnancy. Fluid containing hairs, meconium, and other fetal debris enters the maternal circulation through tears in the uterine or cervical veins. Pulmonary embolization is accompanied by an intense immune response leading to profound cardiovascular collapse.

Pathophysiological effects of pulmonary embolism vary with the method of occurrence, severity of obstruction, and underlying pulmonary and cardiac disease. In general, blood flow distal to the obstruction is impaired. The loss of blood flow results in a decreased number of perfused alveoli, leading to an increase in dead space ventilation and decreased surfactant production. Platelet aggregation at the site of the embolism triggers the release of thromboxane A_2 and serotonin, causing widespread vasoconstriction and pulmonary artery hypertension.

Increased airway resistance leads to increased work of breathing, decreased alveolar ventilation, atelectasis, and hypoxemia as deoxygenated blood is shunted back into the arterial circulation. Increased pulmonary vascular resistance leads to right heart failure, decreased left ventricular filling pressures, and decreased cardiac output.

Assessment

Clinical manifestations vary with the type and severity of pulmonary emboli and the presence of underlying pulmonary or cardiovascular disease (Clinical Findings 4–7). Small pulmonary emboli (<25% of pulmonary vascular bed occluded) may cause little distress in the absence of underlying disease. Large and multiple pulmonary emboli (>50% of pulmonary vascular bed occluded) can lead to severe pulmonary hypertension and cardiovascular collapse in the absence of underlying disease.

POINTS TO REMEMBER

▶ Because pulmonary embolism is a manifestation of other conditions in the body, not a disease process in itself, a thorough nursing history (see Tables 1–1 and 4–1 and Clinical Findings 4–7) is crucial to identify patients at risk and facilitate prophylactic measures per hospital procedure.

▶ Because rapid, early, detection of patients presenting with a pulmonary embolism potentiates a more favorable outcome, in addition to the initial and baseline assessments (see Table 2–1), focused pulmonary and cardiovascular assessments (see Tables 2–1, 4–1, and 5–1), as well as a focused assessment of the underlying disorder should be completed as often as the patient's condition dictates to detect or anticipate and prevent complications such as ARDS (see Clinical Findings 4–1), right heart failure (see Clinical Findings 5–2), shock (see Clinical Findings 12–3), and cardiopulmonary arrest.

▶ Ongoing assessment incorporates the evaluation of responses to diagnostic procedures and therapeutic interventions aimed at improving pulmonary blood flow; it includes collaboration with other members of the health team to promote effective ventilation and prevent further injury.

Clinical Findings 4–7   *Pulmonary Embolism*

I. HISTORY

A. Predisposing factors

1. *Thrombi, air, or fat*
   - Immobility
   - Advanced age
   - Vascular disorders (history of deep venous thrombosis [DVT], clotting disorders, varicose veins)
   - Atrial fibrillation
   - Congestive heart failure
   - Acute myocardial infarction
   - Shock (sepsis)
   - Burns
   - Diabetes mellitus
   - Dehydration
   - Malignancy

- Trauma
- Bone fractures with soft tissue injury
- Postoperative patients (in particular, hip, pelvic, abdominal, neuro, and cardiovascular)
- Invasive venous procedures
- Polycythemia
- Obesity
- Cigarette smoking
- Oral contraceptives
- Estrogen therapy
- Pregnancy

  2. *Amniotic fluid emboli*
  - Amniocentesis
  - Uterine rupture
  - Cesarean section
  - Complicated labor and delivery
  - Advanced maternal age
  - Multiple births

B. Subjective findings
  1. Dyspnea related to increased dead-space ventilation
  2. Fatigue related to the increased work of breathing
  3. Pleuritic chest pain related to inflammation of pleura (worse on inspiration)
  4. Apprehension, anxiety related to sudden onset of symptoms (feeling of impending doom with massive emboli)

II. LABORATORY AND BEDSIDE MONITORING FINDINGS

A. Chest x-ray: Generally not helpful in diagnosis but may show atelectasis, pleural effusion, elevated diaphragm, or distention of pulmonary vessels

B. Ventilation-perfusion scan: Normal ventilation to areas of absent perfusion

C. Pulmonary angiography: Definitive diagnosis for pulmonary embolism

D. Arterial blood gases (see Chapter 13 and Fig. 13–2 for related information on arterial blood gas studies, acid-base balance, and the efficiency of gas exchange)
  1. Hypoxemia (PaO_2 <70 to 80 mm Hg) related to right-to-left shunt
  2. Decreased PaCO_2 (<35 mm Hg) related to tachypnea
  3. Respiratory alkalosis (pH >7.45) related to hyperventilation
  4. Increased PAO_2–PaO_2 gradient reflective of intrapulmonary shunting

    5. Prolonged hypoxemia and increased intrapulmonary shunting eventually leads to tissue hypoxia and metabolic acidosis (pH <7.35), and an increased $PaCO_2$ (>45 mm Hg) and respiratory acidosis

E. Other laboratory studies

    1. Leukocytosis and elevated fibrin degradation products related to the inflammatory process (see Table 13–9 for related information on WBC count)

    2. Elevated serum lipase levels with fat embolism

F. ECG

    1. Sinus tachycardia related to hypoxemia

    2. Dysrhythmias (in particular, premature ventricular contractions) related to right ventricular failure, hypoxemia, or shock (see Table 14–3 for related information on dysrhythmias)

    3. Peaked P wave related to pulmonary hypertension

    4. Transient and nonspecific T wave changes related to sudden right ventricular overload

    5. Right axis deviation related to sudden right ventricular overload and delayed closure of the pulmonic valve

    6. Incomplete or complete right bundle branch block related to sudden right ventricular overload

G. Hemodynamic parameters (see Chapter 14, Table 14–2 and Fig. 14–2, for related information on hemodynamic parameters)

    1. Hypotension related to decreased cardiac output secondary to decreased left ventricular filling pressures

    2. Increased right atrial, right ventricular, and pulmonary artery pressure related to pulmonary artery hypertension and subsequent right ventricular failure

    3. Normal or decreased PCWP related to decreased left ventricular filling secondary to right ventricular failure

    4. Decreased cardiac output related to decreased left ventricular filling secondary to right ventricular failure

III. PHYSICAL ASSESSMENT FINDINGS

A. General observations (inspection)

    1. *Mental status:* Restlessness related to hypoxemia

    2. *Fever:* Low-grade fever related to the inflammatory response

    3. *Skin*

      • Redness, heat, or swelling of extremities related to DVT

      • Petechiae over thorax, axillae, and upper extremities related to hypercoagulopathy or fat emboli

      • Cyanosis related to severe hypoxemia or shock

4. *Respiratory pattern:* Tachypnea related to hypoxemia
5. *Cough and sputum:* Dry cough leading to hemoptysis related to pulmonary irritation, inflammation, or infarction
6. *Respiratory excursion:* Decreased chest expansion on affected side related to pleuritic pain (splinting)
7. *Neck veins:* Jugular venous distention related to increased pulmonary vascular resistance or right ventricular failure (blood is unable to move forward from the right side of the heart to the left side of the heart as it should)

B. Palpation

1. *Skin:* Cool, moist periphery related to decreased peripheral blood flow
2. *Chest wall and thorax*
   - Asymmetrical chest expansion related to splinting
   - Pleural friction fremitus over area of inflamed pleura

C. Auscultation

1. *Abnormal breath sounds:* Decreased breath sounds related to atelectasis
2. *Adventitious sounds*
   - Crackles may be heard with increased pulmonary secretions
   - Wheezing may be heard with bronchoconstriction or increased pulmonary secretions
   - Pleural friction rub related to inflamed pleura
   - Churning noise over right ventricle related to air emboli
3. *Heart sounds*
   - Increased intensity of S_2 or fixed splitting of S_2 related to sudden right ventricular overload and delayed closure of the pulmonic valve
   - Right ventricular S_3, S_4 gallop related to right ventricular failure
   - Murmur related to turbulent blood flow through partially obstructed blood vessel

OBSTRUCTIVE DISORDERS

Obstructive disorders decrease air flow within the lungs. Vital capacity, residual volume, and functional residual capacity may be affected. Obstructive disorders, including chronic bronchitis and emphysema, usually lead to chronic respiratory failure, but episodes of acute respiratory failure can be superimposed. Asthma is a recurrent, reversible obstructive disorder.

Chronic Obstructive Pulmonary Disease (COPD)

(chronic airflow obstruction, chronic airflow limitation)

COPD is a condition characterized by the presence of chronic bronchitis, emphysema, or a combination of both disorders. The majority of patients present with a combination of both disorders.

Pathophysiology

Chronic bronchitis (productive cough 3 months per year for 2 consecutive years) is an inflammatory response to an irritant, primarily smoking. Repeated exposure to the irritant causes airway changes, including mucosal swelling, impaired ciliary function, and hypersecretion of mucus. Thick mucus production and hypertrophied bronchial smooth muscle lead to stagnation of secretions and increased susceptibility to infection.

Inspiratory and expiratory airway obstruction leads to overinflated alveoli, decreased expiratory airflow, and abnormal distribution of ventilation. Eventually, ventilation-perfusion mismatches occur, resulting in hypoxemia and chronic CO_2 retention.

Pulmonary vasoconstriction occurs as a compensatory response to the hypoxemia. The increased pulmonary vascular resistance places an increased workload on the right ventricle and ultimately leads to right ventricular hypertrophy (cor pulmonale) and right ventricular failure (see Clinical Findings 5–2).

Emphysema is characterized by destruction of the alveolar walls and enlargement of the air spaces distal to the terminal bronchioles. Loss of elastic recoil, distention of lung tissue (hyperinflation), and a marked reduction in the surface area available for gas exchange are the primary features.

Alveolar destruction is associated with the release of protease enzymes. These protease enzymes (primarily elastase) break down elastin, a protein found in the connective tissue of alveolar walls. (Protease enzymes are normally kept in check by a protease inhibitor enzyme. Smoking or a genetic deficiency of this antiprotease enzyme predisposes the individual to the development of emphysema.)

The breakdown of elastin leads to loss of elastic recoil of the lung. Loss of elastic recoil, airway narrowing, and increased resistance during expiration lead to decreased air flow, air trapping in the distal alveoli, distended air sacs, and airway collapse.

The loss of alveolar walls and the formation of large air spaces reduce the alveolar diffusing surface and lead to ventilation-perfusion abnormalities. The formation of bullae (large, thin-walled cysts) further decreases the surface area for gas exchange.

Assessment

Clinical manifestations vary with the type and severity of COPD (Clinical Findings 4–8). A clinical presentation purely associated with either chronic bronchitis or emphysema is seldom seen; the disorders most often occur together.

POINTS TO REMEMBER

▶ The critically ill adult may present with acute respiratory failure associated with an exacerbation of COPD.
- In addition to the initial and baseline assessments (see Table 2–1), a focused respiratory assessment (see Tables 2–1 and 4–1) should be completed as often as the patient's condition dictates to detect early changes in respiratory function and facilitate the prevention of further decline.
- As well, a focused cardiovascular assessment should be completed in the presence of cor pulmonale (see Tables 2–1 and 5–1 and Clinical Findings 5–2).

▶ COPD may be an underlying disease associated with an unrelated critical disorder.
- In addition to a focused assessment of the presenting disorder, a thorough nursing history, baseline assessment, and focused respiratory and cardiovascular assessments should be directed at establishing a data base of normals for the patient to serve as a comparison for future reference (see Tables 1–1, 2–1, 4–1, and 5–1 and Clinical Findings 4–8).
- As well, the baseline and focused assessments should be directed at the early detection of infection, heart failure (see Clinical Findings 5–1 and 5–2), or other complications likely to precipitate an episode of acute respiratory failure.

▶ Ongoing assessment incorporates the evaluation of responses to diagnostic procedures and therapeutic interventions aimed at improving oxygenation, conserving energy, and preventing respiratory muscle fatigue; it includes collaboration with other members of the health team to promote effective breathing patterns and increase pulmonary muscle function, and to prevent further decline through complications such as respiratory infection.

Clinical Findings 4–8 *Chronic Obstructive Pulmonary Disease (COPD)*

I. HISTORY

A. Predisposing factors
1. Smoking
2. Environmental pollutants
3. Industrial irritants
· 4. Family history (genetic disposition)

B. Precipitating factors leading to acute respiratory failure include
1. Respiratory infection
2. Myocardial infarction
3. Heart failure
4. Sedatives
5. Dehydration
6. Electrolyte imbalance
7. Physical stress related to other disorders, trauma, or surgery

C. Subjective findings
1. Dyspnea on exertion progressing to dyspnea at rest related to the progression of airway disease
2. Headache related to increased levels of CO_2
3. Fatigue related to increased work of breathing, increased metabolic demands, cor pulmonale
4. Activity intolerance related to breathlessness
5. Anxiety related to difficulty in breathing
6. Hopelessness related to the debilitating nature of the disease

II. LABORATORY AND BEDSIDE MONITORING FINDINGS

A. Pulmonary function studies (see Table 13–1 for related information on pulmonary function studies)
1. Decreased forced expiratory volume with chronic bronchitis and emphysema related to air flow obstruction
2. Decreased vital capacity with emphysema; normal or slight decrease with chronic bronchitis related to degree of hyperinflation
3. Increased residual volume with chronic bronchitis and emphysema related to hyperinflation
4. Increased functional residual volume with emphysema related to hyperinflation; normal or slight increase with chronic bronchitis
5. Increased total lung capacity with emphysema related to increased compliance

6. Increased static lung compliance with emphysema related to loss of elastic recoil

7. Decreased diffusing capacity with emphysema related to loss of surface area for gas exchange

B. Chest x-ray

1. Hyperinflated lungs, presence of blebs or bullae, and low, flat diaphragm with emphysema

2. Enlarged right ventricle related to cor pulmonale (chronic bronchitis)

3. Congested lung fields related to increased pulmonary secretions with chronic bronchitis

C. **Arterial blood gas studies** (see Fig. 13–2 for related information on interpretation of acid-base disorders)

1. In general, as COPD progresses, the PaO_2 decreases (<70 to 80 mm Hg), and the $PaCO_2$ increases (>45 mm Hg), resulting in chronic respiratory acidosis with metabolic alkalosis occurring as compensation

2. The bronchitic patient usually manifests hypoxemia and hypercapnia earlier in the stage of the disease

3. The patient with emphysema is able to maintain a higher minute ventilation and may present with normal oxygenation or moderate hypoxemia and respiratory alkalosis (severe hypoxemia and respiratory acidosis may not be present until endstage disease)

D. **Other laboratory studies**

1. Hematocrit normal with emphysema; polycythemia with chronic bronchitis

2. Elevated WBC count with chronic bronchitis in the presence of infection (see Tables 13–8 and 13–9 for related information on red blood cell (RBC) count, hematocrit, and WBC count)

E. **ECG**

1. In general with COPD, ECG changes may include
   - Tall, peaked P wave ("P pulmonale") related to right atrial enlargement
   - Increased QRS amplitude related to right ventricular hypertrophy
   - Right axis deviation

2. Sinus tachycardia, supraventricular, and ventricular dysrhythmias may be present related to hypoxemia, right ventricular failure, acid-base imbalances, or electrolyte imbalances (see Table 14–3 for related information on dysrhythmias)

III. Physical Assessment Findings

A. **General observations (inspection)**

1. *Mental status*
   - Restlessness, confusion, or agitation may be present, related to hypoxemia

- Drowsiness or lethargy may be present, related to hypercapnia

2. *Skin*
   - May be dusky or cyanotic with chronic bronchitis related to hypoxemia ("blue bloater")
   - May be pink with emphysema related to the ability to maintain oxygen levels ("pink puffer")
   - Cachectic; muscle wasting may be present with emphysema, related to the increased work of breathing and increased metabolic demands

3. *Nails:* Clubbing may be present with chronic bronchitis, related to chronically decreased oxygen levels and associated compensatory polycythemia

4. *Respiratory pattern*
   - Tachypnea may be present with emphysema, related to "air hunger" (use of accessory muscles increases the demand for oxygen) and need to maintain acceptable CO_2 levels
   - Asynchronous breathing may be present with emphysema, related to uncoordinated activity of fatigued respiratory muscles and use of intercostal and abdominal muscles

5. *Respiratory effort*
   - Pursed-lip breathing may be present with emphysema, related to an effort to expel air over a longer period of time (before small airways collapse)
   - Use of accessory muscles may be present with emphysema, related to hyperinflation of the lung and flattening of the diaphragm (neck and abdominal muscles may be used during expiration to assist the diaphragm to rise against gravity)

6. *Cough and sputum*
   - Minimal or absent cough may occur with emphysema (if cough, productive of a minimal amount of mucoid sputum)
   - Chronic cough may be present with bronchitis, productive of excessive, purulent sputum

7. *Respiratory excursion*
   - Increased anteroposterior (AP) diameter (barrel chest) may be present with emphysema, related to hyperinflation of the lungs (enlarged alveoli inhibit the lungs from returning to the normal resting state during expiration) and flattening of the diaphragm
   - Decreased diaphragmatic excursion may be present with emphysema, related to hyperinflation of the lungs and flattening of the diaphragm

8. *Neck veins:* Jugular venous distention may be present with chronic bronchitis related to cor pulmonale or right ventricular failure (blood is unable

to move forward from the right side of the heart to the left side of the heart as it should)

B. Palpation

1. *Skin*
   - Peripheral edema may be present with chronic bronchitis, related to right ventricular failure
   - Warm, cyanotic extremities and bounding pulses may be present with chronic bronchitis, related to hypercapnia or polycythemia (compensatory increase in cardiac output to move more oxygen)

2. *Chest wall and thorax:* Decreased chest expansion may be present with emphysema, related to hyperinflated lungs

C. Percussion

1. May be hyperresonant with emphysema, related to increased lung volumes
2. May be resonant with chronic bronchitis, or dull if areas of consolidation

D. Auscultation

1. *Abnormal breath sounds:* Diminished breath sounds may be present with emphysema, related to an increased AP diameter of the chest

2. *Adventitious breath sounds*
   - Expiratory wheeze may be audible with emphysema, related to narrowed airways, prolonged expiration
   - Crackles, wheezes (rhonchi) may be present with chronic bronchitis, related to increased pulmonary secretions

3. *Heart sounds*
   - Distant heart sounds may be present with emphysema, related to an increased AP diameter
   - Loud S_2 or right-sided S_3; S_4 may be present with chronic bronchitis, related to cor pulmonale or right ventricular failure

Asthma

Pathophysiology

Asthma is characterized by airway inflammation that precipitates contraction of airway smooth muscle. The extent of hyperreactivity and bronchial constriction depends on the degree of inflammation present.

Exposure to a predisposing factor, extrinsic or intrinsic (see Clinical Findings 4–9), causes cells within the airways to become abnormally active and inflamed. Subsequently, inflammatory mediators are released, causing increased capillary permeability, mucosal edema, hypersecretion of thick mucus, bronchial hyperreactivity, and bronchoconstriction of the central and peripheral airways.

Pulmonary function may be normal between attacks, or chronic debilitation may be present with advanced disease. During attacks, the overproduction of mucus and bronchial spasm cause airway narrowing and obstruction to air flow, airtrapping, hyperinflation of the lungs, ventilation-perfusion mismatching, and intrapulmonary shunting. Progressive hypoxemia can lead to compensatory pulmonary vasoconstriction, pulmonary hypertension, and impaired right ventricular function.

Assessment

Clinical presentation varies with the severity and duration of the attack (Clinical Findings 4–9). Acute attacks may vary in severity from mild dyspnea to asphyxiation and death.

POINTS TO REMEMBER

▶ The critically ill adult may present with acute respiratory failure associated with a life-threatening exacerbation of asthma or status asthmaticus:
  • Exhaustion, dehydration, alterations in the level of consciousness, and cardiovascular collapse can occur very quickly.
  • In addition to the initial assessment (see Table 2–1), a thorough baseline and focused respiratory and cardiovascular assessments (see Tables 2–1, 4–1, and 5–1) should be completed as often as the patient's condition dictates to facilitate early detection of complications and urgent intervention.
▶ Asthma may be an underlying disease associated with an unrelated critical disorder:
  • In addition to a focused assessment of the presenting disorder, a thorough nursing history, baseline assessment, and focused respiratory assessment (see Tables 1–1, 2–1, and 4–1 and Clinical Findings 4–9) should be directed at establishing a data base of normals for the patient to serve as a comparison for future reference.
  • As well, the baseline and focused assessments should be directed at early detection of predisposing factors such as viral infections, emotional distress, and other complications likely to precipitate an acute asthmatic attack.
▶ Ongoing assessment incorporates the evaluation of responses to diagnostic procedures and therapeutic interventions aimed at the

reversal of airflow obstruction; it includes collaboration with other members of the health team to improve oxygenation and maintain an effective breathing pattern.

Clinical Findings 4–9   *Asthma*

I. HISTORY

A. Predisposing factors
  1. *Extrinsic (allergens)*
     - Genetic predisposition
     - Dust
     - Pollens
     - Molds
  2. *Intrinsic*
     - Pulmonary irritants (e.g., smoke, aerosols)
     - Occupational irritants (e.g., formaldehyde, engine exhaust)
     - Viral infections
     - Exercise
     - Emotional or physical stress
     - Medications (e.g., aspirin, nonsteroidal anti-inflammatory drugs)
     - Weather changes (e.g., fog, smog)

B. Subjective findings
  1. Dyspnea related to bronchoconstriction and airway obstruction, intrapulmonary shunting, and impaired gas exchange
  2. Fatigue and exhaustion related to the increased work of breathing
  3. Anxiety or fear related to difficulty in breathing

II. LABORATORY AND BEDSIDE MONITORING FINDINGS

A. Pulmonary function studies (see Table 13–1 for related information on pulmonary function studies)
  1. May be normal between attacks
  2. Decreased forced expiratory volume, peak expiratory flow rate (PEFR), and vital capacity related to airway obstruction
  3. Increased residual volume, functional residual capacity, and total lung capacity related to hyperinflation

B. Chest x-ray: Hyperinflation related to increased lung volumes during attacks

C. Arterial blood gas studies (see Chapter 13 and Fig. 13–2 for related information on arterial blood gas studies, interpretation of acid-base disorders, and the efficiency of gas exchange)

1. Mild hypoxemia may be present initially, related to intrapulmonary shunting secondary to underventilated alveoli associated with bronchospasm, increased secretions, and edema; increased dead space may be associated with overinflation of other alveoli
2. Hypocapnia ($Paco_2$ <35 mm Hg) and respiratory alkalosis (pH >7.45) may be present as the attack progresses, related to an increased ventilatory drive secondary to hypoxemia and anxiety
3. Pao_2 <60 mm Hg, and $Paco_2$ >45 mm Hg, and respiratory acidosis (pH <7.35) may be present with progressive severity and duration of the attack, related to increased intrapulmonary shunting and inability of the patient to maintain hyperventilation

D. Other laboratory studies
1. Elevated leukocyte count related to presence of infection
2. Elevated eosinophil count related to allergen, inflammatory response, infection
3. Elevated serum immunoglobulin E (IgE) related to allergens, environmental stimulation, occupational exposure
(see Table 13–9 for related information on WBC count and differential)

E. ECG: Tachycardia related to hypoxemia and anxiety (increased stress response)

III. PHYSICAL ASSESSMENT FINDINGS

A. General observations (inspection)
1. *Mental status*
   - Restlessness, agitation, or confusion related to hypoxemia
   - Fragmented speech or inability to speak related to breathlessness
2. *Skin:* Cyanotic with progressive severe attack, related to peripheral vasoconstriction (stress response), hypoxemia, or decreased blood flow to the tissues
3. *Respiratory pattern*
   - Tachypnea related to hypoxemia and often compounded by anxiety
   - Prolonged expiration with severe respiratory distress related to difficulty of moving air out of lungs
4. *Respiratory effort:* Use of accessory muscles and suprasternal and intercostal retractions related to increased work of breathing
5. *Cough and sputum:* Cough productive of thick, tenacious sputum related to bronchial inflammation and hypersecretion of mucus (cough often aggravates bronchospasm)
6. *Respiratory excursion:* Minimal chest expansion related to hyperinflation

B. Palpation

1. *Skin*
   - Diaphoretic related to heightened stress response
   - Warm with presence of fever
2. *Chest wall and thorax:* Decreased chest expansion with inspiration related to hyperinflation

C. Auscultation

1. *Abnormal breath sounds:* Diminished breath sounds related to decreased air flow, hyperinflation
2. *Adventitious breath sounds*
   - Inspiratory and expiratory wheeze related to bronchoconstriction (the degree of wheezing is not a reliable indicator of the severity of an attack. A decrease in the extent of wheezing may indicate a positive response to treatment or severe deterioration in the patient's condition)
   - The absence of a wheeze may indicate that the patient is unable to move enough air to make a vibration in the narrowed airways

5

Cardiovascular Assessment

FUNCTION OF THE CARDIOVASCULAR SYSTEM

The principal function of the cardiovascular system is transportation of blood to and from the lungs (pulmonary circulation), and to and from the rest of the body (systemic or peripheral circulation). Blood is the medium that supplies oxygen, nutrients, and immunoglobulins to cells; it also collects and transports the by-products of cellular metabolism to elimination points in the respiratory, gastrointestinal, renal, and integumentary systems.

Blood flows in response to pressure gradients from an area of higher pressure to one of lower pressure. Rate and direction of flow are controlled by the following:

- Rhythmic muscular contraction (systole) and relaxation (diastole) of the chambers of the heart
- Action of valves within the heart and blood vessels
- Caliber, compliance, and integrity of heart and blood vessel walls, and
- Amount and composition of circulating blood

Blood flow is described in terms of cardiac output, which is the amount of blood ejected from the left ventricle into the aorta per minute (heart rate × stroke volume). The average minute cardiac output in the healthy, unstressed adult is 5 liters. Cardiac output is influenced by cardiac **inotropy,** or contractility; by **preload,** or the amount of blood in the ventricle at the end of diastole; and by **afterload,** or the vascular resistance the ventricles must overcome during systole in order to move blood into circulation. The **stroke volume** (SV) is the difference between the end-diastolic volume (EDV) and the end-systolic volume (ESV). The **ejection fraction** (SV/EDV) is usually about 60% of the end-diastolic volume.

The heart is regulated intrinsically by stretch receptors that respond, within limits, to changes in the volume of blood with changes in the force of contraction (Frank-Starling law). Specialized conductive tissue in cardiac muscle (sinoatrial and atrioventricular nodes, His' bundles, and Purkinje's fibers) transmits action potentials through cardiac muscle fibers, producing rhythmic, coordinated contraction and relaxation. The heart and blood vessels are regulated extrinsically by the following:

- **Sympathetic** and **parasympathetic** (vagus) nerves of the autonomic nervous system that regulate cardiac rate and vascular resistance through stimulation of cholinergic or adrenergic receptors, respectively
- Sensory nerve terminals called **baroreceptors** located in blood vessel walls (e.g., aortic arch, carotid sinuses) that are sensitive to changes in arterial pressure
- **Chemoreceptors** sensitive to oxygen, carbon dioxide and pH levels
- The **vasomotor center of the lower brain stem** (central nervous system ischemic response), which raises arterial blood pressure in response to cerebral ischemia
- Certain **hormones,** including those of the pituitary, adrenal, and thyroid glands, and the kidney, which have a variety of effects on cardiovascular function.
- Concentrations of **potassium** and **calcium** ions in extracellular fluid, which affect cardiac contractility

The heart is fist-sized, rotated to the left, and tilted on its axis so that the apex (lower area) is close to the chest wall. The heart is a four-chambered organ composed of a specialized muscle layer (myocardium) and three thin inner layers of connective tissue (endocardium). The heart is encased in a pericardial sac. The visceral pericardium (epicardium) covers the heart's outer surface. The parietal pericardium overlays this and is separated from it by a thin layer of serous fluid that reduces friction between the two surfaces. Over this is a tough fibrous layer attached to the sternum and diaphragm that stabilizes the heart in the thoracic cavity.

The direction of blood flow through the four cardiac chambers is determined by the opening and closing of two atrioventricular valves (mitral and tricuspid) and two semilunar valves (aortic and pulmonic) in response to pressure gradients. The right ventricle and left atrium control flow through the pulmonary circulation. The right atrium and left ventricle direct flow through the systemic circulation. Since there is no valve controlling the flow of blood from the vena cavae into the right atrium, increased pressure in the right heart produces signs and symptoms in the neck veins (jugulars), abdomen, and peripheral circulation. Since there is no valve controlling the flow of blood from the pulmonary veins into the left atrium, increased pressure in the left heart produces signs and symptoms in the pulmonary circulation.

Blood flow to the heart itself is provided by the right and left coronary arteries and their branches that arise directly from the aorta. Venous blood returns through coronary veins to the coronary sinus and to the right atrium.

Arteries, arterioles, and arterial capillaries distribute blood to the peripheral and pulmonary areas. Arterial blood pressure is determined by cardiac output and the systemic vascular resistance in the blood vessels. Vascular resistance may be affected by blood viscosity, vessel diameter, and vessel distensibility or compliance. Arteries and veins have three layers: the intima, media, and adventitia. Arteries have more smooth muscle and elastic fibers than veins. Veins, however, have valves that control the direction and volume of blood flow returning to the heart. Capillary walls are only one cell thick to allow for nutrient and waste exchange between the blood and individual cells and interstitium.

In assessing the circulatory system, the nurse must keep in mind all of the systems with which it has a major interface, including respiratory, neurological, gastrointestinal, endocrine, integumentary, and renal.

Changes with Aging

In industrialized societies heart disease is the primary cause of mortality in those 65 and older. Expression of disease, however, depends in large part on genetics and lifestyle behaviors, including physical activity, diet, alcohol consumption, and smoking habits.

Expected structural changes in the heart include a modest increase in left atrial and ventricular size, which remain within normal limits in the absence of cardiac disease. Left ventricular thickening involving a decrease in the number and an increase in the size of cardiac myocytes, fragmentation of elastin, and increased fibrotic tissue contribute to decreased cardiac compliance. The proportion of pacemaker cells in the sinoatrial (SA) node is reduced from 50% to 10%, and fat cells accumulate. Calcification occurs around the atrioventricular (AV) node, ventricular septum, bundle of His, and aortic valve. These structural changes may cause the electrical axis of the heart to shift to the left and slightly prolong the PR and QT intervals.

Changes in large arteries include collagen degeneration and increased fibrosis. Some calcification occurs in the medial layer, especially in vessels of the legs and feet. These changes are enhanced in patients with diabetes and those on long-term corticosteroid therapy. Arteries also become atheromatous with age, causing lumen narrowing. The degree of atherosclerosis depends on the presence of the usual risk factors for cardiac disease. Blood vessel changes lead to an increase in arterial stiffness, or sclerosis, increased peripheral vascular resistance, and some increase in arterial systolic pressure. Stenosis of large arteries (e.g., carotids) may produce a bruit on auscultation.

Cardiovascular changes with aging may prolong the relaxation phase, slow the left ventricular filling rate, increase the end-diastolic volume, and prolong the ejection phase of the cardiac cycle. This may result in a high normal left ventricular end-diastolic filling pressure (measured by pulmonary capillary wedge pressure) and produce a fourth heart sound, common in the elderly population.

β-Adrenergic stimulation of the heart and blood vessels and baroreceptor sensitivity decrease with age. This results in a decreased maximal heart rate (220 − age), a slowed increase in rate in response to stress, and possibly orthostasis. This may lead to an increased incidence of compensatory supraventricular and ventricular premature beats. It may also affect response to inotropic agents frequently prescribed in critical-care situations. Cardiac valve leaflets, especially those of the aortic valve become calcified, frequently resulting in a murmur over the aortic area of the precordium.

Left ventricular hypertrophy, decreased cardiac output, and hypertension are not expected changes with aging. They probably result from a combination of normal and pathologic changes and a decline in functional reserve capacity with age. Symptoms of angina and myocardial infarction in the elderly may be diminished, atypical, or absent. The nurse must anticipate problems through careful initial, baseline, focused, and ongoing assessments.

TABLE 5-1 Cardiovascular Assessment Techniques, Tips, Geriatric Considerations

Technique	Performance Tips	Description/Rationale	Geriatric Considerations
Pertinent History			
1. Related medical history	Review the patient's known medical history for **actual or potential disease states** that can affect cardiovascular function	Cardiovascular function may be affected by diseases or conditions that affect • The heart or blood vessels • The respiratory system • Neurologic innervation of cardiovascular organs • Infectious diseases • Endocrine diseases • Renal disease Cardiovascular function may also be affected by • Electrolyte, acid-base disorders • Immunocompromise • Chest trauma • Multisystem trauma	Coronary artery disease is the major cause of morbidity and mortality in those 65 and older Postmenopausal women have a risk similar to their male counterparts unless they are on hormone-replacement therapy (HRT)

		• Lifestyle behaviors: smoking, high cholesterol, obesity, sedentary lifestyle • Heredity, gender, age • Recent cardiopulmonary resuscitation	
2. Related drug history	Review the patient's recent past and current **drug therapy** for medications that may • Magnify cardiovascular signs and symptoms • Mask cardiovascular signs and symptoms *ASSESSMENT TIPS* 1. Attempt to correlate a new symptom with a recently administered drug or with a recently discontinued drug or changed dose	Drugs taken prior to admission or administered in the critical care setting may affect cardiovascular function in a variety of ways Look for drugs that are expected to mask or relieve certain types of chest pain, such as • Anginal pain: nitrates • Gastric ulceration: gastric acid inhibitors or neutralizers • Pleuritic, pain: anti-inflammatory drugs • Musculoskeletal pain: anti-inflammatory drugs, analgesics	Because of altered pharmacokinetics and pharmacodynamics with aging • Unexpected drug responses may occur at usual doses • Drugs may have a cumulative effect • Drugs may cause an unexpected response (see Chapter 3) Polypharmacy may produce adverse side effects affecting cardiovascular functions

Table continued on following page

TABLE 5-1 Cardiovascular Assessment Techniques, Tips, Geriatric Considerations *Continued*

Technique	Performance Tips	Description/Rationale	Geriatric Considerations
	2. Attempt to correlate improvement of a symptom with a recently administered drug or with a recently discontinued drug or changed dose		
3. Common complaints or observations that indicate the need for a focused assessment of the cardiovascular system	The most common sign and symptom of cardiovascular disease is **pain** *ASSESSMENT TIPS* 1. Interview the alert person about the exact nature of any discomfort	Common sources of chest pain include cardiac, respiratory, gastrointestinal, and musculoskeletal; consider past medical history of such conditions during assessment The most common cause of cardiovascular pain is ischemia caused by diminished oxygen supply to an organ or body area	In the geriatric patient typical chest pain may be diminished, atypical, or nonexistent; a significant number of elderly persons experience silent myocardial infarction, without typical complaints of pain The chest pain of angina or myocardial infarction may present as dyspnea and be difficult to differentiate from CHF or respiratory pathology

2. Use the following mnemonic to assure that all major characteristics of pain have been evaluated: **P** Precipitating factors, prodrome **Q** Quality, quantity **R** Region, radiation **S** Associated symptoms, setting **T** Timing, treatment effects	Also consider a history of cardiotoxic drugs (e.g., cocaine, certain chemotherapeutic agents) that may be affecting cardiac function Chest pain may also be caused by obstructions, inflammation, or trauma Characteristics of chest pain can aid in diagnosis of developing conditions (see Table 5–2, p. 232)	These situations require closer attention to objective data in the aging patient Other common sources of "chest pain" in the elderly include • Hiatal hernia with resultant esophageal reflux, aggravated in the supine position • Degenerative joint disease Careful assessment is required to differentiate new pain from pre-existing pain of multiple chronic diseases
4. Nonverbal behaviors		Changes in nonverbal behavior may be the only sign of change in physical condition in the elderly; classic symptoms of cardiac problems may be absent or atypical (see Chapter 3)
Look for changes in • Activity level • Facial expression • Mental status • Respiratory rate, rhythm, depth, effort • Changes in cardiac hemodynamics	In the poorly responsive or nonverbally responsive patient, such behaviors may be the only or first signs of a change in physical condition or adverse response to medications	

Table continued on following page

TABLE 5-1 Cardiovascular Assessment Techniques, Tips, Geriatric Considerations *Continued*

Technique	Performance Tips	Description/Rationale	Geriatric Considerations
	• Changes in ST segment, T wave		Older persons may underreport pain they attribute to the consequence of aging and disease
			Pain assessment may be complicated by cognitive impairment, sensory impairment, or depression
5. Psychological and cultural considerations	*Look for* • Stoicism, denial • Moaning, crying • Revealing symptom to family member rather than to a health professional	The meaning of pain, perceived intensity, and accepted ways of expression vary among individuals and cultures Nurses also have their own individual and culture expectations of how pain should be accepted and expressed; each nurse needs to evaluate his or her expectations and how they influence assessment and the extent of therapeutic interventions	Culture-specific, pain-related behaviors are likely to persist in first- and second-generation immigrants or may be reverted to in times of crisis by any patient

Physical Examination
*Blood Pressure
Determination*

If a patent arterial line is in place, intra-arterial pressure is generally more accurate than cuff pressure

Blood pressure values can be affected by equipment error or by physiological conditions

- If cuff and arterial pressures vary by more than 10%, consider equipment error as a cause of discrepancies
- If differences are significant, they *may affect treatment decisions*
- Consider anxiety ("white coat" hypertension) and pain as possible causes of elevated blood pressure in the critically ill patient aware of the surroundings
- Look for the presence of target organ disease (e.g., left ventricular hypertrophy, heart failure, renal stenosis) or other risk factors (e.g., diabetes, thyroid disease) in evaluating the significance of any blood pressure value

Elevated blood pressure is a treatable cause of heart failure and of stroke

Table continued on following page

157

TABLE 5–1 Cardiovascular Assessment Techniques, Tips, Geriatric Considerations *Continued*

Technique	Performance Tips	Description/Rationale	Geriatric Considerations

	Cuff size
	• Select by *bladder size* and *arm circumference*
	  – **Length:** Bladder should encircle ≥80% of the limb
	  – **Height:** Bladder should be 40% of the limb circumference
	• Consequences of improperly sized cuff
	  – If too small: Overestimates blood pressure
	  – If too large: Underestimates blood pressure
	Placement and technique
	• Wrap cuff snugly around the *bare arm*
	• Place cuff 1 inch (2.5 cm) above the antecubital fossa
	• Keep patient's arm at heart level (if the arm cannot be positioned at heart level, add or subtract 0.8 mm Hg from readings for each 1 cm the arm is positioned above or below the heart, respectively)
	• Palpate the radial pulse while rapidly inflating the cuff to about 30 mm Hg above the point at which the pulse on the cuffed arm disappears
	• Place the diaphragm of the stethoscope *lightly* over the brachial artery in the antecubital space
		Hypertension in the adult is defined as systolic pressure ≥140 mm Hg and diastolic pressure ≥90 mm Hg
		Hypertension in the elderly is defined as systolic pressure ≥160 mm Hg (isolated systolic hypertension) or combined with a diastolic pressure ≥90 mm Hg
		Age-related systolic hypertension is associated with increased stiffness (decreased compliance) of the cardiovascular structures due to calcification or lipid deposits	

- Deflate cuff steadily at 2 to 3 mm Hg per second
- View gauge straight on at eye level
- *Do not* reinflate the cuff immediately before the gauge has returned to zero; this may produce an erroneously high reading
- *Do not* reinflate the cuff immediately after the gauge has returned to zero; this may produce an erroneously high reading
- Wait 1 to 2 minutes before cuff reinflation on the same arm
- Do not interpret a single elevated reading as a diagnosis of hypertension

ASSESSMENT TIPS

1. Rule out nonpathologic causes of *high* systolic blood pressure readings:
   - Technique (see above)
   - *Pseudohypertension,* especially common in the older patient (see Geriatric Considerations, at right)

Pseudohypertension is caused by the inability of a blood pressure cuff to compress a sclerotic artery

Cuff pressures in the elderly should be measured using the palpation method to avoid misinterpretation of the lower end of an auscultatory gap for systolic blood pressure

Age-related systolic hypertension is associated with calcification of arteries; such calcification may produce an abnormally high systolic reading by cuff

ASSESSMENT TECHNIQUE

- Palpate the radial pulse while the cuff is inflated
- If the radial artery remains palpable, the high reading is likely due to a sclerotic brachial artery

Table continued on following page

159

TABLE 5–1 Cardiovascular Assessment Techniques, Tips, Geriatric Considerations *Continued*

Technique	Performance Tips	Description/Rationale	Geriatric Considerations
			• In this instance use the arterial line pressure for accuracy *ASSESSMENT TECHNIQUE* • Palpate the radial pulse • Inflate the cuff to 30 mm Hg above the point at which the pulse becomes nonpalpable • Deflate the cuff until the pulse returns—this is the accurate systolic pressure
	2. Rule out nonpathologic causes of *low* systolic blood pressure readings: • Technique *(see above)* • *Auscultatory gap*, especially common in the older patient (see Geriatric Considerations, at right)	An *auscultatory gap* is the disappearance of the systolic Korotkoff sound and its reappearance at a lower pressure. This is caused by decreased blood flow through an extremity (e.g., arteriosclerosis, hypertension, aortic stenosis) Cuff pressures in the elderly should be measured using the palpation method to avoid misinterpretation of the lower end of an auscultatory gap for systolic blood pressure	
	3. Control *venous congestion* in the forearm, distal to the cuff placement	*Venous congestion* can be due to heart failure or local obstruction or may be assumed because of poor examiner technique	Venous congestion may persist longer than usual in the elderly patient

- Raise the arm above the head prior to applying the cuff
- Inflate the cuff rapidly
- Deflate the cuff completely between readings
- Allow blood flow to normalize in the extremity between inflations
- Avoid repeated, slow cuff inflations
- Consider arm-to-arm variations in blood pressure
- In the presence of cardiac dysrhythmias, take an average of serial cuff pressures rather than a single pressure

Venous congestion may cause
- Difficulty hearing Korotkoff sounds
- Cuff systolic pressure reading *lower* and diastolic pressure reading *higher* than they actually are

Arm-to-arm variations may be due to
- Supravalvular aortic stenosis
- Aortic insufficiency

Cardiac dysrhythmias can cause fluctuations in blood pressure by varying cardiac output

With aging, atherosclerosis of a scapular or brachial artery may produce lower blood pressure in the affected arm

Table continued on following page

TABLE 5-1 Cardiovascular Assessment Techniques, Tips, Geriatric Considerations *Continued*

Technique	Performance Tips	Description/Rationale	Geriatric Considerations
	• **Document** cuff-pressure averaging to ensure consistency of technique between examiners • Correlate abnormal readings (hypo- or hypertension) with other assessment data	Hypertension may be secondary to another disease or may be primary hypertension with no clearly indentified cause Consider the effects of current medications or those taken prior to admission on blood pressure	Altered pharmacokinetics and pharmacodynamics with aging as well as polypharmacy may affect blood pressure in the elderly (see Chapter 3)
Inspection/Palpation **1. General observations** • Mental status	*Look for* • Restlessness, agitation, anxiety • Confusion • Apprehension, panic	These may be early indications of hypoxic changes that may result from • Changing physical condition • Adverse drug response Restlessness or anxiety may be associated with pain	Changes in level of consciousness and mentation are often the *only* indications of changes in condition; classic symptoms may be absent (see Chapter 3)

	• Feelings of impending doom • Drowsiness, fatigue	Weakness may be due to decreased perfusion of cardiac or skeletal muscles Changes in mentation may also be indicative of decreased cerebral perfusion, hemorrhage, thrombus, or embolism (see Chapter 6)

• Respiratory status	*Look for*
	• Dyspnea
	• Orthopnea
	• Paroxysmal nocturnal dyspnea
	• Tachypnea
	• Cough
		Respiratory distress may indicate
		• General hypoxemia
		• Compromised pulmonary circulation with impaired gas exchange
		  – Respiratory pathology
		  – Cardiovascular pathology
		• Increased intrathoracic blood volume in the supine position (heart failure)
		• Pericarditis with chest pain on deep inspiration or position change, possibly relieved with leaning forward

• Head movements	*Look for* rhythmic head movements (de Musset's sign)	Nodding movements correlated with ventricular systole and arterial Nodding movements must be distinguished from the side-to-

Table continued on following page

TABLE 5-1 Cardiovascular Assessment Techniques, Tips, Geriatric Considerations *Continued*

Technique	Performance Tips	Description/Rationale	Geriatric Considerations
		wave forms probably represent hyperdynamic carotid blood flow (e.g., aortic regurgitation, aortic aneurysm)	side, rolling movements of parkinsonism
		See Chapter 4, Respiratory Assessment	See Chapter 4, Respiratory Assessment
2. Integument (also see respiratory assessment)	*Look at* • General color • Local variations • Vascular areas • Dependent areas		
• Skin color			
• Skin temperature • Skin moisture	*ASSESSMENT TIPS* See Chapter 4, Respiratory Assessment	See Chapter 4, Respiratory Assessment Moderate fever is expected up to 72 hours after myocardial infarction	See Chapter 4, Respiratory Assessment
• Skin turgor	*ASSESSMENT TIPS* 1. Assess by pulling up the skin over the forehead or sternum (presternal tenting); hydrated skin should snap back briskly	A possible indication of state of hydration; tenting of presternal skin suggests dehydration; dehydration affects circulating blood volume and kidney function	Loss of skin elasticity with aging can also cause skin to tent and must be cautiously interpreted as dehydration Consideration should be given to urine specific gravity, cardiac

2. Do not assess skin over the back of the hand, which may produce a false positive result, especially in the elderly
3. Other sites that have been recommended for evaluation of tugor include the neck, abdomen, and thigh; caution should be exercised in using these sites in the elderly or those with severe weight loss (see Geriatric Considerations)

output, and other traditional parameters indicating the state of hydration

Dehydration is a frequent cause or contributor to hypovolemia in the elderly, and its correction is relatively easy if recognized early

Malnutrition and overuse of diuretics are frequent contributors to dehydration in the elderly and should be assessed by history, where possible

• Skin lesions

Look for vascular lesions, including
• Petechiae
• Splinter hemorrhages (see below)

Petechiae are small violet or purple lesions on the skin produced by capillary fragility and hemorrhage

Osler's nodes are small, tender, dermal infarcts on the pads of the fingers or

Petechial lesions are common in the elderly, related to increased capillary fragility with age

Certain drugs also cause petechial lesions as a side effect; including chronic corticosteroid use

Table continued on following page

Technique	Performance Tips	Description/Rationale	Geriatric Considerations
	• Osler's nodes	toes caused by cardiac vegetations or vasculitis associated with circulating immune complexes	Petechial lesions alone are not an indication of infective endocarditis
	• Janeway lesions	Janeway lesions are red, macular lesions on the palms and soles	
		These lesions are often found in combination with a diagnosis of infective endocarditis and are commonly accompanied by a cardiac murmur	
	Look for characteristic lesions in parenteral drug users, patients with valvular disease, and those with invasive lines, especially over prolonged periods		
• Nails	*Look at*	(See Chapter 4, Respiratory Assessment)	
	• Plates, beds, clubbing (see Chapter 4, Respiratory Assessment)		
	• Splinter hemorrhages	Longitudinal dark or red streaks on the distal third of the nailbeds are suggestive of infective endocarditis, trichinosis, or history of manual labor	

	Look for	May suggest	
3. Renal	• Urine output <0.5 ml/kg/h • Increased urine specific gravity • Elevated BUN	May suggest • Decreased circulating blood volume with activation of compensatory mechanisms • Decreased renal perfusion (embolism)	Renal blood flow and glomerular filtration rate may be reduced by 50% with advancing age; this results in a decreased ability to handle fluid, electrolyte, and metabolic changes
	ASSESSMENT TIPS 1. Make certain examination is performed in good light with minimal glare 2. Perform inspection and palpation simultaneously 3. With increasing skill, inspection and palpation can be integrated with auscultation, enhancing the accuracy and efficiency of the examination		
4. The precordium (optional)			
• Pulsations	*ASSESSMENT TIPS* 1. Precordial movements are best seen with light positioned to cast a shadow across the chest; this is best accomplished by shining a light tangentially across the chest from right to left	Cardiac movements are generally not discernible unless severe chamber hypertrophy, cardiomegaly, or valvular damage underlies the disease condition, or unless the person is very thin Newly developing pulsations suggest evolving pathology	In the frail, underweight elderly person, normal cardiac pulsations may be visible because of loss of chest wall muscle and adipose tissue No movement may be visible in the obese or barrel-chested elder

Table continued on following page

TABLE 5-1 Cardiovascular Assessment Techniques, Tips, Geriatric Considerations *Continued*

Technique	Performance Tips	Description/Rationale	Geriatric Considerations

	2. Examination is best performed while standing to the patient's right side
	3. Correlate findings with cardiac anatomy (see Fig. 5-1)
	4. Methodically inspect and palpate five cardiac areas:
	  • **Aortic:** Area of the second intercostal space, right sternal border (2ICS, RSB)
	  • **Pulmonic:** Area of the second intercostal space, left sternal border (2ICS, LSB)
		Marked pulsation suggests conditions involving widened pulse pressure, such as hypertension, thyrotoxicosis, aortic insufficiency
		
		Systolic pulsation in the pulmonic area (2ICS, LSB) may indicate pulmonary hypertension (pulsation caused by closure of the pulmonic valve under pressure)	

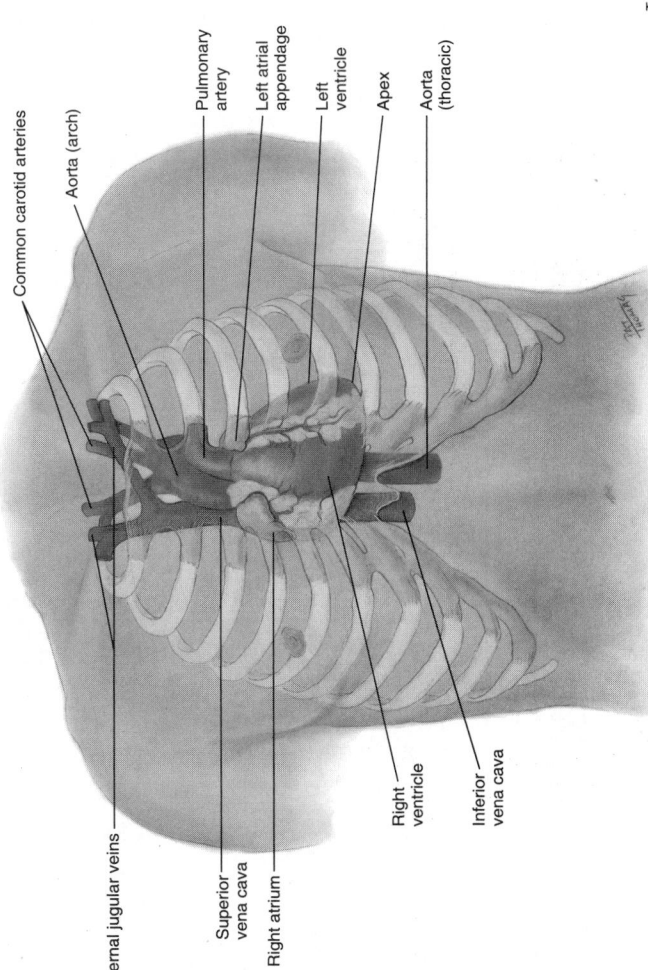

FIGURE 5-1

Position of the cardiac chambers and major blood vessels on the precordium in the healthy adult. (From Jarvis, C. [1996]. *Physical examination and health assessment* [3rd ed., p. 515]. Philadelphia: W. B. Saunders.)

Common carotid arteries

Aorta (arch)

Pulmonary artery

Left atrial appendage

Left ventricle

Apex

Aorta (thoracic)

Internal jugular veins

Superior vena cava

Right atrium

Right ventricle

Inferior vena cava

Table continued on following page

TABLE 5-1 Cardiovascular Assessment Techniques, Tips, Geriatric Considerations *Continued*

Technique	Performance Tips	Description/Rationale	Geriatric Considerations
	• **Tricuspid:** Left lower sternal border (LLSB) • **Mitral (apical):** Area of the fifth intercostal space, left midclavicular line (5ICS, LMCL), or at the cardiac apex • **Epigastric area:** Lower sternal border, midsternal line (LSB, MSL) 5. Visible pulsations are usually best palpated with the pads of the fingers 6. It may help to time pulsation with ventricular systole	See discussion of PMI below. Pulsation of the abdominal aorta may be visible inferior to the xiphoid process in the epigastric region, especially in thin individuals; the pulsatile area is normally vertical and narrow A diffuse pulsatile area or mass in the epigastric region suggests an aortic aneurysm and should be further assessed for bruit, using both stethoscope bell and diaphragm; *avoid deep palpation of the abdomen if an aneurysm is suspected or confirmed;* palpation may extend an aortic dissection or rupture the vessel	

- By palpation: carotid pulsation is slightly behind ventricular systole
- By arterial line: peak of wave is simultaneous with or following ventricular systole, depending on line placement
- By cardiac monitor: ventricular systole follows the QRS complex; atrial systole precedes the PR interval

7. Describe pulsations by area, size, and pulse characteristics

Table continued on following page

171

TABLE 5-1 Cardiovascular Assessment Techniques, Tips, Geriatric Considerations *Continued*

Technique	Performance Tips	Description/Rationale	Geriatric Considerations
• Lifts and heaves	*ASSESSMENT TIP* Use light pressure with the flat of the hand to evaluate the location and intensity of these movements	Lifts and heaves are sustained outward movements of the ventricle during systole that are visible over areas of the precordium • Lift or heave at the apex or lateral to the left midclavicular line (MCL) suggests left ventricular hypertrophy (Fig. 5–2) or cardiomegaly • Lift in the right or left parasternal area accompanied by lateral retraction (RV rock) suggests right ventricular hypertrophy (e.g., pulmonic valve disease, pulmonary hypertension)	

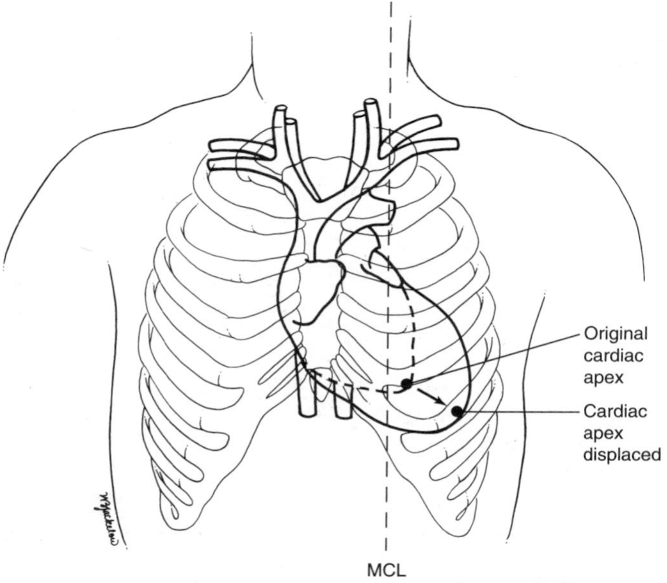

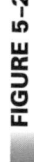

FIGURE 5-2

Position of the apex of the left ventricle with left ventricular hypertrophy. MCL, midclavicular line. (Adapted from Swartz, M. H. [1998]. *Textbook of physical diagnosis* [3rd ed., p. 278]. Philadelphia: W. B. Saunders.)

Original cardiac apex

Cardiac apex displaced

MCL

Table continued on following page

TABLE 5–1 Cardiovascular Assessment Techniques, Tips, Geriatric Considerations *Continued*

Technique	Performance Tips	Description/Rationale	Geriatric Considerations
• Thrills	*ASSESSMENT TIPS* 1. Use light pressure with the flat of the hand 2. Vibrations are best felt with ball and heel of hand, which are very sensitive to such movement 3. This examination may be omitted, as it only confirms a loud murmur that would be easily discernible with auscultation	Thrills are palpable, low-frequency vibrations felt over areas of severe underlying blood turbulence; they are usually associated with loud cardiac murmurs	
• Point of maximal impulse (PMI)	This is also known as the **apical impulse** (this should not be confused with the apical pulse, which is assessed by auscultation rather than inspection and palpation)	The normal PMI identifies the apex of the left ventricle as it rotates outward to the chest wall during ventricular contraction (systole) The normal PMI has these characteristics:	

ASSESSMENT TIPS

1. While best assessed with a person sitting and leaning forward, it can also be assessed if a person is assessed in the supine position; assessment is inaccurate if a person is in the side-lying position, since this displaces the heart

2. Place the flat of the hand, initially, over the lower left precordium; if a pulsation is felt, refine its exact location and characteristics using the index and middle fingertips and pads

3. Describe PMI characteristics as discussed at right

- 1–2 cm diameter (quarter sized)
- <10 cm from MSL (5th ICS, LMCL)
- A light, brisk tap against the finger pad

The laterally displaced PMI is an indication of cardiomegaly and specifically of left ventricular hypertrophy and dilatation (see Fig. 5–2)

A ventricular aneurysm may be present if a PMI is displaced medially and superiorly to its expected location

An abdominal mass or abdominal distention may displace a normal PMI upward by exerting upward pressure on the diaphragm

COPD with lung hyperinflation may displace the normal PMI to the epigastric region at the left sternal border (LSB)

Table continued on following page

TABLE 5-1 Cardiovascular Assessment Techniques, Tips, Geriatric Considerations *Continued*

Technique	Performance Tips	Description/Rationale	Geriatric Considerations
	4. PMI is inaccessible to assessment in 30%–50% of adults	Pneumothorax may displace the normal PMI away from the affected side. In this case also look for tracheal deviation (see Chapter 4) S_3: a second impulse felt after the PMI, caused by rapid filling of the ventricle during early diastole; S_3 may be easier to palpate than to auscultate; a palpable S_3 can be used to confirm an extra heart sound as a suspected S_3	
Cardiac Auscultation	*ASSESSMENT TIPS* Effective auscultation requires the examiner to do the following: 1. **Provide a quiet environment;** for patients on		

mechanical life support or treatment modalities that cannot be silenced, cardiac auscultation will need to be augmented with inspection and palpation techniques, the use of invasive monitoring, and other diagnostic tests

2. **Place earpieces forward in the ears** — This follows the forward curvature of the ear canal, optimizing sound transmission and perception

3. **Block out visual stimuli**, initially, by beginning auscultation with closed eyes — Visual stimuli are stronger than auditory; closing the eyes assists the examiner in focusing on the cardiac sounds

Table continued on following page

TABLE 5-1 Cardiovascular Assessment Techniques, Tips, Geriatric Considerations *Continued*

Technique	Performance Tips	Description/Rationale	Geriatric Considerations
	4. **Ensure direct contact of the stethoscope with the chest wall;** auscultation should not be done over a patient gown	Movement of fabric under the stethoscope may be mistaken for cardiac or respiratory sounds; judgments made based on the quality of such sounds may be in error	
	5. **Press the diaphragm of the stethoscope firmly to the chest** by pressing against the bell, if located directly above it, or by pressing the index and middle fingers firmly on the back of the diaphragm straddling the base of the bell	Firm skin contact allows the diaphragm to better transmit high-frequency heart sounds, such as S_1, S_2, clicks, snaps, and most murmurs	

6. **Press the bell of the stethoscope lightly against the chest,** barely trapping air underneath it; this can be done by holding the tubing immediately proximal to the bell, rather than the bell itself	The purpose of the bell is to transmit low-frequency sounds, such as S_3, S_4, and low-frequency murmurs and bruits If the bell is pressed too firmly against the chest, it acts like a diaphragm, and low-frequency sounds are missed
7. **Listen to only one sound at a time,** describing its characteristics before focusing on the next sound	Sounds have different expected characteristics in different locations on the precordium; changes in the character of sounds or occurrence of sounds in particular areas can aid in accurate diagnosis
8. **Compare each sound as heard in the various auscultatory areas**	
9. In critical care areas **perform auscultation**	In acute and ambulatory settings, cardiac diagnosis also includes auscultation in the sitting position and

Table continued on following page

TABLE 5–1 Cardiovascular Assessment Techniques, Tips, Geriatric Considerations *Continued*

Technique	Performance Tips	Description/Rationale	Geriatric Considerations
	in the supine and left lateral recumbent (LLR), i.e., left side-lying position	leaning forward; these positions are usually not feasible in the critical care setting; the LLR position will bring the ventricle closer to the chest wall for assessment	
	10. **Time the sounds with events in the cardiac cycle** (see Fig. 5–3, pp. 182, 183) by any of the following methods: • Simultaneously palpate the carotid or other peripheral pulse • Time with arterial wave forms • Time with ECG monitor (see above)	Such techniques may help to describe and identify unknown sounds	

11. **Associate sounds with inspiration** by watching the chest rise and fall while auscultating	Sounds originating in the right heart are often exaggerated with inspiration because increased intrathoracic pressure during inspiration enhances blood return to the right heart; increased intrathoracic pressure may produce events such as • Physiologic splitting of S_2 • Sinus dysrhythmia Timing sounds with the respiratory cycle can also help to distinguish • Pathological splitting of S_2 (see below) • Soft murmurs vs. breath sounds • Pericardial vs. pleural friction rub • Murmur of tricuspid insufficiency or stenosis

Table continued on following page

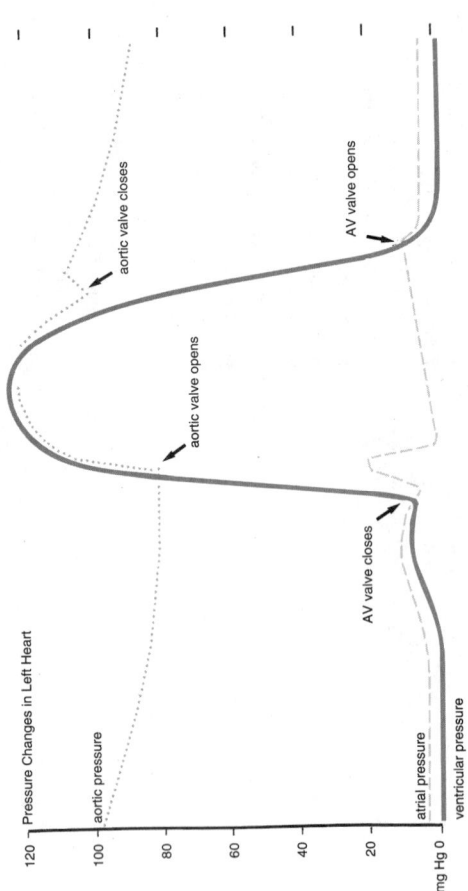

Pressure Changes in Left Heart

120
100
80
60
40
20
mg Hg 0

aortic pressure

aortic valve closes

aortic valve opens

AV valve opens

AV valve closes

atrial pressure

ventricular pressure

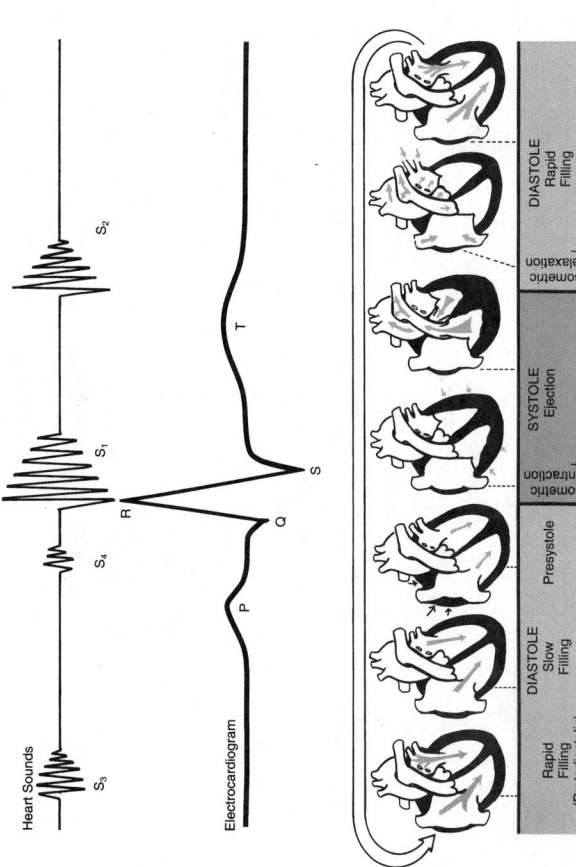

FIGURE 5-3

Timing of heart sounds with events in the cardiac cycle. (From Jarvis, C. [1996]. *Physical examination and health assessment* [3rd ed., p. 518]. Philadelphia: W. B. Saunders.)

TABLE 5–1 Cardiovascular Assessment Techniques, Tips, Geriatric Considerations *Continued*

Technique	Performance Tips	Description/Rationale	Geriatric Considerations
	12. **Auscultate the five cardiac areas where valvular sounds are best heard:** • *Aortic area:* 2nd ICS, RSB • *Pulmonic area:* 2nd ICS, LSB • *Tricuspid area:* LLSB • *Erb's point:* 3rd ICS, LSB • *Mitral area:* 5th ICS, LMCL 13. Recent recommendations suggest a zigzag pattern of auscultation that includes the right parasternal area at the apex of the right ventricle	The two normal heart sounds (S_1 and S_2) are produced by *closure* of the atrioventricular and semilunar valves in the heart; sounds produced by these valves are *not* heard best over their anatomical location but over areas of the precordium that maximize transmission of sounds from each valve; these areas are located downstream, in the direction of normal blood flow from each valve (Note: the aortic valve is anatomically located in the left heart but is auscultated on the right chest; the tricuspid and pulmonic valves are located in the right heart but are auscultated on the left chest) (see Fig. 5–4)	

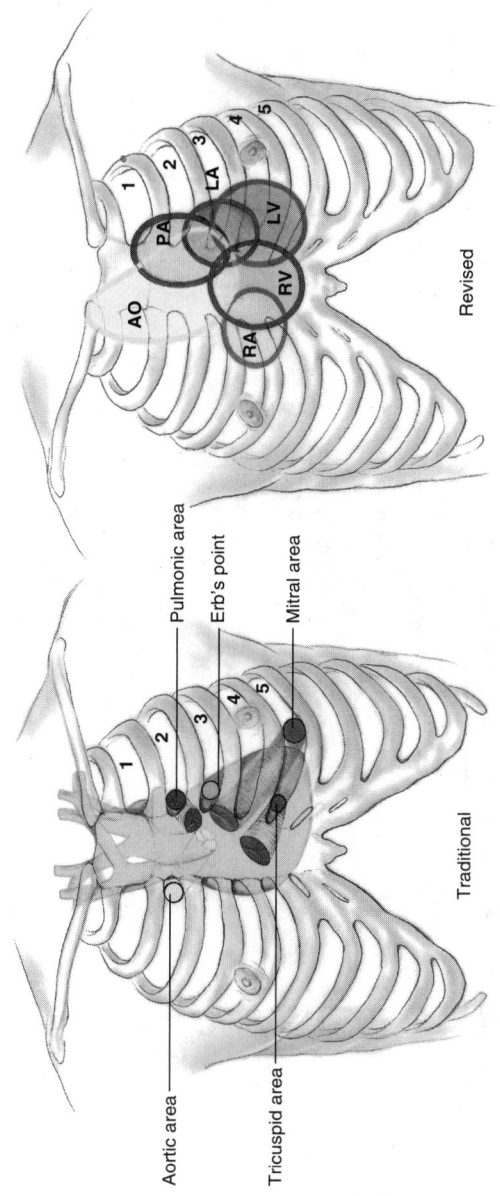

FIGURE 5-4

Auscultatory areas on the precordium. (From Jarvis, C. [1996]. *Physical examination and health assessment* [3rd ed., p. 539]. Philadelphia: W. B. Saunders.)

AUSCULTATORY AREAS

Aortic area

Pulmonic area

Erb's point

Tricuspid area

Mitral area

Traditional

AO

PA

LA

1 2 3 4 5

LV

RV

RA

Revised

Table continued on following page

TABLE 5-1 Cardiovascular Assessment Techniques, Tips, Geriatric Considerations *Continued*

Technique	Performance Tips	Description/Rationale	Geriatric Considerations
	14. *Inch through* these areas first with the diaphragm and then with the bell	Inching allows the examiner to detect subtle changes in each heart sound. It also helps the examiner detect the introduction of an extra heart sound	
	15. **Make certain to place the patient in the LLR position when auscultating the mitral area with the bell**	The S_3 and S_4 heart sounds, if present, are best heard in the mitral area; since they are low-frequency sounds, they are best heard with the bell of the stethoscope; placing the patient in the LLR position optimizes the chances of hearing these often diagnostically significant sounds	

1. General
  • Rate

ASSESSMENT TIPS 1. To establish an accurate baseline heart rate it is important to be familiar with the patient's prehospitalization physical conditioning program, medications, and underlying disease states 2. In critical care settings rate can most efficiently be obtained from cardiac monitoring equipment; looking at wave forms can also enhance your correlation of auscultatory sounds with events in the cardiac cycle	Be particularly attentive to the individual who • Is on a program of regular aerobic exercise (which may slow resting and nonresting heart rates) • Uses β-adrenergic blocking agents; over time, these may slow resting heart rate • Uses drugs that may increase heart rate (e.g., asthma drugs)	*Rate* Resting heart rate does not change with aging except in those who are physically conditioned and in persons whose heart rates are altered by drugs or disease; common conditions in the elderly that affect resting heart rate are • Undiagnosed or uncontrolled thyroid disease (brady- or tachy-rhythm) • Treatment with β-adrenergic blocking agents for control of preexisting disease (e.g., propranolol) Do not assume that the aging person is not physically fit; many seniors engage in fitness programs

Table continued on following page

TABLE 5-1 Cardiovascular Assessment Techniques, Tips, Geriatric Considerations *Continued*

Technique	Performance Tips	Description/Rationale	Geriatric Considerations
	3. Evaluate for a pulse deficit: Simultaneously auscultate the heart and palpate a peripheral pulse	With cardiac dysrhythmia, changes in diastolic filling time may diminish cardiac output enough to weaken the pulsation transmitted to the periphery; in this instance, heart rate must be assessed apically Simultaneous assessment provides data on perfusion in the absence of invasive monitoring equipment	
• Rhythm	*ASSESSMENT TIPS* 1. In a critical care setting, rhythm can most efficiently be evaluated from the ECG monitor; looking at these tracings during auscultation can also enhance your correlation of auscultatory sounds with		*Rhythm* A variety of ectopic beats are common in aging persons and thus may not, in isolation and with only sporadic occurrence, reflect underlying disease or adverse change in condition Because of compromised functional reserve with aging, quicker action

2. Heart sounds
(See Fig. 5–5)

events in the cardiac cycle

2. In situations where an ECG monitor is not yet placed, describe cardiac rhythms as "regular," "regularly irregular," or "irregularly irregular"

ASSESSMENT TIP
Distant or muffled cardiac sounds may be due to
- Examiner's not blocking out visual stimuli
- Increased distance of the heart from chest wall
- Decreased ventricular compliance
- Electromechanical dissociation

to correct symptomatic rhythms may be required
Many elderly persons have been prescribed digoxin before hospitalization; when dysrhythmias occur, consider
- Digitalis toxicity
- Digitalis withdrawal
- Potassium imbalance

Increased distance of the heart from the chest wall may be due to
- Emphysema with hyperinflation of lungs
- Barrel chest
- Well-developed chest musculature
- Truncal obesity
- Decreased ventricular compliance
- Ruptured ventricular aneurysm
- Pericardial effusion, tamponade
- Overriding breath sounds

Table continued on following page

189

TABLE 5-1 Cardiovascular Assessment Techniques, Tips, Geriatric Considerations *Continued*

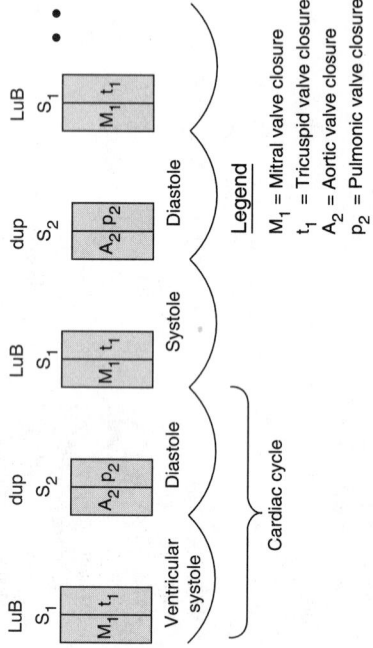

FIGURE 5-5

Schematic presentation of the events in the cardiac cycle.

Legend

M_1 = Mitral valve closure
t_1 = Tricuspid valve closure
A_2 = Aortic valve closure
p_2 = Pulmonic valve closure

- Normal

S_1
- Intensity at each location

S_1 is produced by closure of the mitral (M_1) atrioventricular valve in the left heart and the slightly slower closure of the tricuspid (t_1) atrioventricular valve in the right heart (see Fig. 5–5)

S_1 sounds are loudest in the mitral and tricuspid areas at the apex (bottom) of the heart

- Splitting into its right and left heart components

Occasionally a narrowly split S_1 is heard in the tricuspid area; it is non-pathologic

Wide splitting in the tricuspid area or splitting in the mitral area in the adult may indicate valvular damage (see Fig. 5–6)

S_2
- Intensity at each location

S_2 is produced by closure of the aortic (A_2) semilunar valve in the left heart and the slightly slower closure of the pulmonic (p_2) semilunar valve in the right heart (see Fig. 5–5)

Table continued on following page

191

TABLE 5–1 Cardiovascular Assessment Techniques, Tips, Geriatric Considerations *Continued*

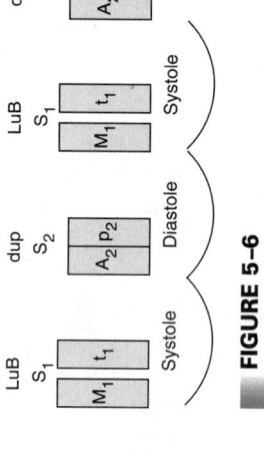

FIGURE 5–6
Splitting of the first heart sound (S_1).

• Splitting into its right and left heart components	S_2 sounds are loudest in the aortic and pulmonic areas at the base (top) of the heart	A split S_2 on inspiration in the elderly patient may indicate a bundle branch block
	Occasionally a narrowly split S_2 is heard in the pulmonic area or at Erb's point, especially in children and young adults; it is called physiologic splitting and occurs on inspiration; it is not pathologic	
	Wide splitting in the pulmonic area or splitting in the aortic area in the adult may indicate cardiac damage	
	Splitting of S_2 on expiration (paradoxical splitting) is also pathologic (see Fig. 5–7)	
• Extra		
S_3 (also called a ventricular gallop)	A low frequency sound produced by rapid filling of ventricles during early ventricular diastole	An S_3 in an aging person strongly suggests ventricular failure or volume overload from a regurgitant valve

Table continued on following page

193

TABLE 5–1 Cardiovascular Assessment Techniques, Tips, Geriatric Considerations *Continued*

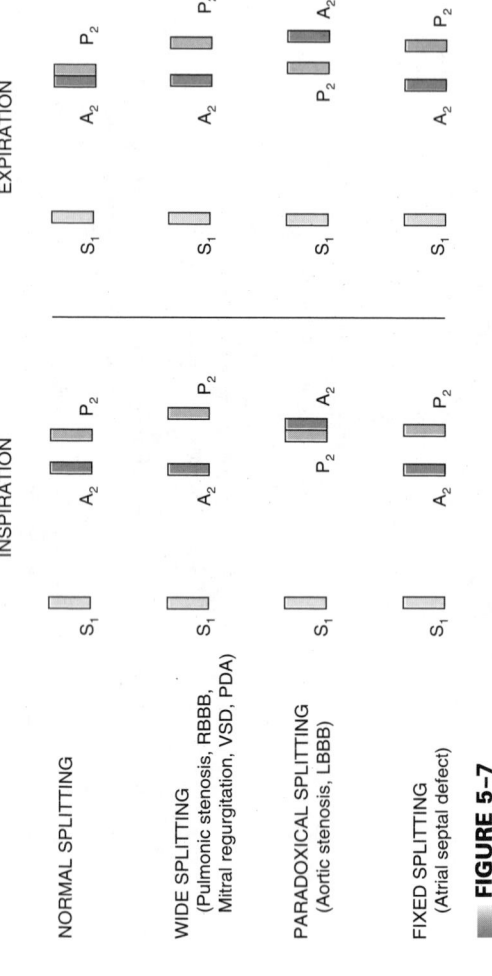

	INSPIRATION	EXPIRATION
NORMAL SPLITTING	S_1 A_2 P_2	S_1 A_2 P_2
WIDE SPLITTING (Pulmonic stenosis, RBBB, Mitral regurgitation, VSD, PDA)	S_1 A_2 P_2	S_1 A_2 P_2
PARADOXICAL SPLITTING (Aortic stenosis, LBBB)	S_1 P_2 A_2	S_1 P_2 A_2
FIXED SPLITTING (Atrial septal defect)	S_1 A_2 P_2	S_1 A_2 P_2

FIGURE 5–7

Abnormalities of splitting of the second heart sound (S_2). RBBB, right bundle branch block; VSD, ventricular septal defect; PDA, patent ductus arteriosus; LBBB, left bundle branch block. (From Swartz, M. H. [1998]. *Textbook of physical diagnosis* [3rd ed., p. 314]. Philadelphia: W. B. Saunders.)

Rapid filling may be due to

- Age or gender: may be normal in children, young adults, women
- High cardiac output states: hyperthyroidism, fever, anemia, pregnancy, trained athlete
- Volume overload: regurgitant valve
- Decreased ventricular compliance: angina, ventricular failure

ASSESSMENT TIPS

1. Heard best with the bell in the mitral area (or possibly at the lower sternal border if the right ventricle is involved)
2. Listen for an S_3 immediately following S_2 (Lub—dup—up) during ventricular diastole (see Fig. 5-8)
3. May be heard best with the person in the LLR position
4. May be associated with a lift or heave in the mitral area
5. The ear easily accommodates to the S_3 sound, so

Table continued on following page

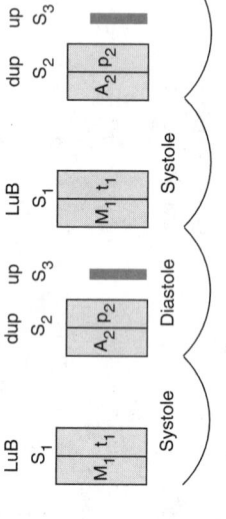

FIGURE 5-8
The third heart sound (S_3).

it is best detected with initial auscultation of the mitral area or lower sternal border with the bell

6. An S_3 that varies with respiration may differentiate right ventricular failure (S_3 heard on inspiration) from left ventricular failure (S_3 heard on expiration), depending on which ventricle is experiencing increased filling pressure

7. Differentiate an S_3 from a split S_2 by location, pitch, and correlation with inhalation

	S_3	Split S_2
Location	Mitral	Pulmonic
	Sternal border	Erb's point
Pitch	Lower than S_2	Same as S_2
Inhalation	Unaffected by or increased with	Varies with

Table continued on following page

TABLE 5–1 Cardiovascular Assessment Techniques, Tips, Geriatric Considerations *Continued*

Technique	Performance Tips	Description/Rationale	Geriatric Considerations
S₄ (also called an atrial gallop) *ASSESSMENT TIPS* 1. Heard best with the bell in the mitral area (or possibly at the left or right lower sternal border) 2. Listen for an S₄ immediately preceding S₁ (lu—Lub—dup) in ventricular diastole (see Fig. 5–9) 3. May be heard best with the person in the LLR position 4. An S₄ which varies with respiration may differentiate right ventricular	A low-frequency sound produced by atrial contraction against resistance late in ventricular diastole Resistance may be due to • Physical conditioning of a trained athlete • Age: may be normal in persons over 40, especially following strenuous exercise • Decrease in ventricular compliance (CAD, cardiomyopathies) • Increased afterload (systemic hypertension, aortic stenosis) • Increased preload (pulmonary hypertension, pulmonary stenosis)	An S₄ auscultated in geriatric patients commonly is due to aortic sclerosis with reduced ventricular compliance Aortic sclerosis may also produce a brief, soft systolic murmur in the aortic area Sudden appearance of an S₄ or murmur more likely signals an acute change of condition

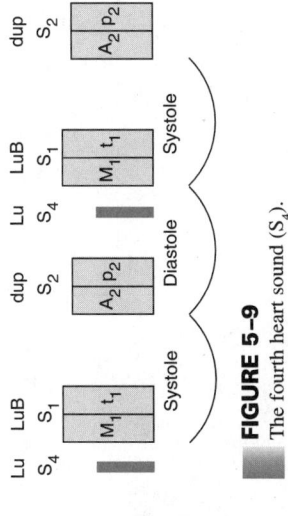

FIGURE 5-9
The fourth heart sound (S₄).

The fourth heart sound (S$_4$).

TABLE 5-1 Cardiovascular Assessment Techniques, Tips, Geriatric Considerations *Continued*

Technique	Performance Tips	Description/Rationale	Geriatric Considerations
	failure (S_4 heard on inspiration) from left ventricular failure (S_4 heard on expiration) depending on which ventricle has decreased compliance 5. Differentiate S_4 from a split S_1 by location and pitch		

	S_4	Split S_1
Location	Mitral	Tricuspid
	Sternal border	Mitral (rare)
Pitch	Lower than S_1	Same as S_1

(see Fig. 5–10)

Summation gallop (S_1, S_2, S_3, S_4)

ASSESSMENT TIP
Sound like a galloping horse with either three or four sounds, depending on cardiac rate

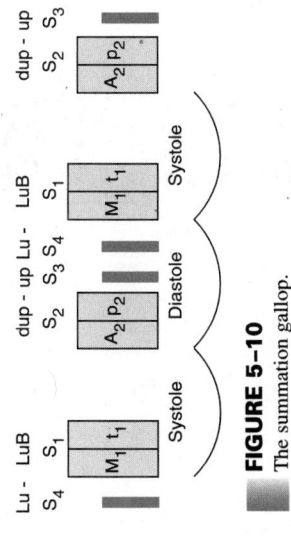

FIGURE 5-10
The summation gallop.

Table continued on following page

TABLE 5–1 Cardiovascular Assessment Techniques, Tips, Geriatric Considerations *Continued*

Technique	Performance Tips	Description/Rationale	Geriatric Considerations
(Identification of the following sounds requires practice; diagnostic tests such as the echocardiogram, if available, will confirm suspected diagnoses; in that case, auscultation provides confirmation and allows the examiner to enhance cardiac auscultation skills)	**Opening snaps (OS)** (diastolic sound; see Fig. 5–11) *ASSESSMENT TIPS* 1. Though heard best in the same areas as the S₃, this is a sharp, high-pitched, snapping sound, best heard with the diaphragm, unlike the S₃, which is generally more muted 2. The snap is usually accompanied by the diastolic murmur of mitral or tricuspid stenosis (see below)	Produced in early ventricular diastole (following S₂); snaps are produced by the *opening of a stenotic atrioventricular valve* (mitral, tricuspid)	

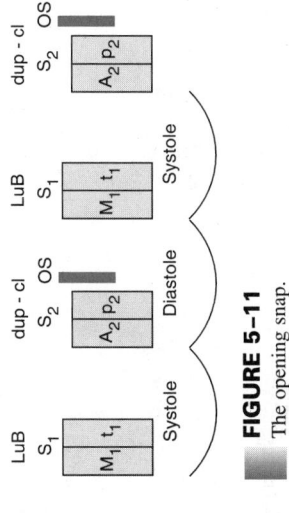

FIGURE 5-11
The opening snap.

Table continued on following page

TABLE 5-1 Cardiovascular Assessment Techniques, Tips, Geriatric Considerations *Continued*

Technique	Performance Tips	Description/Rationale	Geriatric Considerations
	Clicks (systolic sounds; see Fig. 5-12) • Ejection clicks (EC) • Midsystolic clicks (MSC)	**Ejection clicks** are heard early in ventricular systole (following S_1) and are produced by *opening of a stenotic semilunar valve* (aortic, pulmonic)	

ASSESSMENT TIPS

1. These are sharp, high-pitched, clicking sounds best heard with the diaphragm
2. The aortic click is heard early in ventricular systole, both in the aortic and mitral areas
3. The pulmonic click is heard early in ventricular systole, in the pulmonic area, and may be softer with inspiration

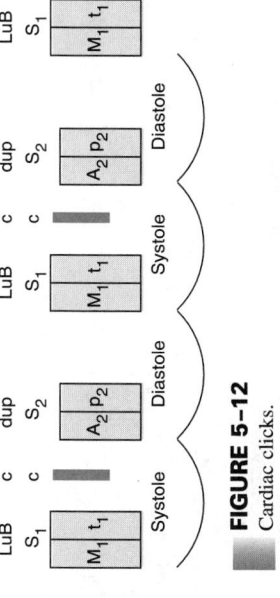

FIGURE 5-12
Cardiac clicks.

Table continued on following page

TABLE 5-1 Cardiovascular Assessment Techniques, Tips, Geriatric Considerations *Continued*

Technique	Performance Tips	Description/Rationale	Geriatric Considerations
	4. The click produced by a prolapsed valve is heard later in ventricular systole in the mitral or tricuspid areas 5. The click produced by a prolapsed valve is usually accompanied by the systolic murmur of mitral or tricuspid prolapse	**Midsystolic clicks** occur, as the name implies, later in systole and are caused by the ballooning of a *prolapsed mitral or tricuspid valve* into the respective atrium during ventricular systole	
	Iatrogenic heart sounds *ASSESSMENT TIP* Confirm with patient history of prosthetic valve or pacemaker placement	These are sounds produced by prosthetic valves; they have a sharp, mechanical sound	
3. Murmurs	*ASSESSMENT TIPS* 1. It may help in identifying murmurs in ventricular	Murmurs are produced by turbulent blood flow; cardiac murmurs can be produced by	

systole or diastole to listen while palpating a peripheral pulse or watching the cardiac monitor

2. Cardiac murmurs and bruits in large blood vessels may be mistaken for breath sounds
   - Ask the cooperative patient to hold his breath briefly to aid in differentiation
   - With the noncooperative patient, coordinate the sound with events in the cardiac cycle as displayed on the cardiac monitoring equipment, with visible respirations, or by

- Forward flow through stenotic valves that do not fully open
- Backward flow through incompetent (regurgitant, insufficient) valves that do not fully close
- Enlarged or ballooning chambers
- Septal defects, ruptures
- Transient high output states (fever, thyrotoxicosis)

Sounds produced by turbulent blood flow in large blood vessels are called bruits; these can be produced by

- Narrowing
- Dissection
- Iatrogenic shunting (dialysis access)

Table continued on following page

TABLE 5–1 Cardiovascular Assessment Techniques, Tips, Geriatric Considerations *Continued*

Technique	Performance Tips	Description/Rationale	Geriatric Considerations
	simultaneously palpating the carotid artery 3. Murmurs may obliterate normal and extra heart sounds 4. Low-frequency murmurs may only be heard with the bell of the stethoscope 5. In a critical care setting the most important characteristics of a murmur to describe are the timing, location, and radiation; other characteristics are of more diagnostic than treatment importance:	Classic characteristics of murmurs include • **Timing** (systole, diastole, continuous) • **Location** (auscultatory area where sound is heard the loudest) • **Radiation** (neck, axillae, abdomen); this is usually downstream in the direction of blood flow	

- The murmur of mitral stenosis (diastolic) may only be heard in the LLR position
- Some murmurs can only be diagnosed with the patient sitting upright or leaning forward; this may be impractical in critical care settings

- **Loudness:** graded I/VI to VI/VI
  - I/VI: Barely audible; often missed initially
  - II/VI: Audible, but faint
  - III/VI: Clearly audible
  - IV/VI: Loud, with palpable thrill
  - V/VI: Loud with stethoscope barely on the chest, with palpable thrill
  - VI/VI: Heard with stethoscope off the chest, with palpable thrill

- **Frequency** (pitch): high, medium, low (i.e., is it heard with diaphragm, bell, both)
- **Pattern of sound** (see Fig. 5–13)
- **Quality** (blowing, rumbling, musical, etc.)

Table continued on following page

TABLE 5-1 Cardiovascular Assessment Techniques, Tips, Geriatric Considerations *Continued*

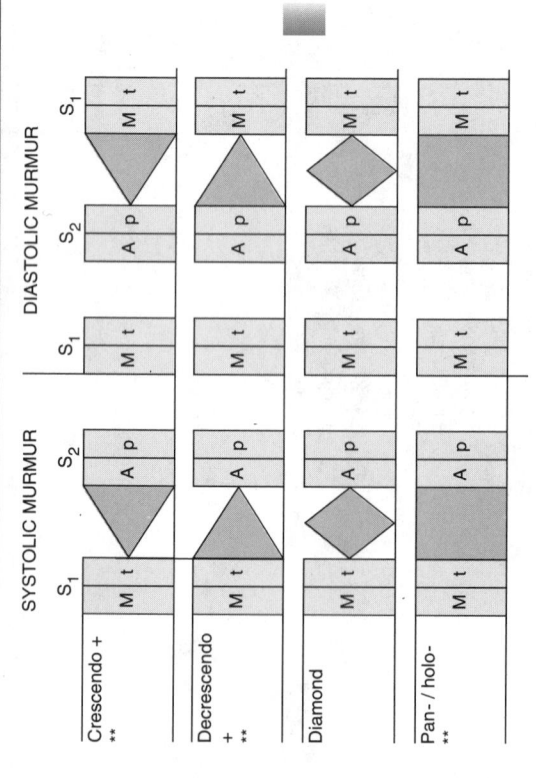

FIGURE 5-13

Patterns of sound produced by cardiac murmurs.

+   The murmur may begin early, middle or late systole or diastole.
** The murmur may obliterate the first (S₁) or second (S₂) heart sound.

6. Sudden development of or change in a murmur indicates a changing cardiac condition and should be aggressively evaluated	Suddenly appearing murmurs may suggest • Altered cardiac output • Right or left heart failure • Cardiac ischemia, infarct • Ruptured interventricular septum • Ruptured papillary muscle	The older person frequently has a brief, soft, early systolic murmur in the aortic area produced by aortic sclerosis; it is frequently accompanied by an S_4 heart sound
7. While some systolic murmurs are nonpathologic, it is best to initially consider all systolic murmurs pathologic	Children and young adults may have an innocent or functional soft systolic murmur in the pulmonic area that comes and goes with position change	Sudden changes in or development of a murmur indicate an acute change in condition
8. Consider all diastolic murmurs to be pathologic	High output states may produce transient murmurs due to turbulent blood flow; these disappear with correction of the underlying problem	

Table continued on following page

211

TABLE 5-1 Cardiovascular Assessment Techniques, Tips, Geriatric Considerations *Continued*

Technique	Performance Tips	Description/Rationale	Geriatric Considerations

Systolic Murmur

Heard between or including S_1 and S_2 during ventricular systole when

The mitral (M_1) and tricuspid (t_1) valves are closed . . .

Condition	Location of Systolic Murmur	Radiation	Shape
Mitral insufficiency	Mitral area (possibly with click)	Left axilla	Pansystolic
Tricuspid insufficiency	Tricuspid area (+ with inspiration) (possibly with click)	—	Pansystolic

. . . and the aortic (A_2) and pulmonic (p_2) valves are open

Condition	Location of Systolic Murmur	Radiation	Shape
*Aortic stenosis**	Aortic area (possibly with click)	Neck, LSB, apex	Diamond, ejection
Pulmonic stenosis	Pulmonic area (possibly with click)	Right neck	Diamond, ejection

*It is common to hear an early systolic murmur in the aortic area in the aging person; this may be associated with aortic sclerosis, a benign condition caused by fibrosis and calcification; sclerosis can lead to a pathologic aortic valve stenosis

Diastolic Murmur

Heard between or including S_2 and the following S_1, during ventricular diastole when
The aortic (A_2) and pulmonic (p_2) valves are closed . . .

Condition	Location of Diastolic Murmur	Radiation	Shape
Aortic insufficiency	Aortic area, Erb's point (sitting forward)	—	Decrescendo
Pulmonic insufficiency	(difficult to assess)	—	Decrescendo

. . . and the mitral (M_1) and tricuspid (t_1) valves are open

Condition	Location of Diastolic Murmur	Radiation	Shape
Mitral stenosis	Mitral area (LLR position)	—	Crescendo
Tricuspid stenosis	Tricuspid area (+ with inspiration)	—	Crescendo

Table continued on following page

TABLE 5-1 Cardiovascular Assessment Techniques, Tips, Geriatric Considerations *Continued*

Technique	Performance Tips	Description/Rationale	Geriatric Considerations
	Continuous Murmur Heard in both systole and diastole	Produced by combination of conditions or septal defect • A mammary soufflé may be heard in the breasts and right and left midsternum in the late stage of pregnancy and during lactation; this may have both systolic and diastolic components or only a systolic component • A machinery or in-out murmur is usually without interruption and associated with a septal defect or rupture	
4. Pericardial Friction Rub	*ASSESSMENT TIPS* 1. Produces a leathery, sandy, or grating sound 2. Has one systolic and two diastolic components:	Produced by inflammation of the pericardial sac with roughening of visceral and parietal surfaces	

- Ventricular systolic sound (heard following the S_1 sound)
- Ventricular diastolic sound (heard following the S_2 sound)
- Atrial systolic sound (heard following the S_2 sound)

3. It may be heard throughout the precordium or may be isolated to the actively moving cardiac apex (mitral area)

4. May be best heard with patient sitting with breath held in exhalation

5. Commonly accompanied by chest pain somewhat relieved by sitting forward

Table continued on following page

TABLE 5–1 Cardiovascular Assessment Techniques, Tips, Geriatric Considerations *Continued*

Technique	Performance Tips	Description/Rationale	Geriatric Considerations

	6. In its subtler form it may be mistaken for a cardiac murmur
	7. It may be differentiated from a pleural friction rub by
	  • Having a cooperative patient hold the breath briefly while you auscultate
	  • Coordinating the sound with the events in the cardiac cycle as displayed before you on the cardiac monitoring equipment or by palpating a carotid pulse or watching respirations		

Evaluation of Large Blood Vessels

1. Inspection and palpation
- Carotid arteries

ASSESSMENT TIPS

1. Palpate each artery in the vertical groove of the neck just medial to the sternomastoid muscle
2. Palpate low in the neck (not near the jaw line) to avoid accidental massage of the carotid sinuses, which can lower blood pressure and heart rate in susceptible individuals
3. Palpate simultaneously with the pads of the second, third, and fourth fingers to maximize poten-

in the uncooperative or comatose patient

The carotid arteries arise from the aortic arch shortly beyond the coronary arteries; they are the vessels of choice for evaluating arterial circulation by palpation

The common carotid arteries are deep in the neck anterior to each sternomastoid muscle; they bifurcate superior and lateral to the thyroid cartilage in the area of the carotid sinuses into the internal and external carotid arteries

Visible pulsations of the carotid artery may occur in hyperdynamic states and with aortic regurgitation

Carotids and other peripheral blood vessels may feel ropelike because of calcification

With aging the carotid arteries may kink, producing a pulsatile mass low in the neck; this is due to lengthening and weakening of the carotid wall

Changes in carotid pulse characteristic of aortic stenosis or insufficiency are common; such changes may be obliterated by generalized stiffness of the carotids with aging

Table continued on following page

TABLE 5–1 Cardiovascular Assessment Techniques, Tips, Geriatric Considerations *Continued*

Technique	Performance Tips	Description/Rationale	Geriatric Considerations
	tial for finding the pulsation		
	4. If the artery is difficult to assess, turn the neck toward the side being palpated; this will relax the sternomastoid muscle		
	5. Palpate each artery separately to avoid diminishing arterial circulation to the brain		
	6. Use carotid pulsation to aid assessment of events in cardiac cycle (see cardiac auscultation)		
	7. The carotid artery is usually the best choice for assessing pulselessness		

	in an unmonitored patient or a patient with an equivocal wave form	
• Jugular veins	Jugular veins reflect right atrial pressure and right ventricular function • External jugular veins are fullest in the supine position, and should be flattened in the normovolemic person in a sitting position	A tortuous aorta can raise the venous pressure in the left jugular vein by inhibiting drainage into the vena cava
	ASSESSMENT TIPS 1. Serves as a nonspecific indicator of volemic changes. Central venous pressure monitoring is more accurate 2. Best assessed in the right neck 3. Use tangential light to highlight venous movement 4. Evaluate the height of movement in the internal jugular vein (this may be difficult to distinguish from a carotid pulsation; see Table 5-3, p. 233)	• Flat veins in the supine person are indicative of hypovolemia or acute vasodilatation • Full veins suggest fluid overload, right ventricular failure, increased

Table continued on following page

TABLE 5-1 Cardiovascular Assessment Techniques, Tips, Geriatric Considerations *Continued*

Technique	Performance Tips	Description/Rationale	Geriatric Considerations
	5. It may be easier to identify the point above which the external jugular vein collapses; this vein overlies the sternomastoid muscle 6. If the external jugular vein is difficult to identify, apply finger pressure across the sternomastoid muscle, which will cause obstruction and vein engorgement 7. During unobstructed flow, measure fullness in the vein, which should	pulmonary vascular resistance, pericardial effusion, or tamponade • Jugular venous distention may be associated with increased right ventricular end-diastolic pressure	

	be less than 3 cm above the sternal angle	Gravity influences emptying of blood from the low-pressure venous system
	8. Look for changes in the jugular vein as the person is moved from supine to semi–Fowler's position	
	9. Look for normal variations in the jugular veins with respirations:	Decreased left ventricular volume with inspiration allows increased return of blood from the periphery to the right heart
	• Deep inspiration lowers the movement	
	• Deep expiration increases the movement	
	10. Look for changes with dysrhythmias	Pulsations diminish with atrial fibrillation and increase with flutter
	ASSESSMENT TIPS	
	1. Patient should be supine, relaxed, and breathing through the mouth	
– Special Test: Hepatojugular reflux		An indication of right ventricular function
		Persons with right ventricular failure have dilated liver sinusoids; pres-

Table continued on following page

TABLE 5-1 Cardiovascular Assessment Techniques, Tips, Geriatric Considerations *Continued*

Technique	Performance Tips	Description/Rationale	Geriatric Considerations
	2. Apply firm, sustained pressure to the liver by pushing in and upward in the right upper abdominal quadrant at the costal margin 3. Sustain pressure for 30 to 60 seconds	sure over the liver pushes blood into the vena cavae and jugular veins Since the Valsalva maneuver increases venous pressure, the patient must be breathing with open mouth and must be warm and relatively pain free Pressure over the abdomen must be sustained for at least 30 seconds because the initial physiologic response to the test is transient jugular distention Results: • Transient jugular vein distention is normal • Jugular venous distention that persists throughout the application of pressure over the liver suggests right ventricular failure	

2. Carotid auscultation

ASSESSMENT TIPS

1. Get into the habit of performing this assessment with cardiac auscultation for efficiency

2. Auscultate with diaphragm and bell listening for a bruit

3. It may be necessary to have the cooperative patient hold the breath since bronchial breath sounds in the neck area can be mistaken for a bruit

4. Remember that bruits auscultated in the neck may be radiations from a cardiac murmur; carotid bruits, on the other hand, do not radiate to the heart

Bruits over a carotid artery suggest narrowing of the artery with atherosclerotic plaque

Elderly persons may have a carotid bruit while maintaining adequate cerebral circulation; the presence of an asymptomatic carotid bruit, however, indicates generalized atherosclerosis

Table continued on following page

223

TABLE 5–1 Cardiovascular Assessment Techniques, Tips, Geriatric Considerations *Continued*

Technique	Performance Tips	Description/Rationale	Geriatric Considerations
Peripheral Vasculature in the Extremities **1. Inspection**	*Look for* • General color • Discolorations	The general condition of peripheral circulation is an indication of systemic circulatory status Local changes may indicate arterial or venous insufficiency or occlusion due to thrombus formation, aneurysm, embolism, coagulopathies, cellulitis, or phlebitis Condition of extremities may also provide clues to preexisting systemic disease (e.g., diabetes) or local disease (e.g., Raynaud's disease) **Redness:** inflammation, superficial thrombophlebitis **Brown coloration at ankle, calf:** deposits of hemosiderin and melanin following destruction of red blood cells with venostasis and capillary rupture	Alert geriatric patients may not experience typical pain or discomfort in lower extremities with pathology because of subtle diminishing of sensations of light touch, temperature, and vibration with aging; this requires the nurse to rely more heavily on physical findings than on patient complaints Superficial veins tend to be visible and tortuous

Pallor: limb pallor in supine position or rubor with dependent positioning suggests arterial occlusion

Rubor: dilation of superficial blood vessels with arterial insufficiency; especially prominent with the extremity in the dependent position

Cyanosis: decreased arterial circulation from occlusive disease or venostasis

Look for
- Hair growth
- Nail condition

Absence of hair growth on toes and lower leg (except at sock line) may indicate chronic arterial insufficiency

Thickened toenails may indicate chronic arterial insufficiency

These signs alone are not diagnostic in the elderly

With advancing age, hair growth diminishes on extremities in the absence of clinical disease

With advancing age toenails thicken and may harbor chronic fungal infection with peeling

Table continued on following page

TABLE 5-1 Cardiovascular Assessment Techniques, Tips, Geriatric Considerations *Continued*

Technique	Performance Tips	Description/Rationale	Geriatric Considerations
2. Palpation • Pulses	*ASSESSMENT TIPS* 1. Palpate contralateral pulses simultaneously to detect differences in contour and amplitude	Occlusion of arterial circulation can cause impairment or loss of an extremity The contour and amplitude of an arterial pulse assessed by palpation or arterial line are indicative of certain cardiac and respiratory abnormalities (see Fig. 5–14) Weak or absent pulse suggests partial or complete occlusion of the vessel, as may occur with thrombus or embolus formation Pulses may be difficult to palpate in the obese person	Pedal pulses may be more difficult to palpate

Type of pulse	Characteristics	Possible causes
Normal	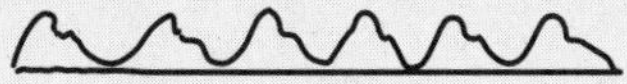	
Weak	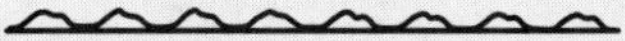	Hypovolemia Diminished cardiac output Aortic stenosis
Full, bounding	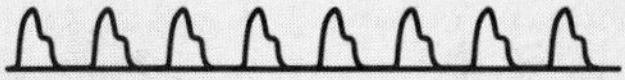	Fever, anxiety, exertion Hyperthyroidism Arteriosclerosis
Anacrotic	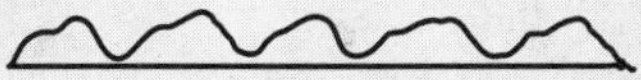	Aortic stenosis
Water-hammer (Corrigan's)	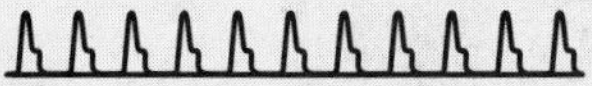	Aortic regurgitation
Bigeminal	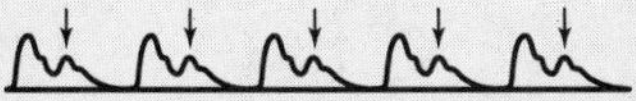	Dysrhythmia: bigeminal, coupled rhythms

Bisferiens		Aortic regurgitation
		  (also with stenosis)
		Idiopathic hypertrophic
		Subaortic stenosis
		  (IHSS)

Alternans	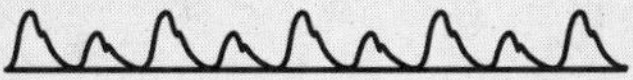	Left ventricular failure
Paradoxical	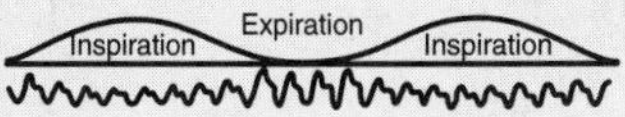	Constrictive pericarditis Cardiac tamponade COPD

FIGURE 5–14

Variations in arterial pulsations and possible causes.

TABLE 5–1 Cardiovascular Assessment Techniques, Tips, Geriatric Considerations *Continued*

Technique	Performance Tips	Description/Rationale	Geriatric Considerations
	2. Evaluate for a pulse deficit: simultaneously auscultate the heart and palpate a peripheral pulse 3. Several descriptive scales exist to describe the strength of a peripheral pulse; they should be used with caution and only if all staff clearly understand the scale values in use: it is often better to report pulse strength descriptively (e.g., bounding, full, strong, weak, diminished, absent)	With cardiac dysrhythmia, changes in diastolic filling time may diminish cardiac output enough to weaken the pulsation transmitted to the periphery; in this instance heart rate must be assessed apically; simultaneous cardiac auscultation and palpation of a peripheral pulse provides data on perfusion in the absence of invasive monitoring equipment	

4. Check collateral arterial pulses in any extremity prior to and during use of any peripheral arterial line to assure limb oxygenation	*Allen's Test* • Have patient clench fist tightly for several seconds to blanch skin of palms (nurse should do this for unresponsive or uncooperative patient) • Compress radial (or ulnar) artery • With artery still compressed, open palm to a relaxed position • Palm will regain color quickly if the noncompressed ulnar or radial artery is patent	
• Temperature	Localized warmth suggests inflammation Localized coolness suggests partial or complete arterial occlusion	It is not uncommon for a patient to have cool extremities bilaterally
• Edema	*ASSESSMENT TIPS* 1. Assess for edema in extremities, sacrum, scrotum, and other dependent areas, and in the periorbital area	Increased venous pressure (systemic or local) causes transudation of fluid to dependent areas and to areas where skin is thin with minimal muscular and connective tissue support (e.g., periorbital, scrotal)	Pedal edema should be interpreted cautiously as a sign of right heart failure in the elderly Pedal edema may be due to chronic venous insufficiency with venous tortuosity and valve collapse; this

Table continued on following page

229

TABLE 5-1 Cardiovascular Assessment Techniques, Tips, Geriatric Considerations *Continued*

Technique	Performance Tips	Description/Rationale	Geriatric Considerations
	2. Assess for edema by compressing skin against underlying bone for 5 seconds; observe for pitting on release 3. Describe edema clearly in terms of extent, type (pitting, nonpitting), depth or duration of any pitting 4. Descriptive scales should be used with caution and only if all staff clearly understand scale values in use: it is better to report characteristics of pitting edema descriptively in terms of location, depth, and duration of pitting	Improvement or extension of edematous areas mark the outcome of treatment Assessments for change are often not performed by the same nurse; this requires that descriptors be clear to all	is often accompanied by stasis pigmentation (mottled brown) Pedal edema may also be secondary to lymphatic obstruction or hypoalbuminemia

• Calf tenderness

5. Assess for ascites secondary to right ventricular failure (see Chapter 7)

ASSESSMENT TIP
Perform either of the two maneuvers below, *making sure that the foot is flexed 90 degrees at the knee* before starting:
- Gently compress the calf against the bone, palpating for an area of firmness or tenderness
- Briskly dorsiflex the ankle by pushing up against the sole of the foot; this maneuver should not normally produce calf pain (Homan's sign).

Performing an assessment for calf tenderness with the knee in extension may produce a false positive result in the alert and cooperative patient because of stretching of the Achilles tendon with dorsiflexion of the foot

Calf pain or pain behind the knee produced by either of these maneuvers may be an indication of thrombosis in the extremity

In the uncooperative patient, arterial occlusion must be evaluated by other signs discussed above

The nurse should regularly assess for thrombosis in the critical care patient who is at high risk due to immobility

The elderly are at high risk for development of thrombi and emboli related to immobility

TABLE 5–2 Differential Diagnosis of Chest Pain in the Acutely Ill Patient

Central or Bilateral Chest Pain	Right or Left Chest Pain
Cardiovascular	**Cardiovascular**
Anginas	Anginas
Myocardial infarction	Myocardial infarction
Acute pericarditis	Acute or chronic pericarditis
Valvular disease	After myocardial infarction
Acute dissecting aneurysm	Cardiotomy
After cardiac resuscitation	After cardiac trauma
Sickle cell crisis	After cardiac resuscitation
Vascular, cardiac access devices	Vascular, cardiac access devices
Respiratory	**Respiratory**
Hyperventilation	Pneumonias
Pulmonary edema	Pneumothorax
Pneumothorax	Pulmonary embolism or infarction
Tracheobronchitis	Pleurisy
Pulmonary embolism	Empyema
Gastrointestinal	Lung or pleural tumor
Esophageal disorders	Tuberculosis
Swallowing disorders	**Gastrointestinal**
Gastroesophageal reflux	Pancreatitis
Esophagitis	Cholecystitis
Esophageal rupture	**Musculoskeletal**
Gastric distension	Chest muscle pain, inflammation
Peptic ulceration	Costochondritis
Pancreatitis	Intercostal neuritis
Cholecystitis	Rib fracture
Musculoskeletal	Rheumatoid arthritis
Chest muscle pain, inflammation	Cervical, thoracic disc disease
Costochondritis	Degenerative, inflammatory disease of shoulder
Cervical, thoracic disc disease	
Miscellaneous	**Miscellaneous**
Mediastinitis	Herpes zoster
Mediastinal tumor	Subdiaphragmatic abscess
Chest surgery, procedures	Chest surgery, procedures
Anxiety	Breast pain

Data from Wiener, S. L. (1993). *Differential diagnosis of acute pain by body region.* New York: McGraw-Hill.

TABLE 5–3 Differentiating the Normal Characteristics of Carotid and Internal Jugular Pulsations

Characteristic	Carotid	Internal Jugular
Location	High in the neck	Low in the neck
	Medial to the sternomas-toid muscle	Lateral or beneath the sternomastoid muscle
Palpability	Palpable as a single, strong pulsation slightly later than ventricular systole	Not palpable
		Visible as a 2–3 component, diffuse, undulating waveform with each cardiac cycle
	Pulsation remains palpable with moderate pressure	Visible components are easily obliterated with light pressure
Effect of respiration	None	Waveform is diminished in height and volume with inspiration due to decreased intrathoracic pressure
Effect of positioning	None	Waveform is diminished in height and volume as the patient assumes a sitting position*

*External jugular veins that overlay the sternomastoid muscle may normally appear full in supine and semi–Fowler's positions. If they are fully distended above a sitting position of 45 degrees, this is strongly suggestive of increased central venous pressure (CVP). True distention, however, must be differentiated by evaluation of the waveform. Some thin individuals and those with well-developed sternomastoid muscles may simply have prominent external jugular veins without true distention.

CARDIOVASCULAR DISORDERS
Heart Failure

Heart failure is defined as insufficient cardiac output to meet the metabolic needs of the tissues and organs of the body. Causes of heart failure include any clinical condition that impairs the ability of the myocardial fibers to contract and relax, or any clinical condition that leads to excessive myocardial workload (increased volume, or preload, or increased pressure, or afterload). Classifications of heart failure include left ventricular failure, right ventricular failure, high output failure, low output failure, systolic failure, and diastolic failure.

Left and Right Ventricular Failure

Types of disorders that may culminate in left ventricular failure include myocardial infarction (coronary artery disease), valvular disease, and systemic hypertension. Right ventricular failure is usually the result of left ventricular failure (biventricular failure), but other causes include right ventricular myocardial infarction and pulmonary hypertension.

High-Output Failure

High-output failure is associated with hyperdynamic states such as anemia, hyperthyroidism, and septicemia. In anemia and hyperthyroidism, the cardiac output rises to meet accelerated metabolic demands and prevent metabolic acidosis. In septicemia, vasodilation lowers the systemic vascular resistance, and fever increases the metabolic rate. Cardiac output increases to maintain blood pressure and prevent metabolic acidosis.

Low-Output Failure

Low-output failure is usually associated with myocardial disease such as cardiomyopathy or constrictive pericarditis. The myocardium may be unable to increase contractility (systolic dysfunction), or diastolic filling may be impaired (diastolic dysfunction). Decreased contractility may lead to biventricular failure and a decline in cardiac output, or impaired diastolic filling may increase the left ventricular end-diastolic pressure and result in pulmonary and venous congestion as well as a decline in cardiac output.

Systolic Failure and Diastolic Failure

Heart failure may occur during systole or diastole, or reflect both systolic and diastolic dysfunction (see low-output failure). In systolic failure, a decrease in contractility reduces the stroke volume and increases the end-diastolic volume. In diastolic failure, a decrease in compliance restricts ventricular filling, which decreases the end-diastolic volume and reduces the stroke volume. Decreased compliance may be secondary to conditions such as ventricular hypertrophy, myocardial ischemia, pericardial effusion, pericardial tamponade, and positive pressure ventilation.

Acute and Chronic Heart Failure

Heart failure may be acute or chronic. Chronic heart failure may become acute at any time. The most serious complication of heart failure is cardiogenic shock (see Chapter 12 and Clinical Findings 12–3).

POINTS TO REMEMBER

▶ Previously diagnosed thyroid conditions (usually controlled with thyroid medication) may be missed in the critically ill adult unless past medical and medication history is carefully reviewed.

▶ Hypothyroidism is common in the elderly population. Previously undiagnosed and untreated thyroid disease may become apparent with decompensation and the stress of illness. At this time, thyroid disease may manifest itself as a cardiac dysrhythmia or as an alteration in cardiac output.

▶ Heart failure in the elderly is usually a combination of right and left ventricular failure (biventricular failure).

Left Ventricular Failure

Pathophysiology

In left ventricular failure, decreased contractility or excessive myocardial workload (increased preload or afterload or both) reduces the left ventricular ejection fraction, causing the stroke volume to decrease. The decline in stroke volume has both backward and forward effects (see Fig. 5–15).

Backward Effects of Left Ventricular Failure

As less blood is ejected into the systemic circulation, the ejection fraction decreases, and the left ventricular filling pressure or left ventricular end-diastolic pressure (LVEDP) rises. The increased LVEDP is transmitted backward to the left atrium, pulmonary veins, and pulmonary capillaries.

Increased capillary hydrostatic pressure forces fluid into the lung tissue and alveoli, resulting in pulmonary edema (see Clinical Findings 4–2). If the pulmonary edema and left heart failure are not controlled, pulmonary vascular resistance (PVR) will increase, resulting in right ventricular failure (see Clinical Findings 5–2).

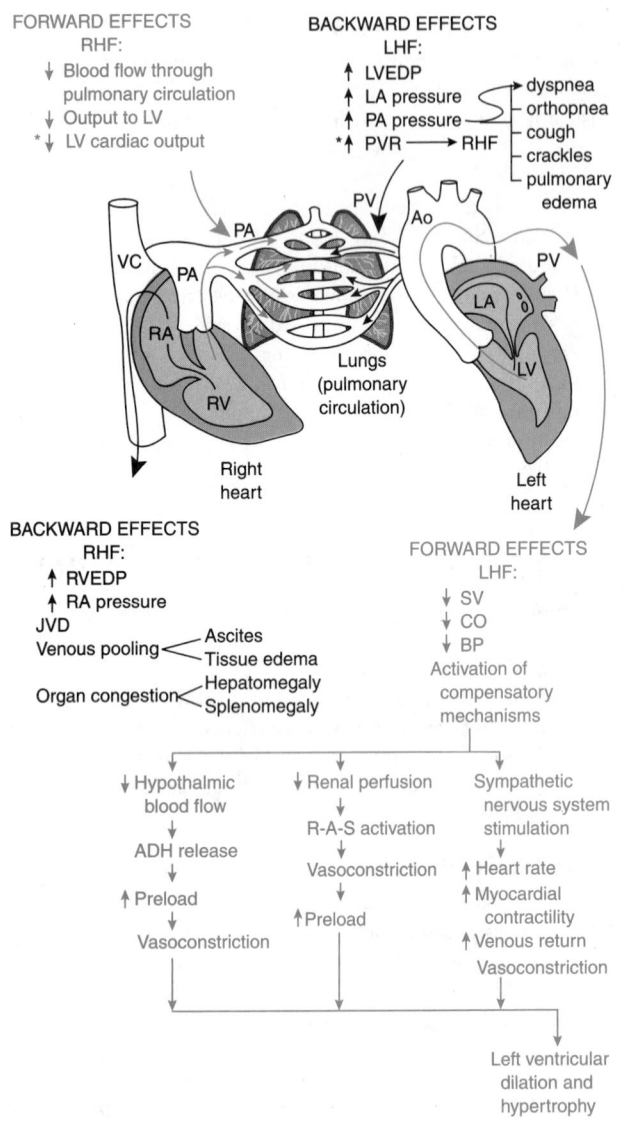

FORWARD EFFECTS
RHF:
↓ Blood flow through pulmonary circulation
↓ Output to LV
*↓ LV cardiac output

BACKWARD EFFECTS
LHF:
↑ LVEDP
↑ LA pressure
↑ PA pressure ⎬→ dyspnea
*↑ PVR ——→ RHF — orthopnea
— cough
— crackles
— pulmonary edema

VC
PA
RA
RV
PA
Lungs (pulmonary circulation)
PV
Ao
PV
LA
LV

Right heart

Left heart

BACKWARD EFFECTS
RHF:
↑ RVEDP
↑ RA pressure
JVD
Venous pooling ⎬— Ascites
— Tissue edema
Organ congestion ⎬— Hepatomegaly
— Splenomegaly

FORWARD EFFECTS
LHF:
↓ SV
↓ CO
↓ BP
Activation of compensatory mechanisms

↓ Hypothalamic blood flow
↓
ADH release
↓
↑ Preload
↓
Vasoconstriction

↓ Renal perfusion
↓
R-A-S activation
↓
Vasoconstriction
↓
↑ Preload

Sympathetic nervous system stimulation
↑ Heart rate
↑ Myocardial contractility
↑ Venous return
Vasoconstriction

Left ventricular dilation and hypertrophy

FIGURE 5–15
Backward and forward effects of heart failure.

Forward Effects of Left Ventricular Failure

As less blood is ejected into the systemic circulation, the stroke volume decreases, and the cardiac output falls. The drop in cardiac output triggers a number of compensatory mechanisms. These compensatory mechanisms initially increase cardiac output, but eventually they lead to cardiac decompensation.

Compensatory Mechanisms

See Figure 5–15.

Sympathoadrenergic Activation

Baroreceptors in the aortic arch and carotid arteries detect a fall in systemic blood pressure. The sympathetic nervous system (SNS) is stimulated and responds by releasing epinephrine and norepinephrine:

- Activation of β_1 receptors produces an increase in heart rate and myocardial contractility in an effort to improve stroke volume and cardiac output.
- Activation of α_1 receptors promotes arterial vasoconstriction in an effort to maintain blood pressure.
- Venoconstriction redistributes blood flow and enhances venous return in an effort to increase preload and cardiac output.

Renin-Angiotensin-Aldosterone Activation

Decreased blood flow to the kidneys activates the renin-angiotensin-aldosterone cascade:

- Angiotensin II intensifies arterial vasoconstriction.
- Aldosterone promotes the renal tubular reabsorption of sodium and water in an effort to expand plasma volume and increase preload.

Arginine Vasopressin

The hypothalamus responds to the decrease in blood flow by stimulating the posterior pituitary to release antidiuretic hormone (ADH):

- ADH (vasopressin) further increases water reabsorption and increases plasma volume.
- In addition, ADH contributes to vasoconstriction.

Atrial Natriuretic Factor (ANF)

ANF is a vasodilating hormone with natural diuretic properties that is released from the atria in response to atrial stretch: As heart failure worsens, ANF levels rise in an effort to counteract the damaging effects of increased preload and vasoconstriction.

Ventricular Dilation and Hypertrophy (Ventricular Remodeling)

- Ventricular dilation occurs in response to the increase in preload: The increased end-diastolic volume causes the myocardial fibers to stretch during diastole, enhancing the force of contraction during systole (Frank-Starling law of the heart).
- Ventricular hypertrophy occurs over time as a result of increased diastolic stress (increased preload), or increased systolic stress (increased afterload): The increase in wall thickness provides more muscle mass and results in an increase in the force of contraction.

Decompensation
Sympathoadrenergic Activity

As heart failure progresses, inhibitory signals from the baroreceptors (parasympathetic stimulation) are depressed. SNS activity continues in the presence of vasoconstriction and increased volume. The high circulating levels of catecholamines reduce or desensitize β_1 receptors (β-receptor down-regulation), and the myocardium becomes less responsive to sympathetic stimulation:

- Tachycardia impairs ventricular filling and relaxation and contributes to increased preload, myocardial wall tension, myocardial workload, ventricular hypertrophy, and oxygen consumption.
- Decreased diastolic filling times may lead to decreased perfusion of the coronary arteries and contribute to an ischemic-induced decrease in contractility.
- Impaired ability of the myocardium to respond to inotropic stimulation contributes to decreased contractility, and increased myocardial workload and oxygen consumption.
- Persistent arterial vasoconstriction contributes to increased afterload, myocardial wall tension, myocardial workload, ventricular hypertrophy, and oxygen consumption. (Endothelin, a potent vasoconstrictive substance produced by the vascular epithelium, is thought to contribute to the profound vasoconstriction.)

Atrial Natriuretic Factor

The beneficial effects of ANF are exceeded by the antagonistic effects of the sympathetic nervous system and the renin-angiotensin-aldosterone cascade:

- If present, right ventricular failure may be exacerbated by increased preload.
- If right ventricular function is intact, a greater volume of blood will be ejected into the lungs, contributing to pulmonary edema and increasing the PVR.
- As well, a greater volume of blood will reach the left side of the heart, increasing left ventricular filling pressures and contributing to increased myocardial workload and ventricular hypertrophy.
- Intense vasoconstriction leads to a massive increase in systemic vascular resistance (SVR), increased myocardial workload, ventricular hypertrophy, and oxygen consumption.

Ventricular Remodeling

Ventricular hypertrophy becomes maladaptive. The myocardial structure is altered to the point that pumping efficiency is impaired and contractility decreases:

- β-receptor down-regulation and increased circulating catecholamines contribute to intracellular calcium overload of the mitochondria, causing a reduction in mitochondrial function and decreased adenosine triphosphate (ATP) production.
- The myocardium becomes stiff (noncompliant) and unable to generate enough energy to perfuse itself or other tissues and body organs.

Assessment

The clinical presentation of left ventricular failure varies with the degree of left ventricular failure and the underlying disorder (see Clinical Findings 5–1). Physical findings may be absent in the presence of severe disease, or the critically ill adult may present with physical findings indicative of moderate or extreme ventricular dysfunction.

POINTS TO REMEMBER

▶ Because left ventricular failure is a manifestation of underlying disease, a thorough nursing history (see Tables 1–1 and 5–1 and Clinical Findings 5–1) is crucial to identify patients at risk.

▶ Because decreased cardiac output reduces the delivery of oxygen and nutrients to peripheral body tissues and organs and increased LVEDP causes pulmonary congestion, in addition to the initial and baseline assessments (see Table 2–1), focused respiratory and cardiovascular assessments (see Tables 2–1, 4–1, and 5–1), as well as focused assessments of the underlying pathology, should be completed as often as the patient's condition dictates to detect or anticipate and prevent complications such as pulmonary edema (see Clinical Findings 4–2), right heart failure (see Clinical Findings 5–2), renal failure (see Clinical Findings 8–1), and cardiogenic shock (see Clinical Findings 12–3).

▶ Ongoing assessment incorporates the evaluation of responses to diagnostic procedures and therapeutic interventions aimed at improving cardiac output and oxygen supply to tissues and organs; it includes collaboration with other members of the health team to reduce myocardial oxygen consumption and prevent further deterioration.

Clinical Findings 5–1 *Left Ventricular Failure*

I. HISTORY

A. Predisposing factors

1. Myocardial infarction (anterior in particular because of potential for more extensive damage to the left ventricle)
2. Valvular disorders
3. Ventricular septal defect
4. Cardiomyopathy
5. Cardiac tamponade
6. Constrictive pericarditis
7. Systemic hypertension
8. Tachydysrhythmias
9. Hyperdynamic states (e.g., anemia, thyrotoxicosis, sepsis)

B. Subjective findings

1. Dyspnea exacerbated by exertion related to pulmonary congestion
2. Orthopnea or paroxysmal nocturnal dyspnea related to increased intrathoracic blood volume in the supine position
3. Fatigue related to the increased work of breathing
4. Fatigue or weakness related to decreased blood flow to skeletal muscles

5. Chest pain related to myocardial ischemia, inflammation, or pressure from surrounding structures
6. Palpitations related to dysrhythmias
7. Dizziness, syncope related to decreased cerebral blood flow
8. Anxiety related to fear of the unknown or death

II. LABORATORY AND BEDSIDE MONITORING FINDINGS

A. **Chest x-ray**

1. Left ventricular or left atrial enlargement may be present, depending on the degree of left ventricular failure (right ventricular or right atrial enlargement may be present, depending on the nature of the underlying disorder; a widened mediastinum may be indicative of cardiac tamponade)
2. Pulmonary congestion may be present, depending on the degree of left ventricular failure

B. **Arterial blood gases** (see Chapter 13 for related information on acid-base disorders, the efficiency of gas exchange, and serum lactate levels, and see Chapter 14 and Table 14–1 for related information on oxygen delivery and consumption parameters)

1. PaO_2 may be <60 to 70 mm Hg related to intrapulmonary shunting secondary to pulmonary edema (see Clinical Findings 4–2)
2. $PaCO_2$ may be <35 mm Hg related to tachypnea
3. pH may be >7.45 reflective of tachypnea and respiratory alkalosis
4. pH may be <7.35 reflective of decreased peripheral blood flow and reduced oxygen delivery to the tissues (metabolic acidosis)
5. HCO_3 may be <22 mEq/L reflective of metabolic acidosis
6. Base deficit may be <−2 mEq/L reflective of metabolic acidosis
7. Serum lactate levels may be >2 mEq/L reflective of tissue oxygen deficits

C. **Other laboratory studies**

1. Blood urea nitrogen (BUN) may be >20 mg/dl, and creatinine may be >1.2 mg/dl related to decreased blood flow to the kidneys (see Table 13–6 for related information on BUN and creatinine)
2. Electrolyte imbalances may include (see Table 13–5 for related information on electrolyte imbalances)
   - Dilutional hyponatremia (Na <135 mEq/L) related to increased aldosterone production and vasopressin release
   - Hypokalemia (K <3.5 mEq/L) related to increased aldosterone production or the use of diuretics
   - Hyperkalemia (K >5 mEq/L) related to decreased renal perfusion

3. Liver function studies may show elevated results related to decreased blood flow to the liver or liver congestion secondary to right ventricular failure (see Clinical Findings 5–2 for related information on right ventricular failure and Table 13–4 for related information on liver function studies)
4. Hemoglobin may be <12 g/dl, reflective of anemia related to the underlying disorder
5. Hematocrit may be <36%, reflective of anemia related to the underlying disorder, or dilutional related to an increased volume (see Table 13–8 for related information on hemoglobin and hematocrit)

D. ECG (abnormalities often reflective of underlying disorder or predisposing factor)

1. Left atrial hypertrophy (broad and bipeaked P waves) or left ventricular hypertrophy (increased amplitude of the QRS complex)
2. Conduction defects (a prolonged QT interval may be associated with cardiomyopathies, which may predispose the patient to polymorphic ventricular tachycardias such as torsades de pointes)
3. Bundle branch blocks
4. Myocardial ischemia, injury, or infarction (see Table 5–4 for related information on ECG changes during myocardial infarction)
5. Dysrhythmias such as sinus tachycardia, atrial fibrillation, and premature ventricular contractions may be related to increased levels of circulating catecholamines (sympathetic stimulation), myocardial ischemia, acid-base and electrolyte imbalances, and increased pressure in atria or ventricle (see Table 14–3 for related information on dysrhythmias)

E. Hemodynamic parameters (see Chapter 14, Table 14–2, and Fig. 14–2 for related information on hemodynamics, including formulas for calculation of parameters such as systemic vascular resistance and left ventricular stroke work index)

1. Blood pressure may be low related to decreased cardiac output (CO), or it may be normal or increased related to compensatory mechanisms and vasoconstriction (compensation may be less pronounced in the elderly)
2. Widened pulse pressure may be present, associated with aortic regurgitation
3. Narrow pulse pressure may be present, associated with cardiomyopathy, constrictive pericarditis, or pericardial tamponade
4. Pulmonary capillary wedge pressure (PCWP) may be >15 to 18 mm Hg, and left atrial pressure (LAP) may be >10 mm Hg, related to an increased LVEDP (giant V waves may be present, related to increased left atrial volume and pressure associated with mitral regurgitation)

TABLE 5-4 Correlation of Site of Infarction with Coronary Artery Affected

Coronary Artery Affected	Area or Structure Supplied	Type of Infarction and ECG Indicators
Right coronary artery	Right atrium SA node (55% of population) AV node (90% of population) Bundle of His Inferior or posterior left ventricular wall (in most of the population the right coronary artery creates the posterior descending artery and supplies posterior third of septum and a portion of posterior left ventricle; otherwise these areas are supplied by left circumflex artery) Right ventricle	Inferior infarction: • Indicative changes in leads II, III, and aVF • Reciprocal changes in leads I, aVL, and V_{1-4} Right ventricular infarction: ST segment elevation in leads V_1 and right precordial leads V_3R-V_6R
Left anterior descending coronary artery	Anterior and apical portions of left ventricle Anterior two thirds of septum Bundle of His Right bundle branch Anterior and posterior branches of left bundle	Anterior infarction: • Indicative changes in leads V_{3-4} • Reciprocal changes in leads II, III, and aVF Anteroseptal infarction: • Indicative changes in leads V_{1-4} • Reciprocal changes in leads I and aVL Anterolateral infarction: • Indicative changes in leads I, aVL, and V_{3-6} • Reciprocal changes in leads II, III, and aVF

Table continued on following page

TABLE 5–4 Correlation of Site of Infarction with Coronary Artery Affected *Continued*

Coronary Artery Affected	Area or Structure Supplied	Type of Infarction and ECG Indicators
Left circumflex coronary artery	Left atrium Lateral wall of left ventricle SA node (45% of population) AV node (10% of population) Posterior portion of left ventricle	Extensive anterior: • Indicative changes in leads I, aVL, and V_{1-6} • Reciprocal changes in leads II, III, and aVF Lateral wall infarction: • Indicative changes in leads I, aVL, and V_{5-6} • Reciprocal changes in leads II, III, aVF True posterior infarction: Tall R wave in leads V_{1-2}

- **Changes indicative of infarction** include T wave inversion, ST segment elevation, and Q waves in the ECG leads over the involved area
- **Reciprocal changes** include ST segment depression, tall R waves, and tall T waves in the leads opposite the involved area
- **Non-Q-wave changes** of infarction include ST segment depression and inverted T waves in the leads facing the epicardial surface over the area of infarction

5. SVR may be >1200–1500 dyne/s/cm^{-5} related to increased afterload (vasoconstriction)
6. CO may be <4 L/min/m^2 and cardiac index (CI) may be <2.5 L/min/m^2 related to decreased stroke volume (pulmonary artery pressure [PAP], RVEDP, right atrial pressure [RAP], and central venous pressure [CVP] may be elevated, depending on the nature of the underlying disorder and associated right ventricular failure)

III. PHYSICAL ASSESSMENT FINDINGS

A. General observations (inspection)

1. *Mental status:* Restlessness and confusion may be present, related to decreased cerebral blood flow

2. *Head and neck*
   - Nodding of head (de Musset's sign) may occur with aortic regurgitation
   - Visible pulsation of carotid artery may occur with aortic regurgitation
3. *Speech:* Hoarseness or dysphagia related to compression of the pharyngeal nerve by an enlarged left atrium or dilated pulmonary artery may occur with mitral stenosis
4. *Respiratory pattern:* Tachypnea may be present, related to pulmonary congestion and impaired gas exchange
5. *Cough:* Cough productive of blood-tinged or pink, frothy sputum may be present related to increased fluid in the lungs (see Clinical Findings 4–2 for physical findings associated with pulmonary edema)
6. *Skin and mucous membranes:* Cyanosis may be present related to decreased blood flow or peripheral vasoconstriction
7. *Nails*
   - Capillary refill may be >2 seconds, related to decreased peripheral blood flow
   - Positive Quinke's sign (visible capillary pulsation of nailbed when pressure is exerted on fingertip) may occur with aortic regurgitation
8. *Urine*
   - Urine output may be decreased and concentrated with a high specific gravity, related to decreased renal perfusion and activation of compensatory mechanisms
   - Nocturia may be present, related to redistribution of blood flow and increased renal perfusion in the supine position

B. Palpation

1. *Skin:* Cool and moist extremities may be present, related to decreased blood flow to the tissues or compensatory sympathetic nervous system response (diaphoresis and peripheral vasoconstriction)
2. *Peripheral pulse* (see Table 5–1 and Fig. 5–14 for related information on arterial pulses)
   - Peripheral pulses may be weak, related to decreased cardiac output, or irregular, related to dysrhythmias
   - Pulsus alternans (alternating left ventricular stroke volumes related to changes in compliance and contractility) may be present with severe left ventricular failure
   - Water-hammer pulse (greater volume than normal with sharp decline) may occur with aortic regurgitation
   - Pulsus paradoxus (>10 mm Hg) may be present with pericardial tamponade

3. *Precordium*
   - Lift or heave at apex or lateral to midclavicular line may be present, related to left ventricular hypertrophy
   - Laterally displaced apical impulse may be present, related to left ventricular hypertrophy (see Fig. 5–2)
   - Forceful diffuse apical impulse may occur with aortic regurgitation
   - Forceful sustained apical impulse may occur with aortic stenosis
   - Systolic or diastolic thrill may be associated with a loud murmur

C. Auscultation (see Table 5–1 and Figs. 5–6 to 5–13 for related information on heart sounds and murmurs)

   1. *Heart sounds*
      - Tachycardia may be present, related to increased sympathetic stimulation
      - Muffled heart sounds may indicate pericardial tamponade
      - Soft first sound associated with premature closure of the mitral valve may occur with increased left ventricular pressure
      - Split-second sound associated with shortened ventricular ejection may occur with mitral regurgitation
      - S_3 on expiration may be present, related to increased filling pressure in the left ventricle
      - S_4 on expiration may be present, related to decreased left ventricular compliance
      - Summation gallop rhythm may be present, related to severe left ventricular failure

   2. *Murmurs*
      - Pansystolic murmur may be present with mitral regurgitation, related to turbulent blood flow in a reverse direction (left ventricular dilation may cause or accentuate)
      - Diastolic murmur may be present with aortic regurgitation, related to turbulent blood flow in a reverse direction (back flow from aorta to left ventricle)
      - Opening snap and diastolic murmur may be present with mitral stenosis, related to turbulent blood flow through a narrowed opening
      - Systolic murmur and ejection click may be present with aortic stenosis, related to turbulent blood flow through a narrowed opening

   3. *Breath sounds:* Crackles (basilar not clearing with cough) may be present, related to pulmonary congestion

Right Ventricular Failure

Pathophysiology

Usually right ventricular failure is a consequence of left ventricular failure (increased pressure progresses backward from the left heart and lungs, resulting in biventricular failure). However, pure right ventricular failure can result from right ventricular infarction or a respiratory disorder.

Right ventricular infarction causes damage to the right ventricle and decreases contractility. Pulmonary disease increases the pulmonary vascular resistance, and the right heart has to work harder to eject blood into the pulmonary vascular circuit.

Regardless, in right ventricular failure decreased contractility or excessive myocardial workload (increased preload or afterload or both) reduces the right ventricular ejection fraction, causing the stroke volume to decrease. The decline in stroke volume has both backward and forward effects (see Fig. 5–15).

Backward Effects of Right Ventricular Failure

As less blood is ejected from the right ventricle into the pulmonary circulation, the right ventricular ejection fraction decreases, and the right ventricular pressure, or preload (RVEDP) rises. The increased RVEDP is transmitted backward through the right atrium, vena cava, and systemic venous system, causing venous pooling and organ congestion.

Excess fluid volume and venous pooling increase the capillary hydrostatic pressure, causing fluid to shift from the vascular system to the tissues and resulting in peripheral edema. Edema is usually apparent in the dependent areas (lower extremities when standing or sitting, sacrum or scrotal edema with bedrest).

Liver congestion (hepatomegaly) may increase hydrostatic pressure in the portal circulation and cause fluid to shift from the portal system to the peritoneal cavity, resulting in ascites. The increased pressure in the portal system may be reflected back to the spleen, causing congestion (splenomegaly), and to the gastrointestinal tract.

Renal congestion may decrease the glomerular filtration rate and lead to fluid retention. Impaired venous drainage from the head and neck may impair mental functioning.

Forward Effects of Right Ventricular Failure

As the right ventricular stroke volume decreases, less blood flows through the pulmonary circuit to the left heart. The left ventricular filling pressure decreases, and the cardiac output drops. The decline in cardiac output triggers a number of compensatory mechanisms and a clinical presentation related to the forward effects of left ventricular failure (see Clinical Findings 5–1).

Assessment

The clinical presentation of right ventricular failure varies with the degree of right ventricular failure (see Clinical Findings 5–2), associated left ventricular failure (see Clinical Findings 5–1), the underlying disorder, and the presence of underlying respiratory disease. Because right ventricular failure often follows left ventricular failure, the predisposing factors for right ventricular failure should include all the predisposing factors for left ventricular failure (see Clinical Findings 5–1).

POINTS TO REMEMBER

▶ Right ventricular failure decreases blood flow through the pulmonary circuit. Pulmonary congestion is the result of left ventricular failure, or an underlying respiratory disorder.

▶ Because right ventricular failure is commonly associated with left ventricular failure, and left ventricular failure is a manifestation of a number of underlying disorders, a thorough nursing history (see Tables 1–1 and 5–1 and Clinical Findings 5–1 and 5–2) is crucial to identifying patients at risk.

▶ Because systemic venous congestion may impair function of the liver, portal system, spleen, gastrointestinal tract, kidneys, brain, and subcutaneous tissue, in addition to the initial and baseline assessments (see Table 2–1), focused respiratory and cardiovascular assessments (see Tables 2–1, 4–1 and 5–1), as well as focused assessments of the underlying pathology should be completed as often as the patient's condition dictates to detect or anticipate and prevent complications such as renal failure (see Clinical Findings 8–1) and liver failure (see Clinical Findings 7–2).

▶ Ongoing assessment incorporates the evaluation of responses to diagnostic procedures and therapeutic interventions aimed at the reduction of venous congestion and myocardial oxygen consumption; it includes collaboration with other members of the health team to improve right ventricular stroke volume and cardiac output.

Clinical Findings 5–2   *Right Ventricular Failure*

I. HISTORY

A. Predisposing factors
1. Left ventricular failure (see Clinical Findings 5–1)
2. Right ventricular myocardial infarction
3. Valvular disorders
4. Atrial or ventricular septal defect
5. Pulmonary hypertension (chronic obstructive pulmonary disease [COPD], pulmonary embolism, adult respiratory distress syndrome [ARDS])

B. Subjective findings
1. Dyspnea related to increased abdominal girth (ascites), or pulmonary congestion associated with left ventricular failure or an underlying respiratory disorder
2. Anorexia or abdominal pain related to gastrointestinal and abdominal congestion
3. Weakness or fatigue related to malnutrition or decreased muscle perfusion
4. Weight gain related to fluid retention
5. Oliguria related to renal congestion and decreased glomerular filtration rate or decreased renal perfusion

II. LABORATORY AND BEDSIDE MONITORING FINDINGS

A. Chest x-ray
1. Right atrial enlargement or right ventricular enlargement (left atrial or left ventricular enlargement may be present, depending on the degree of right ventricular failure, associated left ventricular failure, and underlying disorder)
2. Pulmonary congestion may be present, related to associated left ventricular failure or an underlying respiratory disorder

B. Arterial blood gases (see Chapter 13 for related information on acid-base disorders and serum lactate levels, and Chapter 14 and Table 14–1 for related information on oxygen delivery and consumption parameters)
1. Respiratory alkalosis ($PaCO_2$ <35 mm Hg, pH >7.45) may be present related to tachypnea

2. Metabolic acidosis (HCO_3^- <22 mEq/L, pH <7.35) may be present related to decreased blood flow and oxygen delivery to the tissues or to a decreased ability of congested tissues to utilize oxygen
3. Serum lactate may be >2 mEq/L related to tissue oxygen deficits

C. Other laboratory studies

1. Serum albumin may be <3.5 g/dl, related to malnutrition (decreased protein intake)
2. Liver function studies (see Table 13–4) may be elevated, related to hepatic congestion or decreased arterial blood flow to the liver
3. Electrolyte imbalances (see Table 13–5) and an elevated BUN and creatinine (see Table 13–6) may be present, related to renal congestion or decreased arterial blood flow to the kidney (activation of compensatory mechanisms)

D. ECG

1. Right atrial hypertrophy (tall peaked P wave, "P pulmonale") or right ventricular hypertrophy (increased amplitude of QRS complex)
2. Dysrhythmias (see Clinical Findings 5–1 for related information)

E. Hemodynamic parameters (see Chapter 14, Table 14–2, and Fig. 14–2 for related information on hemodynamics, including formulas for calculation of parameters such as pulmonary vascular resistance and right ventricular stroke work index)

1. Blood pressure may be variable (see Clinical Findings 5–1 for related information)
2. RAP may be >6 mm Hg (CVP >12 cm H_2O), related to increased right ventricular end-diastolic pressure.
3. PAP may be >25/15 mm Hg, related to increased pulmonary congestion resulting from left ventricular failure or an underlying respiratory disorder
4. PVR may be >250 dyne/s/cm^{-5} related to increased afterload (pulmonary hypertension)
5. Normal or low PCWP (<15 to 18 mm Hg) may be present in the absence of left ventricular failure
6. PCWP may be >18 mm Hg with associated left ventricular failure
7. CO may be <4L/min/m^2, and CI may be <2.5 L/min/m^2, related to decreased forward flow from the right ventricle to the left ventricle or the presence of left ventricular failure

III. Physical Assessment Findings

A. General observations (inspection)

1. *Mental status:* Memory loss or confusion may be present, related to cerebral congestion or cerebral ischemia (decreased blood flow to the brain)

2. *Respiratory status:* Tachypnea may be present, related to an increased abdominal girth (ascites), the presence of left ventricular failure (see Clinical Findings 5–1), or an underlying respiratory disorder

3. *Neck veins:* Jugular venous distention may be present, reflective of an increased RVEDP (an indication that blood is not moving forward from the right side of the heart to the left side of the heart as it should)

4. *Hepatojugular reflux* (HJR): A positive HJR may be present, related to liver congestion (jugular venous distention persists throughout the application of pressure over the liver, reflecting liver congestion related to right ventricular failure)

5. *Abdominal distention:* Bulging flanks in the supine position may be present, related to accumulation of fluid in the peritoneal cavity (ascites)

B. Palpation

1. *Skin:* Peripheral edema (may be pitting) may be present, related to venous congestion and fluid accumulation in the gravity-dependent areas of the body

2. *Precordium*
   - A left parasternal lift may be present, related to cardiomegaly
   - A right ventricular lift may be present, related to pulmonary hypertension (right ventricular hypertrophy)
   - A laterally displaced apical impulse may be present, related to cardiomegaly
   - A systolic or diastolic thrill may be present, related to an associated loud murmur

B. Percussion: With ascites, in the supine position the dependent part of the abdomen will be dull to percussion (fluid), and the upper part will be tympanic (air); in the side lying position the dullness (fluid) will shift to the dependent side (see Fig. 7–5 for related information)

C. Auscultation

1. *Heart sounds* (see Table 5–1 and Figs. 5–6 to 5–13 for related information)
   - Split S_2 may occur with pulmonary hypertension
   - S_3 on inspiration may be present, related to increased right ventricular filling pressure
   - S_4 on inspiration may be present, related to decreased right ventricular compliance

2. *Murmurs*
   - Systolic murmur of tricuspid regurgitation may be present, associated with a dilated right ventricle
   - Diastolic murmur of pulmonic regurgitation may be present, associated with pulmonary hypertension

3. *Breath sounds:* Clear unless left ventricular failure (see Clinical Findings 5–1), or an underlying respiratory disorder

Cardiomyopathy

Pathophysiology

Cardiomyopathy is a subacute or chronic disorder of the cardiac muscle. Myocardial dysfunction may be caused by unknown etiology (idiopathic or primary) or known etiology (secondary). Cardiomyopathies are commonly categorized as dilated, hypertrophic, or restrictive.

Dilated Cardiomyopathy. Dilated or congestive cardiomyopathy is characterized by dilation of both ventricles (rapid cellular destruction prevents hypertrophy) and impairment of systolic function. Decreased contractility reduces the ejection fraction, causing the stroke volume to decrease. The decline in stroke volume has both backward and forward effects (see Fig. 5–15).

Hypertrophic Cardiomyopathy. Hypertrophic cardiomyopathy (idiopathic hypertrophic subaortic stenosis) is characterized by hypertrophy of the ventricles (primarily the left) and the ventricular septum. Small chamber size and a noncompliant ventricle result in impaired diastolic filling and increased LVEDP. The hypertrophied septum may cause mechanical obstruction of the aortic outflow tract and a subsequent reduction in stroke volume and cardiac output.

Restrictive Cardiomyopathy. Restrictive cardiomyopathy is characterized by noncompliant fibrotic ventricles with chambers that cannot expand or contract. Restricted ventricular filling causes increased LVEDP and RVEDP, resulting in pulmonary and systemic venous congestion. Decreased left ventricular filling reduces the cardiac output and eventually causes circulatory collapse.

Assessment

Dilated Cardiomyopathy. The clinical presentation of dilated cardiomyopathy is one of progressive biventricular heart failure (see Clinical Findings 5–1 and 5–2). As the myocardial workload and oxygen demands escalate, activity tolerance is severely compromised, and cardiac transplantation is often the only option for treatment.

Hypertrophic Cardiomyopathy. The patient with hypertrophic cardiomyopathy may be asymptomatic for a number of years, or any situation impairing venous return, intensifying resistance to systolic ejection, or requiring an increase in cardiac output (strenuous activity) may precipitate sudden death. Primary symptoms may include exertional dyspnea, syncope, angina, and dysrhythmias.

Restrictive Cardiomyopathy. The patient with restrictive cardiomyopathy is unable to increase cardiac output during periods of exertion primarily because of restricted ventricular filling. The clinical course becomes one of low output failure with pulmonary and systemic venous congestion (see Clinical Findings 5–1 and 5–2).

POINTS TO REMEMBER

▶ The term *cardiomyopathy excludes* endstage myocardial dysfunction related to coronary artery disease, valvular disease, hypertensive heart disease, or any other congenital, ischemic, or inflammatory myocardial disorder.

▶ The critically ill adult may present with primary (idiopathic) or secondary cardiomyopathy. As well, the critically ill adult is susceptible to the development of secondary cardiomyopathy.

▶ A thorough nursing history (see Tables 1–1 and 5–1) is crucial to identify the cause of secondary cardiomyopathy or to identify patients at risk for the development of secondary cardiomyopathy.

▶ Predisposing factors for secondary cardiomyopathy include

• Viral, bacterial, fungal, parasitic, or protozoal infections, which may cause myocarditis, a hypersensitivity, or an autoimmune response

• Toxins such as alcohol, lead, arsenic, cobalt, and copper, some chemotherapeutic agents that may directly cause cell toxicity, and some drugs such as penicillin, sulfonamides, and tetracyclines that may cause hypersensitivity reactions

• Peripartal events causing cardiac failure in the last month of pregnancy or up to five months postpartum

• Genetic component (particularly hypertrophic cardiomyopathy)

• Metabolic disorders, including hyperthyroidism, hypothyroidism, hypokalemia, hyperkalemia, hemochromatosis, nutritional deficiencies

- Neuromuscular disorders, including Friedreich's ataxia, muscular dystrophy, congenital atrophies
- Infiltrative disorders, including leukemias, neoplasms, sarcoidosis
- Immunologic disorders, including post-transplant
- Connective tissue disorders, including lupus erythematosus and rheumatoid arthritis
- Storage disorders, such as those involving glycogen and mucopolysaccharide deposition

▶ In addition to the initial and baseline assessments (see Table 2–1), focused respiratory and cardiovascular assessments (see Tables 2–1, 4–1, and 5-1), as well as focused assessments of the underlying pathology should be completed as often as the patient's condition dictates to detect or anticipate and prevent complications such as dysrhythmias (see Table 14–3), acute pulmonary edema (see Clinical Findings 4–2), and decreased tissue and organ perfusion.

▶ Ongoing assessment incorporates the evaluation of responses to diagnostic procedures and therapeutic interventions aimed at the enhancement of myocardial function and the reduction of myocardial workload and oxygen demand; it includes collaboration with other members of the health team to prevent further myocardial cell damage and death.

Valvular Disorders

Pathophysiology

Valves control the unidirectional movement of blood through the heart. Congenital malformations or acquired disorders can damage the endocardial and valvular structures and interfere with blood flow. Valvular disorders are functionally categorized as regurgitation and stenosis.

Regurgitation

Failure of a valve to close completely is referred to as **regurgitation** or insufficiency. Blood is allowed to flow in a reverse direction (backward across the valve). Blood volume and pressure behind the valve increase (backward effect), and forward flow (forward effect) decreases. Regurgitant disorders primarily associated with the critically ill adult are mitral and aortic regurgitation.

Mitral Regurgitation. In mitral regurgitation, blood flow is bidirectional. Blood flows from the left atria to the left ventricle during ventricular diastole, and blood flows back across the mitral valve during ventricular systole. Mitral regurgitation may be chronic or acute.

Chronic Mitral Regurgitation. The regurgitant blood increases the left atrial volume and pressure, and the left atrium dilates and hypertrophies to compensate for the extra volume that it is required to pump. The left ventricle also dilates and hypertrophies to maintain an effective stroke volume and systolic pressure. As the amount of regurgitant stroke volume increases, the ejection fraction may be severely reduced, leading to a decline in cardiac output and left ventricular failure (see Clinical Findings 5–1).

Acute Mitral Regurgitation. The left atrium and left ventricle may not have sufficient time to compensate for the extra volume through dilation and hypertrophy. The increased volume and pressures are transmitted back through the pulmonary circuit to the right ventricle and may result in right ventricular failure. The left ventricular stroke volume decreases, and the cardiac output may decline, leading to left ventricular failure (see Fig. 5–15 and Clinical Findings 5–2 and 5–1).

Aortic Regurgitation. In aortic regurgitation, regurgitant blood from the aorta flows back into the left ventricle during diastole. The excess volume of blood (regurgitant blood plus the usual amount of blood received from the left atrium) results in left ventricular volume overload. Aortic regurgitation may be chronic or acute.

Chronic Aortic Regurgitation. The left ventricle dilates and hypertrophies to compensate for the excess volume it is required to pump, and a stronger-than-normal contraction results in an increased stroke volume. An increased systolic pressure stimulates the baroreceptors, and sympathetic outflow is decreased, resulting in systemic arterial vasodilation. This leads to a decrease in diastolic pressure and a reduction in afterload, which may diminish the aortic regurgitation. Eventually however, the excessive myocardial workload and increased myocardial oxygen demand may lead to left ventricular failure (see Fig. 5–15 and Clinical Findings 5–1).

Acute Aortic Regurgitation. The left ventricle may not have sufficient time to compensate for the excess volume through dilation and hypertrophy. The heart rate increases to maintain cardiac output. Tachycardia decreases the length of diastole, and myocardial ischemia may result from decreased coronary artery perfusion. Excessive myocardial workload and increased myocardial oxygen demand may lead to left ventricular failure. The increased left ventricular end-diastolic volume causes the mitral valve to close prematurely, and the left atrial volume and pressure increase. The increased volume and pressure are transmitted backward through the pulmonary circuit to the right ventricle and may result in right ventricular failure (see Fig. 5–15 and Clinical Findings 5–1 and 5–2).

Stenosis

Failure of a valve to open completely is referred to as **stenosis.** Greater pressure is required to open the valve and move the blood forward. Forward flow decreases (forward effect), and blood volume and pressure behind the valve increase (backward effect). Stenotic disorders primarily associated with the critically ill adult are mitral and aortic stenosis.

Mitral Stenosis. In mitral stenosis, forward flow of blood from the left atrium to the left ventricle is impaired. Left atrial volume and pressure increase, and the increased workload leads to left atrial hypertrophy. The elevated volume and pressures may be transmitted back through the pulmonary circuit and result in pulmonary hypertension, right ventricular hypertrophy, and right ventricular failure. Decreased left ventricular preload may lead to decreased stroke volume and left ventricular failure (see Fig. 5–15 and Clinical Findings 5–1 and 5–2).

Aortic Stenosis. In aortic stenosis, forward flow of blood from the left ventricle to the aorta is impaired. Left ventricular volume and pressure increase, and the increased myocardial workload leads to left ventricular hypertrophy. Left ventricular hypertrophy causes the left ventricular end-diastolic pressure to increase, and left atrial workload is increased. Continued stenosis may cause left ventricular dilation and failure, and increased strain on the left atrium (see Fig. 5–15 and Clinical Findings 5–1 and 5–2).

Assessment

The clinical presentation of a valvular disorder varies with the type and progression of valvular dysfunction. Valvular dysfunction may affect more than one valve at the same time (for example, aortic stenosis may be associated with mitral regurgitation or mitral stenosis), and one valve may be associated with both regurgitation and stenosis. Auscultation of the precordium generally reveals a characteristic murmur (see Table 5–1 and Clinical Findings 5–1 and 5–2).

Mitral Regurgitation

The critically ill adult with chronic mitral regurgitation may be asymptomatic but is at risk for atrial and ventricular dysrhythmias, particularly atrial fibrillation, related to the increased pressure in the chambers. Also, sluggish blood flow may lead to thrombus formation and the potential for embolism (see Clinical Findings 4–7). The critically ill adult with chronic or acute mitral regurgitation may exhibit clinical manifestations of acute pulmonary edema (see Clinical Findings 4–2), left ventricular failure (see Clinical Findings 5–1), and right ventricular failure (see Clinical Findings 5–2).

Aortic Regurgitation

The critically ill adult with chronic aortic regurgitation may be asymptomatic but is at risk for an increase in the severity of regurgitation associated with increased sympathetic stimulation (vasoconstriction may increase afterload). The critically ill adult with chronic or acute aortic regurgitation may exhibit clinical manifestations of left ventricular failure (see Clinical Findings 5–1).

Mitral Stenosis

The critically ill adult with mitral stenosis is at risk for dysrhythmias such as atrial fibrillation related to excessive volume and increased pressure in the chamber, and the subsequent formation of thrombus and pulmonary embolism (see Clinical Findings 4–7). The critically ill adult with mitral stenosis may exhibit clinical manifestations of pulmonary congestion (see Clinical Findings 4–2), right ventricular failure (see Clinical Findings 5–2), or left ventricular failure (see Clinical Findings 5–1).

Aortic Stenosis

The critically ill adult with aortic stenosis may exhibit clinical manifestations of left ventricular failure (see Clinical Findings 5–1). Clinical manifestations of right ventricular failure may be apparent as left ventricular failure progresses (see Clinical Findings 5–2).

POINTS TO REMEMBER

▶ Congenital deformities may affect any valve.
▶ Predisposing factors for acquired valvular disorders include the following:

Predisposing Factor	Valvular Disorder
Marfan's syndrome (Myxomatous changes in the mitral valve leaflets may cause severe mitral valve prolapse, often referred to as "floppy mitral valve"; myxomatous changes in the aortic valve leaflets may cause prolapse or tearing with aortic dilation)	Mitral regurgitation Aortic regurgitation
Mitral valve prolapse	Mitral regurgitation
Rheumatic heart disease (Postinflammatory scarring or calcification of leaflets, chordae tendineae, papillary muscles, or annulus)	Mitral regurgitation Aortic regurgitation Mitral stenosis Aortic stenosis
Infective endocarditis (Bacterial, viral, or fungal, infection may cause fibrosis, scarring, or calcification of leaflets; vegetative lesions may occlude valve orifices.)	Mitral regurgitation Aortic regurgitation Mitral stenosis Aortic stenosis
Acute myocardial infarction (Dysfunction or rupture of chordae tendineae or papillary muscle)	Acute mitral regurgitation
Left ventricular dilation (Distortion of the annulus)	Mitral regurgitation
Lupus erythematosus (Immobilization of the posterior mitral valve leaflet)	Mitral regurgitation
Rheumatoid spondylitis or syphilis (Aortic dilation separates leaflets of valve)	Aortic regurgitation

Predisposing Factor	Valvular Disorder ·
Idiopathic calcification (Calcification of the leaflets of the valve may occur with aging)	Aortic stenosis
Atherosclerosis (Changes may affect valves or the aorta)	Aortic stenosis
Trauma (Blunt chest trauma associated with deceleration accidents may cause aortic tears and dissection; penetrating wounds may tear the aorta or annulus)	Acute aortic regurgitation
Dysfunction of a mitral or aortic valve prosthesis	Mitral regurgitation Aortic regurgitation Mitral stenosis Aortic stenosis

▶ Because the critically ill adult is susceptible to the development of an acquired valvular disorder (a newly developed or changing heart murmur may indicate acute mitral or aortic regurgitation), a thorough nursing history (see Tables 1–1 and 5–1 and Predisposing Factors listed above) is crucial to identify patients at risk.

▶ In addition to the initial and baseline assessments (see Table 2–1), focused respiratory and cardiovascular assessments (see Tables 2–1, 4–1, and 5–1), as well as focused assessments of the underlying pathology should be completed as often as the patient's condition dictates to detect or anticipate and prevent complications such as dysrhythmias (see Table 14–3), pulmonary embolism (see Clinical Findings 4–7), acute pulmonary edema (see Clinical Findings 4–2), and inffective endocarditis.

▶ Ongoing assessment incorporates the evaluation of responses to diagnostic procedures and therapeutic interventions aimed at enhancing cardiac output and organ perfusion; it includes collaboration with other members of the health team to prevent further injury and infection.

Acute Infective Endocarditis

Pathophysiology

Vegetative lesions entrapped in fibrin deposits attach themselves to the heart valves and adjacent endocardial surfaces. The infectious process may lead to valvular erosion, scarring, calcification, and embolization of vegetative fragments.

Assessment

Clinical manifestations of acute infective endocarditis are related to the systemic response to infection, valvular dysfunction, and possible embolization. Physical assessment findings may include

- Fever, chills, night sweats, and fatigue
- Valvular regurgitation or stenosis associated with the involved valves (symptoms may include a newly developed or changing heart murmur and manifestations of left or right ventricular failure or of both; see Clinical Findings 5–1 and 5–2)
- Systemic embolization
  - *Cerebral:* Sudden blindness, alteration in level of consciousness, transient ischemic attack, or cerebrovascular accident (see Clinical Findings 6–5)
  - *Renal:* Flank pain with radiation to the groin accompanied by hematuria or oliguria (see Clinical Findings 8–1)
  - *Extremities:* Cold limbs with decreased or absent pulses
  - *Peripheral manifestations*
    ○ Petechiae (small red, flat lesions found on the conjunctiva, mucous membranes, palate, chest and neck)
    ○ Roth's spots (round or oval white spots surrounded by areas of hemorrhage found in the retina)
    ○ Splinter hemorrhages (black longitudinal lines or small red streaks found on the distal third of the nailbed)
    ○ Osler's nodes (tender, raised, erythematous lesions with a white center found on the pads of the fingers, hands, and toes)
    ○ Janeway lesions (nontender, flat, erythematous lesions found on the fingers, toes, nose, or earlobes)
  - Pulmonary embolism may be associated with embolization of vegetative fragments from the right heart (see Clinical Findings 4–7)

POINTS TO REMEMBER

▶ Because of compromised immune systems and numerous invasive procedures, the critically ill adult is susceptible to the development of acute infective endocarditis. A thorough nursing history is crucial to identify patients at risk (see Tables 1–1 and 5–1).

▶ In addition to the initial and baseline assessments (see Table 2–1), focused assessments of all systems (see Tables 2–1, 4–1, 5–1, 6–1, 7–1, 8–1, and 11–1), as well as ongoing assessment of responses to diagnostic procedures and therapeutic interventions should be continuously directed at detecting or anticipating and preventing infection, and facilitating rapid intervention. Prevention of acute infective endocarditis through prophylactic antibiotic therapy should be a major consideration for the critically ill adult with a known valvular disorder or prosthetic valve.

Angina Pectoris

Pathophysiology

Angina pectoris is chest pain resulting from an imbalance between myocardial oxygen supply and myocardial oxygen demand (transient myocardial ischemia). The imbalance can occur from a decrease in coronary blood flow, an increase in myocardial workload, or a fall in the blood oxygen content.

The most common cause of angina is a decrease in coronary blood flow due to atherosclerotic heart disease. Angina may be classified as stable angina, unstable angina, or Prinzmetal's angina.

Stable Angina

Stable, or classic, angina (also referred to as chronic exertional) is characterized by the inability of atherosclerotic coronary arteries to dilate and increase myocardial perfusion in the presence of physical or emotional exertion. The pain is generally predictable, may last from 1 to 5 minutes, and is usually relieved by rest or nitroglycerin.

Unstable Angina

Unstable, or crescendo, angina (also referred to as pre-infarctional) is characterized by new onset chest pain or an increase in the frequency, severity, and duration of attacks. The pain may occur at rest or with minimal exertion and may last longer than 10 minutes.

Prinzmetal's Angina

Prinzmetal's angina generally occurs at rest. The decreased coronary blood flow is usually due to coronary vasospasm.

Assessment

Ischemic pain may be described as burning, squeezing, tightness, or substernal pressure. The pain may radiate to the jaw and teeth, neck, left shoulder, left arm extending down to the fourth and 5th fingers, upper back, or upper abdomen (same sensory neurons) and may be accompanied by nausea, vomiting, anxiety, restlessness, or a feeling of exhaustion.

Respirations may be labored related to anxiety or pulmonary congestion associated with decreased contractility (ischemic-induced). In the aging and diabetic population, dyspnea may be the first sign of ischemia because of diminished pain perception related to peripheral neuropathy.

POINTS TO REMEMBER

▶ Angina is a clinical manifestation of myocardial ischemia: Myocardial ischemia may occur in the presence or absence of coronary artery disease (CAD).

▶ The critically ill adult is susceptible to the development of myocardial ischemia because of preexisting CAD or alterations in oxygen supply and demand. A thorough nursing history (see Tables 1–1, 5–1, and Predisposing Factors that follow) is crucial to identify patients at risk.

▶ Predisposing factors that may precipitate angina in the critically ill adult include the following:

- CAD (associated risk factors include heredity, advancing age, male sex, postmenopausal women, hyperlipidemia, hypertension, diabetes mellitus, obesity, smoking, and sedentary life style)
- Myocardial infarction
- Heart failure
- Cardiomyopathies
- Valvular disorders
- Dysrhythmias
- Hypertension
- Hypotension
- Shock syndrome
- Septic syndrome
- Anemia
- Thyrotoxicosis
- ARDS (pulmonary hypertension)
- Pumonary embolism

▸ Because myocardial ischemia may lead to complications such as dysrhythmias (see Table 14–3) and acute myocardial infarction (see Clinical Findings 5–3), in addition to the initial and baseline assessments (see Table 2–1), focused respiratory and cardiovascular assessments (see Tables 2–1, 4–1, and 5–1) should be completed as often as the patient's condition indicates to detect or anticipate and prevent such complications, and facilitate immediate intervention.

▸ Ongoing assessment incorporates the evaluation of responses to diagnostic procedures and therapeutic interventions aimed at increasing oxygen supply and decreasing oxygen demand; it includes collaboration with other members of the health team to prevent prolonged ischemia and myocardial injury.

Myocardial Infarction

Pathophysiology

Acute myocardial infarction (MI) results from disruption of blood flow to myocardial tissue. Subsequent oxygen deprivation causes irreversible damage to myocardial cells. Myocardial infarctions may be classified as transmural or nontransmural.

Transmural Infarctions

- Transmural infarctions usually involve the full thickness of the myocardium and are associated with abnormal Q waves and with ST and T wave changes on the ECG.
- The most common cause of transmural infarctions is coronary artery occlusion.
- Causes of coronary artery blockage include atherosclerotic plaque formation and rupture, thrombosis, platelet aggregation, and spasm.
- Factors precipitating plaque rupture and thrombus formation include the risk factors for the development of coronary artery disease (see preceding Points to Remember) and severe physical or emotional stress.

Nontransmural Infarctions

- Nontransmural infarctions (subendocardial, non-Q wave) generally involve partial thickness of the myocardium and may be

associated with several causative factors, including atherosclerotic heart disease, microemboli, and oxygen supply-and-demand imbalances:
- The coronary arteries enter the epicardial surface of the heart and transverse through the myocardium before reaching the subendocardial surface.
- Consequently, the subendocardium is particularly vulnerable to low perfusion states such as hypovolemic shock.
• Nontransmural infarctions may extend across the myocardium and progress to transmural infarctions.

Ischemia, Injury, and Death of Myocardial Tissue

In general, the lack of oxygen to the area of myocardium supplied by the involved artery results in ischemia, injury, and tissue death (necrosis). Ischemic myocardial cells are temporarily deprived of oxygen and may resume normal function. Injured myocardial cells surround the area of necrosis and may be salvaged through collateral circulation. Necrotic myocardial cells have received permanent damage and contribute to abnormal contraction, reduced ejection fraction and stroke volume, and increased LVEDP. The amount of tissue death depends on the extent, duration, and severity of decreased blood flow and oxygen supply, and the workload demands on the myocardium.

Site of Myocardial Infarction

The majority of infarctions involve the left ventricle or intraventricular septum. Right ventricular involvement can occur with inferior infarction. Isolated right ventricular infarction is less common. (Table 5–4, p. 243, provides related information on the site of myocardial infarction, associated coronary artery, and ECG changes.)

Assessment

Clinical manifestations vary with the type and extent of myocardial infarction (see Table 5–4 and Clinical Findings 5–3). In general, anterior infarctions damage more of the left ventricle than inferior infarctions and therefore are associated with a higher incidence of left ventricular failure and ectopy, more dismal prognosis, and higher mortality rate.

Clinical manifestations of infarction may also vary with sympathetic and parasympathetic nervous system stimulation. Sympathetic nervous stimulation is usually more common with anterior infarction.

Unfortunately, the increased heart rate, increased contractility, and vasoconstriction may add to the compromised left ventricular workload and oxygen consumption. The increased level of catecholamines may also contribute to ectopy. Parasympathetic stimulation is usually more common with inferior infarction.

POINTS TO REMEMBER

▶ Because acute myocardial infarction and/or sudden death may be the first indication of CAD in the critically ill adult, a thorough nursing history (see Tables 1–1 and 5–1, p. 262, and Clinical Findings 5–3) is crucial to identify patients at risk.

▶ Because myocardial damage may lead to dysrhythmias (see Table 14–3), decreased cardiac output, decreased arterial blood flow to the tissues and tissue and organ ischemia, heart failure (see Clinical Findings 5–1 and 5–2), rupture of the interventricular septum, papillary muscle rupture, ventricular aneurysm or rupture, and cardiogenic shock (see Clinical Findings 12–3), in addition to the initial and baseline assessments (see Table 2–1), focused respiratory and cardiovascular assessments (see Tables 2–1, 4–1, and 5–1) should be completed as often as the patient's condition dictates to detect or anticipate and prevent such complications, and facilitate immediate intervention. Necrotic areas greater than 40% of the myocardium greatly increase the risk of cardiogenic shock and death.

▶ Ongoing assessment incorporates the evaluation of responses to diagnostic procedures and therapeutic interventions aimed at the reduction of myocardial oxygen consumption and the restoration of myocardial oxygen supply; it includes collaboration with other members of the health team to optimize cardiac output and systemic blood flow to the tissues while preventing further myocardial injury.

Clinical Findings 5–3   *Myocardial Infarction*

I. HISTORY

A. Predisposing factors

1. CAD and associated risk factors (see p. 262)
2. Previous history of MI increases the risk of successive infarctions, particularly in the presence of hypotensive episodes (decreased blood flow through the coronary arteries), hypertensive episodes (increased

myocardial workload), and severe physical or emotional stress (increased myocardial workload)

B. Subjective findings

1. *Chest pain of variable presentation*
   - Substernal chest pain that may be localized or radiate to the neck, jaw and teeth, shoulder, down the left arm to the fourth and fifth fingers, upper back or upper abdomen
   - The pain may be described as crushing, burning, squeezing, or as a pressure or weight sitting on the chest
   - The pain may be described as epigastric discomfort or indigestion
   - In general, the pain is usually more severe than in angina, is constant, lasts longer than 15 to 20 minutes, and is not relieved by rest or nitroglycerin
2. *Associated symptoms*
   - Anxiety related to severe chest pain
   - Fear (severe apprehension) related to sense of impending doom
   - Dyspnea related to pain, anxiety, fear (sympathetic nervous system stimulation), or pulmonary congestion associated with decreased left ventricular contractility
   - Weakness related to decreased peripheral blood flow

II. LABORATORY AND BEDSIDE MONITORING FINDINGS

A. Arterial blood gases (see Chapter 13 for related information on acid-base disorders and serum lactate levels and Chapter 14 and Table 14–1 for related information on oxygen delivery and consumption parameters)

1. Respiratory alkalosis (Pco_2 <35 mm Hg and pH >7.45) may be present, related to hyperventilation
2. Metabolic acidosis (HCO_3^- <22 mEq/L and pH <7.35) may be present, related to decreased arterial blood flow to the tissues
3. Serum lactate may be >2 mEq/L, related to tissue oxygen deficits

B. Serum enzymes (see Table 13–3 for onset, peaks, and duration): Elevated serum levels of creatinine kinase (CK), lactic dehydrogenase (LDH), and aspartate aminotransferase (AST, serum glutamic oxaloacetic transaminase [SGOT]) may reflect myocardial cell death; however, these enzymes alone are not specific for diagnosing an acute MI

C. Cardiac isoenzymes (see Table 13–3 for onset, peaks, and duration)

1. An elevated CK-MB (creatinine kinase-myocardial muscle) is related to myocardial cell death (primary diagnostic enzyme for acute MI)
2. An elevated LDH-1 and a ratio of LDH-1 to LDH-2 greater than 1.0 is strongly related to myocardial cell death (highly indicative of an acute MI)

D. Other laboratory studies

1. An elevated erythrocyte sedimentation rate (ESR) and white blood cell count (WBC count) may be present, related to myocardial inflammation (see Table 13–9)

2. An elevated serum cholesterol, low-density lipoprotein (LDL) and triglycerides, and possibly decreased high-density lipoprotein (HDL) may be present, related to presence of CAD (see Table 13–2)

E. ECG (see Table 5–4 for information related to ECG changes and site of infarction)

1. T wave elevation in hyperacute phase followed by inversion related to myocardial ischemia

2. ST segment elevation related to myocardial injury

3. Q wave formation related to death of myocardial tissue

F. Dysrhythmias (general information)

1. Sinus bradycardia and transient first- and second-degree heart blocks are more common with inferior infarctions related to susceptibility to parasympathetic nervous system stimulation and possible involvement of SA and AV nodes (see Table 5–4)

2. Bundle branch blocks and second- and third-degree heart blocks are more common with anterior and anteroseptal infarctions related to possible damage to bundle branches and septum (see Table 5–4)

3. Ventricular dysrhythmias may occur with all types of infarctions in association with ventricular irritability related to bradycardias, hypoxic or ischemic myocardial tissue, acidosis, electrolyte imbalances, and heart failure

4. Ventricular tachycardias may occur with all types of infarction and are life-threatening

5. Sinus tachycardia is more common with anterior MIs, related to susceptibility to sympathetic nervous stimulation but may occur with all types of infarction in association with pain, anxiety, fever, and hypotension

6. Supraventricular tachycardias (including sinus tachycardia, atrial tachycardia, atrial fibrillation, and atrial flutter) are dangerous in the post-MI patient, because rapid ventricular response rates can decrease coronary artery filling times and create an imbalance between oxygen supply and demand, jeopardizing viable myocardial cells (see Table 14–3 for related information on dysrhythmias)

G. Hemodynamic parameters (see Chapter 14, Table 14–2, and Fig. 14–2 for related information on hemodynamics, including formulas for calculation of parameters such as right ventricular stroke work index and left ventricular stroke work index)

1. Hypotension may be present, related to bradycardia and increased parasympathetic nervous stimulation, or associated with decreased stroke volume and decreased cardiac output
2. Hypertension may be present, related to increased sympathetic nervous system stimulation
3. SVR may be >1200–1500 dyne/s/cm^{-5}, related to increased sympathetic nervous system compensatory response (vasoconstriction) or hypertension
4. A RAP >6 mm Hg (CVP >12 cm H_2O) with a low or normal PCWP (<12 mm Hg) may indicate right ventricular (RV) infarction
5. A PCWP >12 to 18 mm Hg with a low CO (<4 L/m^2) and a low CI (<2.5 L/m^2) may indicate left ventricular failure (see Clinical Findings 5–1)
6. An arterial pressure <90 mm Hg systolic, an SVR >2000 dyne/s/cm^{-5}, a PCWP >18 mm Hg, and a CI <2.2 L/min/m^2 may indicate cardiogenic shock (see Chapter 12 and Clinical Findings 12–3 for related information on cardiogenic shock)

III. PHYSICAL ASSESSMENT FINDINGS

A. General observations (inspection)

1. *Mental status*
   - The critically ill adult may be grimacing, sitting forward, and clutching or massaging the chest with a closed fist (Levine's sign), because of severe chest pain
   - The critically ill adult may be listless and motionless with little energy, related to poor cardiac output
   - Restlessness and agitation may be present, related to severe chest pain or decreased cerebral blood flow secondary to decreased cardiac output
   - Confusion, light-headedness, or syncope may be present, related to decreased cerebral blood flow secondary to poor cardiac output associated with impaired left ventricular contractility, or to dysrhythmias such as heart blocks, bradycardias, and tachycardias
2. *Respiratory pattern:* Tachypnea may be present, related to anxiety or to pulmonary congestion secondary to left ventricular failure
3. *Skin*
   - May be normal in color with uncomplicated myocardial infarction
   - May be pale, gray, or cyanotic related to poor cardiac output and decreased arterial blood flow or vasoconstriction (sympathetic nervous system stimulation)
4. *Nails:* Capillary refill may be >2 seconds related to poor cardiac output and decreased arterial blood flow or vasoconstriction (sympathetic nervous system stimulation)

5. *Nausea and vomiting:* Usually more common with inferior infarction related to parasympathetic nervous system stimulation

6. *Hiccups:* May be present with inferior infarction related to parasympathetic stimulation and diaphragmatic irritation

7. *Neck veins*
   - Jugular venous pressure is usually normal in the uncomplicated MI patient
   - Jugular venous distention may be present, related to biventricular failure (see Fig. 5–15 and Clinical Findings 5–1 and 5–2), or right ventricular infarction
   - Flat neck veins in the horizontal position may be present, related to hypotension associated with parasympathetic stimulation in the inferior MI or to hypovolemia

8. *Urine output:* May be decreased related to poor cardiac output and decreased blood flow to the kidney

9. *Fever*
   - Body temperature may be elevated 24 to 48 hours following infarction, related to the inflammatory response and tissue death
   - Low-grade fever 2 to 4 days following infarction may be present, related to pericarditis (the chest pain differs from angina in that it is positional, exacerbated with respiration, and accompanied by a transient pericardial friction rub): Dressler's syndrome, or postmyocardial infarction syndrome, is usually not seen in the critically ill adult as symptoms appear 2 to 10 weeks following myocardial infarction (clinical manifestations include low-grade fever, leukocytosis, pericardial friction rub, and pleuropericardial chest pain)

B. Palpation

1. *Skin*
   - May be warm and dry with uncomplicated myocardial infarction
   - Cool and clammy extremities may be related to poor cardiac output and decreased systemic arterial blood flow or to vasoconstriction (sympathetic nervous system stimulation)

2. *Peripheral pulse* (see Table 5–1 and Fig. 5–14 for related information on arterial pulses)
   - Pulse volume may be weak, related to decreased cardiac output, or full and bounding, related to increased sympathetic nervous system stimulation
   - Pulsus alternans (alternating weak and strong volumes) may be present, related to left ventricular failure
   - Pulse may be irregular, related to dysrhythmias such as ventricular ectopy

- Bigeminal pulse may be present, related to dysrhythmias such as ventricular bigeminy
- Pulse deficit may be present, related to dysrhythmias such as atrial fibrillation

3. *Precordium:* Systolic pulsation or bulge (occurring most often at the apex) in the patient with an anterior infarction may be related to the development of a left ventricular aneurysm

C. Auscultation (see Table 5–1 and Figs. 5–6 to 5–13 for descriptions of heart sounds, murmurs and rubs)

1. Muffled heart sounds may be related to decreased ventricular compliance, or ruptured ventricular aneurysm
2. S_4 may be present on expiration, related to decreased left ventricular compliance (if right ventricular infarction, S_4 may be heard on inspiration)
3. S_3 may be present on expiration, related to increased filling pressure of left ventricle (if right ventricular infarction, S_3 may be heard on inspiration)
4. Summation gallop may be present, related to severe infarction (the presence of S_3 or a summation gallop is associated with an increased mortality rate)
5. Sudden onset of a pansystolic murmur accompanied by a thrill and heard best at the apex may be related to papillary muscle rupture
6. Sudden onset of a pansystolic murmur heard loudest at the left and right sternal borders may be related to rupture of the interventricular septum: New onset murmurs in the acute MI are a medical emergency and should be investigated immediately
7. Pericardial friction rub may be heard related to pericarditis

D. Adventitious breath sounds

1. Crackles may be present, related to increased LVEDP or left ventricular failure
2. Lungs are usually clear on auscultation with right ventricular infarction (unless there is underlying cardiac or respiratory disorder)

Pericarditis

Pathophysiology

Inflammation of the pericardium (fibrous tissue surrounding the heart) may result in acute pericarditis. An inflammatory exudate often leads to an effusion of fluid (serous, fibrinous, purulent, hemorrhagic, or caseous) into the pericardial space (pericardial effusion). A small pericardial effusion may be asymptomatic. If the effusion is large, external compression of the heart chambers may lead to decreased ventricular filling and a reduction in stroke volume (see Pericardial Tamponade, below, for related information).

Chronic inflammation may progress to constrictive pericarditis. In constrictive pericarditis, fibrous scarring occurs over a period of time. The pericardium becomes rigid, preventing adequate filling of the ventricles. Pulmonary and systemic venous pressures increase, and cardiac output decreases (see Restrictive Cardiomyopathy, above, for related information).

Assessment

The clinical manifestations of acute pericarditis are related to the extent of pericardial damage and the systemic effects of inflammation. Rubbing of visceral and parietal surfaces may cause chest pain. The chest pain may be described as sharp or stabbing (dull with effusion) and may increase with coughing, swallowing, movement, and respiration. (Decreased respiratory excursion and dyspnea may be present related to splinting.) The pain may radiate to the back and is usually accompanied by a pericardial friction rub (see Table 5–1 for a description of a pericardial friction rub). Epicardial injury may be reflected on the ECG as ST segment elevation. General signs of inflammation such as chills, fever, fatigue, leukocytosis, and an elevated sedimentation rate may also be present.

The clinical manifestations of constrictive pericarditis are related to increased left ventricular and right ventricular end-diastolic pressures, and decreased cardiac output (see Clinical Findings 5–1 and 5–2). A rise in the central venous pressure may be seen with inspiration (Kussmaul's sign) related to restriction of ventricular filling and volume expansion.

POINTS TO REMEMBER

▶ Pericarditis may be idiopathic or related to a variety of underlying disorders. Predisposing factors include
- Acute myocardial infarction (Dressler's syndrome)
- Cardiac surgery (postcardiotomy syndrome)
- Anticoagulation therapy
- Infection (viral, bacterial, fungal, protozoal, tuberculosis)
- Radiation
- Uremia
- Chest trauma
- Malignant neoplasms

- Connective tissue disorders such as rheumatic fever, rheumatoid arthritis, systemic lupus erythematosus, and scleroderma
- Drug-hypersensitivity reactions, including procainamide, minoxidil, hydralazine, phenytoin, phenylbutazone, penicillin, and daunorubicin.

▶ Because the critically ill adult may present with acute or constrictive pericarditis and because the critically ill adult is also susceptible to the development of acute pericarditis, a thorough nursing history (see Tables 1–1 and 5–1) is crucial to identify the underlying cause of pericarditis or to detect patients at risk for the development of pericarditis.

▶ In addition to the initial and baseline assessments (see Table 2–1), focused respiratory and cardiovascular assessments (see Tables 2–1, 4–1, and 5–1), as well as focused assessments of the underlying pathology should be completed as often as the patient's condition dictates to detect or anticipate and prevent complications such as pericardial effusion (see Clinical Findings 4–5) and cardiac tamponade (see below).

▶ Ongoing assessment of acute pericarditis incorporates the evaluation of responses to diagnostic procedures and therapeutic interventions aimed at the reduction of chest pain; it includes collaboration with other members of the health team to reduce the progression of inflammation.

▶ Ongoing assessment of chronic pericarditis incorporates the evaluation of responses to diagnostic procedures and therapeutic interventions aimed at the reduction of symptoms of right ventricular and left ventricular failure (see Clinical Findings 5–2 and 5–1), it includes collaboration with other members of the health team to improve cardiac contractility.

Pericardial Tamponade

Pathophysiology

Pericardial tamponade results from a sudden or large accumulation of fluid in the pericardial sac. Normally, the pericardial sac holds only 30 to 50 ml of clear fluid.

Cardiac tamponade compresses the chambers of the heart, affecting both ventricular filling and emptying. Restricted right ventricular filling increases the RVEDP and leads to systemic venous congestion.

Restricted left ventricular filling increases the LVEDP and leads to pulmonary venous congestion. Restricted ventricular emptying leads to a reduction in stroke volume, cardiac output, and cardiovascular collapse.

Assessment

The clinical manifestations of pericardial tamponade include increased CVP, jugular venous distention, and the clinical manifestations associated with right ventricular failure (see Clinical Findings 5–2). As well, hypotension and the clinical manifestations associated with left ventricular failure (see Clinical Findings 5–1) may be present.

In addition, changes in intrathoracic pressure during respiration affect ventricular filling and may cause a drop in systolic blood pressure >10 mm Hg during inspiration (pulsus paradoxus). Also, the increased intrapericardial pressure may cause the intracardiac pressures (PCWP, PAS, PAD, CVP) to equalize (see Fig. 14–2).

Muffled heart sounds and a decrease in ECG amplitude may be present, related to the increase in fluid around the heart. As well, a chest x-ray may reveal cardiac enlargement and possible widened mediastinum related to the accumulation of fluid.

POINTS TO REMEMBER

▶ Pericardial tamponade is a life-threatening emergency. Rapid decompensation may result in cardiogenic shock (see Chapter 12 and Clinical Findings 12–3).

▶ Because the critically ill adult may present with pericardial tamponade associated with injuries such as chest trauma, or develop pericardial tamponade secondary to an underlying condition such as pericarditis or cardiac surgery, a thorough nursing history (see Tables 1–1 and 5–1 and Clinical Findings 12–2) is crucial to identify the cause of pericardial tamponade or to identify patients at risk for the development of pericardial tamponade.

▶ In addition to the initial and baseline assessments (see Table 2–1), focused respiratory and cardiovascular assessments (see Tables 2–1, 4–1, and 5–1), as well as focused assessments of the underlying pathology, should be completed as often as the patient's condition dictates to detect or anticipate and prevent complications such as cardiovascular collapse.

▶ Ongoing assessment incorporates the evaluation of responses to diagnostic procedures and therapeutic interventions aimed at the restoration of cardiac output; it includes collaboration with other members of the health team to decrease the amount of fluid accumulation around the heart.

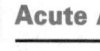

Acute Aortic Dissection

Pathophysiology

Acute aortic dissection results from a tear in the intimal lining of the arterial wall that creates a false lumen for blood flow (the medial layers become separated by a column of blood, which may cause splitting in both directions from the leak). The weakened vessel is susceptible to rupture.

Dissections may be classified according to the origin of the tear and the extent of the involvement of the aorta (De Bakey's classification). Type I dissections involve a tear in the proximal aorta with dissection into the ascending and descending aorta. Type II dissections involve a tear in the proximal aorta with dissection confined to the ascending aorta. Type III dissections involve a tear distal to the left subclavian artery with dissection confined to the descending aorta.

Assessment

Clinical manifestations vary with the location and extent of the aortic dissection and the arterial circulation compromised (see Clinical Findings 5–4). In general, proximal dissection with involvement of the aortic valve may lead to aortic regurgitation and left ventricular failure (see Clinical Findings 5–1), proximal dissection with extension into the pericardium may lead to pericardial tamponade (see above) or cardiogenic shock (see Clinical Findings 12–3), proximal dissection with obstruction of the coronary arteries may lead to myocardial ischemia or infarction (see Clinical Findings 5–3), and proximal dissection with extension into the carotid arteries may lead to a cerebrovascular accident (see Clinical Findings 6–5). Distal dissection with obstruction of the renal artery may lead to acute tubular necrosis (see Clinical Findings 8–1), distal dissection with obstruction of the mesenteric artery may lead to ileus or bowel infarction, distal dissection with gastrointestinal hemorrhage may lead to hypovolemic shock (see Clinical Findings 7–1 and 12–3), and distal dissection with obstruction of blood supply to the spinal nerves may lead to paraplegia (see Clinical Findings 6–7).

POINTS TO REMEMBER

▶ Acute aortic dissection is a life-threatening emergency (rapid progression or rupture of the dissection can lead to exsanguination).

▶ Because the critically ill adult may present with acute aortic dissection associated with injuries such as multiple trauma, or may develop acute aortic dissection associated with an underlying disorder such as hypertension, a thorough nursing history (see Tables 1–1 and 5–1 and Clinical Findings 5–4 and 12–2) is crucial to identify the underlying cause of the dissection or to identify patients at risk for the development of acute aortic dissection.

▶ In addition to the initial and baseline assessments (see Table 2–1) and a focused assessment of the underlying pathology, a focused cardiovascular assessment (see Tables 2–1 and 5–1), as well as a focused assessment of each system affected by the dissection, should be completed as often as the patient's condition dictates to detect or anticipate and prevent complications such as heart failure (see Clinical Findings 5–1 and 5–2), cardiac tamponade, shock (see Clinical Findings 12–3), cerebrovascular accident (see Clinical Findings 6-5), renal failure (see Clinical Findings 8–1), and paraplegia (see Clinical Findings 6–7).

▶ Ongoing assessment incorporates the evaluation of responses to diagnostic procedures and therapeutic interventions aimed at stabilization of the dissection; it includes collaboration with other members of the health team to maintain adequate tissue perfusion and prevent further progression of the dissection and possible rupture of the vessel.

Clinical Findings 5–4   *Acute Aortic Dissection*

I. **HISTORY**

A. **Predisposing factors**
  1. Hypertension (arteriosclerosis, pheochromocytoma, Cushing's disease, cocaine)
  2. Cystic medial necrosis
  3. Marfan's syndrome
  4. Coarctation of the aorta
  5. Pregnancy (hormone changes, increased blood volume, and hypertension especially during third trimester or labor)

6. Crushing or tearing injuries associated with blunt chest or abdominal trauma and rapid deceleration accidents
7. Invasive procedures involving aortic clamping or cannulation

B. Subjective findings

1. Severe chest, epigastric, or back pain, which may be described as ripping, tearing, or stabbing and may reach a peak almost immediately:
   - Anterior chest pain is more commonly associated with proximal dissections
   - Back pain is more commonly associated with distal dissections
2. Dizziness or syncope related to involvement of the carotid artery and cerebral ischemia

II. LABORATORY AND BEDSIDE MONITORING FINDINGS

A. Chest x-ray: Widened mediastinum related to extravasation of blood

B. CT scan: May clearly reveal the intimal tear and extension into the proximal and distal aorta as well as collection of fluid in the pericardial, pleural, and mediastinal spaces

C. Laboratory studies

1. Elevated BUN and creatinine may be present, associated with renal dysfunction related to obstruction of renal blood flow (see Table 13–6 for related information on BUN and creatinine)
2. Elevated cardiac isoenzymes may be present, associated with an acute MI related to involvement of the coronary arteries (see Table 13–3 for related information on cardiac isoenzymes)
3. Decreased hemoglobin may be present, related to blood loss
4. Decreased hematocrit may be present, related to blood loss or hemolysis (see Table 13–8 for related information on hemoglobin and hematocrit)

D. ECG

1. Left ventricular hypertrophy (increased amplitude of QRS complex) may be present, related to preexisting hypertension
2. Changes indicative of ischemia, injury, or infarction may be present, related to progression of the dissection and involvement of the coronary arteries (see Table 5–4)

E. Hemodynamic parameters (see Table 14–2 and Fig. 14–2 for related information on hemodynamic parameters)

1. Hypertension rapidly progressing to hypotension may be related to rupture of the dissection
2. Hypotension may be related to hemorrhage and hypovolemic shock or to cardiac tamponade

3. Unequal blood pressure in each arm may be related to brachiocephalic artery obstruction
4. Thigh blood pressure less than arm blood pressure may be related to descending progression of the dissection

III. PHYSICAL ASSESSMENT FINDINGS

A. General observations (inspection)

1. *Mental status*
   - Alterations in the level of consciousness may be present, related to carotid artery obstruction and cerebral ischemia or to decreased cerebral blood flow related to decreased cardiac output secondary to hypovolemia or cardiac tamponade
   - Restlessness may be present, related to decreased cerebral blood flow associated with shock
2. *Skin:* Cyanosis or pallor may be present, related to decreased systemic arterial blood flow secondary to hypovolemia (hemorrhage), cardiac tamponade, or peripheral vasoconstriction
3. *Nails:* Capillary refill may be >2 seconds related to decreased systemic arterial blood flow
4. *Neck veins*
   - Jugular venous distention may be present, related to pericardial tamponade
   - Flat neck veins in the horizontal position may be present, related to hypovolemia
5. *Abdomen:* Abdominal distention or a pulsating abdominal mass may be present with involvement of the abdominal aorta
6. *Extremities:* There may be ischemia in any extremity, related to the obstruction of blood flow
7. *Urine:* Oliguria or anuria may be present, related to renal artery obstruction, or decreased blood flow to the kidney secondary to shock
8. *Stool:* Melena may be present, related to involvement of the mesenteric artery

B. Palpation

1. *Skin:* May be cool and clammy, related to decreased systemic arterial blood flow secondary to hypovolemic shock, cardiac tamponade, or peripheral vasoconstriction
2. *Peripheral pulses:* Absent or unequal pulses may be related to obstruction of carotid, brachiocephalic, or iliac artery

  3. *Abdomen:* Abdominal tenderness may be present, related to an abdominal
     mass or mesenteric artery obstruction

C. Auscultation

  1. *Heart sounds* (see Table 5–1 and Figs. 5–6 to 5–13 for related informa-
     tion on heart sounds, murmurs, and rubs)
     - Heart sounds may be distant or muffled, related to pericardial tamponade
     - Tachycardia may be present, related to hypovolemic shock, or cardiac
       tamponade
     - New diastolic murmur of aortic regurgitation may be present, related to
       the progression of the dissection into the aortic valve
     - Pericardial friction rub may be present, related to involvement of the
       pericardium and pericardial effusion
  2. *Abdomen*
     - Bowel sounds may be hyperactive, related to the involvement of the
       mesenteric artery
     - Bowel sounds may be hypoactive, related to hypovolemic shock and
       gastrointestinal shunting

6

Neuromuscular Assessment

FUNCTION OF THE NEUROMUSCULAR SYSTEM

The principal functions of the nervous system are

- **Interpretation** of stimuli from the internal and external environment
- **Response** to stimuli from the internal and external environment
- **Control and coordination** of activities of most body organs

These functions are accomplished through specialized cells called neurons that receive *sensory,* or *afferent,* input from peripheral nerves or sensory organs; transmit *motor,* or *efferent,* output to effector cells and organs; or store information for future response as cognitive, emotive, or motor activities. Functions are accomplished through a series of electrochemical reactions. Electrical impulses travel along nerve fibers: dendrites going towards cell bodies and axons going away from cell bodies. A myelin sheath surrounds most axons to increase the speed of impulse transmission. At fiber junctions chemical reactions occur that involve neurotransmitters, which transport impulses across synaptic gaps from presynaptic to postsynaptic fibers. Those with excitatory effects include acetylcholine, norepinephrine, and glutamate. Those with inhibitory effects include dopamine, glycine, γ-aminobutyric acid (GABA), and serotonin.

The two divisions of the nervous system are the central nervous system (CNS) and the peripheral nervous system (PNS). The **central nervous system** includes the cerebrum, cerebellum, diencephalon, brain stem, and spinal cord. It is encased in a rigid skull and vertebral column and protected by suspension in cerebrospinal fluid produced within the four ventricles of the brain. Cerebrospinal fluid is absorbed into the venous circulation through the arachnoid villi. The brain and spinal cord are covered by three fibrous layers, or meninges, the inner *pia mater,* middle *arachnoid,* and outer *dura mater.* The outer layer of the brain dura mater becomes the periosteum of the skull. The inner layer folds once longitudinally to form a separation between the two cerebral hemispheres called the *falx cerebri.* It fuses with a second transverse fold, the *tentorium cerebri* that separates the occipital lobes and the cerebellum. These folds form the anterior, middle, and posterior fossae. Space-occupying pathology in the CNS increases intracranial pressure. Resulting compression and possible herniation of brain contents become life-threatening events.

The *cerebrum* (encephalon) has an outer layer, or cortex, of gray matter (cell bodies and synapses for impulse transmission to and from the periphery) and an inner layer of white matter (ascending sensory and descending motor pathways or bundles of myelinated fibers). Its main divisions include right and left frontal, parietal, temporal, and occipital lobes; the limbic system; and the central basal ganglia. Various areas are concerned with cognition, emotion, sensate interpretation, and voluntary motor response (Fig. 6–1). As a general rule each hemisphere controls sensory and motor functions on the contralateral (opposite) side of the body. The *cerebellum,* situated behind the brain stem, integrates sensory and motor information to coordinate voluntary muscle activities.

The diencephalon (thalamus and hypothalamus) is sometimes considered as part of the brain stem. The thalamus relays information to and from the cerebrum, and the hypothalamus regulates many autonomic and endocrine functions of the body. The rostral to caudal (upper to lower) divisions of the *brain stem* are the mesencephalon (midbrain), pons, and medulla. The brain stem is contiguous with the spinal cord. Arousal requires integrity of the reticular activating system (RAS) of the upper brain stem. Full consciousness and cognition require interaction between an intact cerebral hemisphere and the upper brain stem. The brain stem also influences vital functions, including breathing, circulation, and temperature control.

Arterial blood supply to the brain is through the vertebral and internal carotid arteries. Their terminal branches become the basilar and cerebral arteries, which anastomose to form the cerebral arterial circle of Willis. Venous drainage is accomplished through dural sinuses to the internal jugular veins.

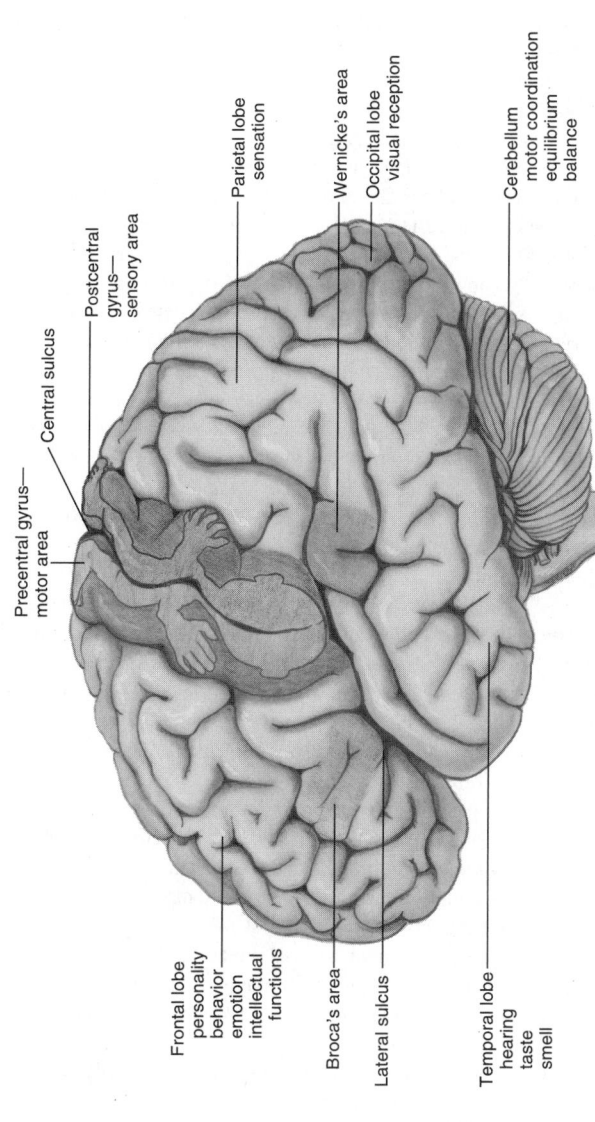

Precentral gyrus—
motor area

Central sulcus

Postcentral
gyrus—
sensory area

Parietal lobe
sensation

Wernicke's area

Occipital lobe
visual reception

Cerebellum
motor coordination
equilibrium
balance

Frontal lobe
personality
behavior
emotion
intellectual
functions

Broca's area

Lateral sulcus

Temporal lobe
hearing
taste
smell

FIGURE 6–1

The functional areas of the cerebral cortex. (From Jarvis, C. [1996]. *Physical examination and health assessment* [3rd ed., p. 710]. Philadelphia: W. B. Saunders.)

The *spinal cord* is the extension of the brain stem. Anatomically the spinal cord consists of central H-shaped gray cellular matter and peripheral white matter containing ascending tracts to the sensory cortex and descending tracts from the motor cortex. These tracts cross from one side of the spinal cord to the other. Injury to the nervous system may therefore produce ipsilateral (same side) or contralateral loss of function. The spinal cord ends at the level of the first lumbar vertebra (L1). Below this level peripheral nerves form the *cauda equina,* or horse's tail, and exit the vertebral column at their respective vertebrae (L2–5 and S1–5).

The second division of the nervous system is the **peripheral nervous system** (PNS). Cell bodies of these nerves are located outside the central nervous system in congregations called *ganglia.* It includes the 12 pairs of *cranial nerves,* which exit the central nervous system at the level of the brain stem and control sensory and motor function on the ipsilateral (same) side of the head and neck. Assessment of end organs for these cranial nerves provides information on brain-stem integrity. The PNS also includes the 32 pairs of *spinal nerves,* which exit the spinal column through each intervertebral foramen. These paired spinal nerves are identified by the area of the cord they exit: 8 cervical, 12 thoracic, 5 lumbar, 5 sacral, and 2 or more coccygeal nerves (Fig. 6–2). Each spinal nerve has a dorsal sensory (afferent) root in the posterior horn of the gray matter and a ventral motor (efferent) root in the anterior horn at its respective level in the cord. Assessment of dermatomes, specific skin surfaces, and skeletal muscles provides information on PNS function and its integrity with the central nervous system. A network of *peripheral nerves* complements spinal nerve function and helps compensate for some losses.

Sensations are transmitted to the sensory cortex via two tracts. The *posterior columns* conduct sensations of position, vibration, and discrete touch. The *spinothalamic tracts* conduct sensations of light and nonlocalized touch (anterior tracts) or pain and temperature (lateral tracts). Because these tracts occupy different locations in the spinal cord and their fibers cross from one side to another at different levels, sensory testing can provide valuable information about the location and extent of injury, based on the presence or absence of specific sensations in different body areas.

Impulses from the **motor cortex** are transmitted principally along the *corticospinal, or pyramidal, tract* to effector muscles. Motor neurons with cell bodies located in the ventral gray matter of the spinal

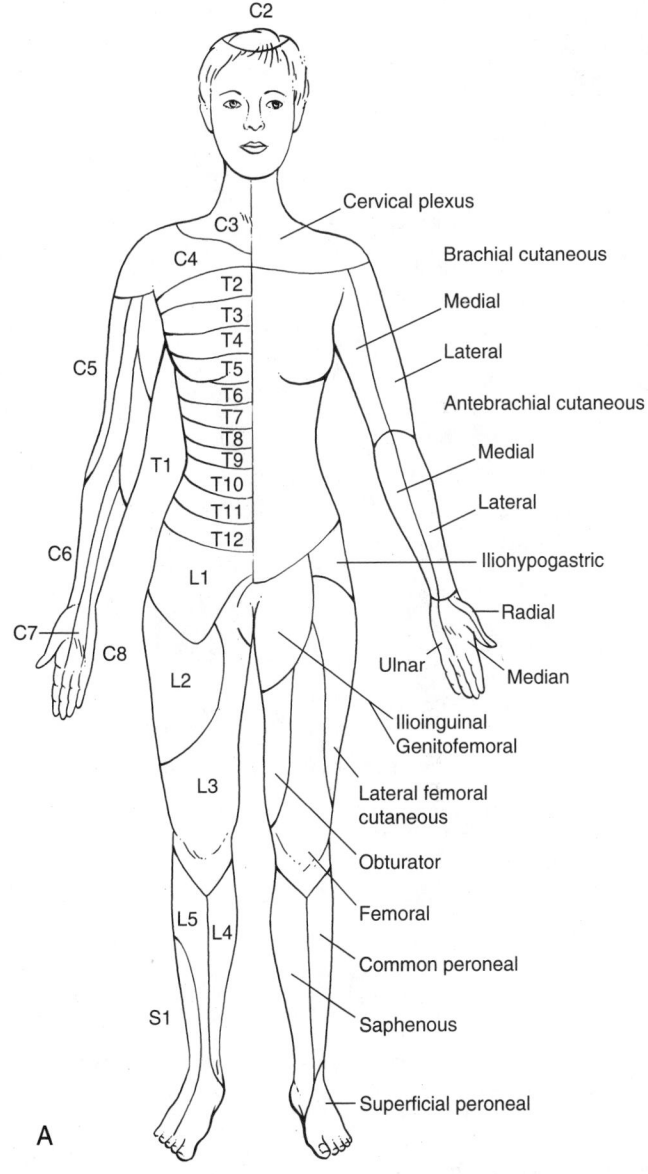

FIGURE 6-2

Segmental distribution of the spinal nerves. **A,** Distribution in the front.

Figure continued on following page

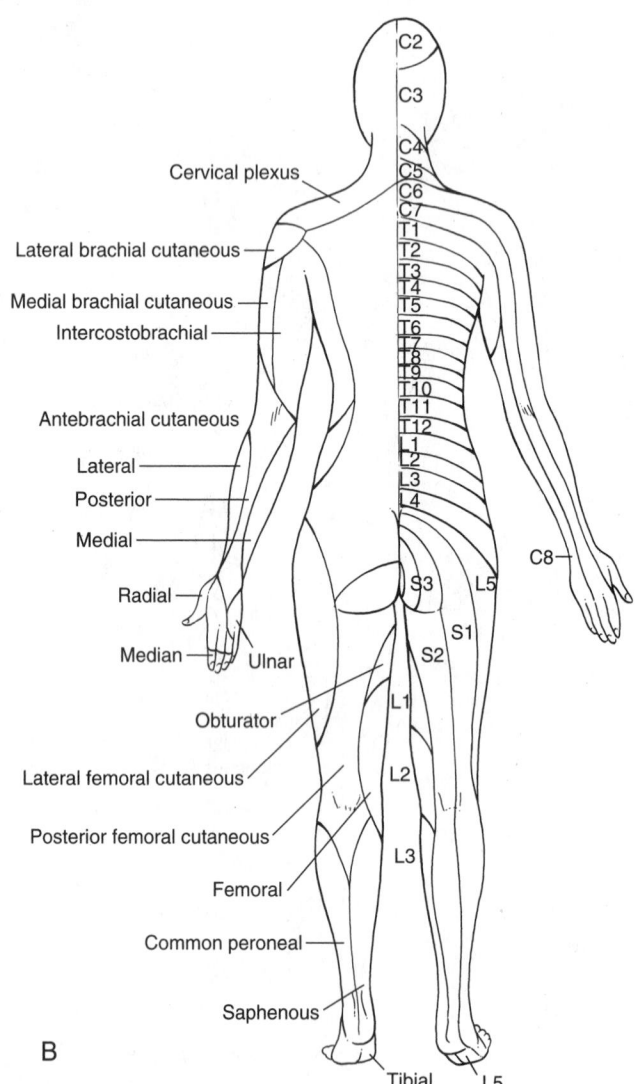

FIGURE 6–2 *Continued*

B, Distribution in the back. (From Swartz, M. H. [1998]. *Textbook of physical diagnosis* [3rd ed., p. 537]. Philadelphia: W. B. Saunders.)

cord that terminate in peripheral nerves innervating skeletal muscles are called *lower motor neurons.* Motor neurons located in the cerebral cortex or brain stem that send axons to lower motor neurons are called *upper motor neurons. Extrapyramidal tracts* primarily coordinate balance and equilibrium and include all other routes in the brain that are involved in motor control.

The PNS also includes the *autonomic nervous system* (ANS). Autonomic nerves innervate all smooth muscle, cardiac muscle, and glands. *Sympathetic* nerves originate in the lower spinal cord (T1–L2) and have an excitatory effect. *Parasympathetic* nerves originate in both sacral and cranial nerve areas, and act in a complementary manner to inhibit function.

Changes with Aging

Neurons do not reproduce. The majority of injured or destroyed cells are replaced by neuroglial cells, which form the support tissue of the nervous system. Lifetime neuronal loss is estimated to be modest in the absence of disease, but it can be severe in the presence of Alzheimer's disease. Losses vary by brain area and may be partially compensated for by dendrite branching. Overall, however, there is some loss of dendrites with normal aging, an imbalance of neurotransmitters, and a decrease in myelin lipids that regulate impulse conduction velocity. These changes combine to affect the communication between neurons and the efficiency and speed of impulse transmission.

The brain diminishes in weight with normal aging. With Alzheimer's disease, brain size decreases and ventricles enlarge. These circumstances may provide some separation between the brain and skull. This allows for greater movement of the brain in acceleration and deceleration injury. Because of these changes, signs and symptoms of space-occupying lesions of the central nervous system may appear subtly, more slowly, and later in the course of injury in the older person.

On autopsy the aged brain shows deposits of amyloid, lipofuscin, senile plaques, and neurofibrillary tangles. These substances are present in those with Alzheimer's disease and also in those with few or no symptoms of dementia. There is some loss of recent memory, especially for large amounts of data, an easier distractibility, quicker fatigue when concentration is required, and slower speed of learning. Cognitive losses, however, are also influenced by social and personality factors, as well as by activity level and disease state.

Pupil size in the elderly person may be smaller than in younger persons, and reaction to light and accommodation may be slower. Visual acuity is also affected by changes in the cornea and lens. Visual fields become limited with loss of periorbital fat and drooping of eyelids. High-frequency hearing loss (presbycusis) occurs. Swallow, gag, and cough reflexes may be less coordinated. Muscle stretch reflexes (see Table 6–5) usually remain intact, except for the Achilles' tendon reflex, which may be absent. There may also be a slowed reflex response to plantar and abdominal stimuli. Sensory discrimination for pressure, pain, and vibration may be diminished, especially in the lower extremities.

Assessments of motor and sensory reactions in any patient, but especially the elderly, must take into consideration several factors that influence the integrity of the neuromuscular system, including the following:

- **Drugs** (CNS stimulants or depressants, sympathetic or parasympathetic stimulants or depressants)
- Diseases that affect **musculoskeletal structures** and motor function such as arthropathies
- **Neurologic diseases,** such as transient ischemic attack (TIA), brain stroke, Parkinson's disease
- **Endocrine diseases** such as thyroid dysfunction or diabetes complications
- **Cardiovascular disease** such as carotid stenosis.

The nurse must carefully evaluate the responses of the elderly patient during initial, focused, and ongoing assessment to differentiate those that indicate evolving pathology from those that represent the effects of underlying disease or drug therapy.

• • •

Physical assessment of the structures of the nervous system in acute and critical care areas requires adaptation of screening techniques used in other clinical settings. Many traditional assessment techniques, because they require the cooperation of a patient who is conscious and cooperative, are not practical in critical care areas. The structure of this section, therefore will be modified to discuss those techniques appropriate for the fully conscious (awake and aware) patient, who is able to receive and follow directions, and those appropriate for the patient with altered consciousness (not awake or unaware), who is unable to follow directions.

Additionally, assessment techniques cannot be organized under the traditional headings of inspection, palpation, percussion, and auscultation. Techniques are organized to proceed from assessments of the highest level of human functioning (cognitive) to the lowest level of human functioning (reflex activity). Such assessments provide a baseline indication of the level and severity of a lesion or injury. Periodic reassessments provide an indication of the progress of a lesion or injury through its effects on function. Finally, it is important when assessing temperature, sensation, movement, and reflex activity to look for changes in response at different levels on the same side of the body (ipsilateral) and to compare responses to identify changes on the opposite (contralateral) side of the body.

The purposes of neurological assessment in the critically ill person are to

- Establish a **baseline** of the individual's BEST neurologic responses to stimulation.
- Determine **early variations** in baseline functioning in order to detect deteriorations in condition at the **earliest stage** possible for effective intervention.
- Aid in **localization of evolving lesions** of the nervous system.

The responsibilities of the nurse for the neurological assessment are to

- Perform assessments that are comprehensive, precise, accurate, and reproducible.
- Record assessments accurately, so that changes in condition may be identified.

TABLE 6–1 Neuromuscular Assessment Techniques, Tips, Geriatric Considerations*

Technique	Performance Tips	Description/Rationale	Geriatric Considerations

1. Vital functions	Injuries extending within the rigid bony structures of the skull and vertebral column are evaluated through their effects on the function of organs they innervate
	
	Look for variability from normal or baseline levels of function; this may indicate changes in the level of injury or the effects of ischemia
	
	Changes in vital functions will vary with the level of the lesion; any of the following findings can be significant
		Causes of injury or extension may include
		• *Solid or vascular lesions or extensions* with resultant increased intracranial pressure and herniation of the brain (e.g., neoplasias, physical trauma, emboli, thrombi, hemorrhage, cerebral edema)
		• *Hypoxia*
		• *Metabolic alterations* such as
		  – Endocrine disorders
		  – Infections or inflammations
		  – Toxins such as drugs or poisons
		  – Prescribed medications having therapeutic or side effects on vital functions
			Assessment of the geriatric patient must take into consideration normal changes with aging in the function of each body system as well as underlying pathologies that may be present in addition to the presenting problem

	Look for	
• **Respiratory function**	• Changes in respiratory rate, depth, and rhythm (see Fig. 6-3) • Loss of respiratory muscle use (see Fig. 6-3)	Changes in respiratory function may be due to • Damage to the cardiorespiratory center in the brain stem • Respiratory disorders • Cardiovascular disorders • Metabolic disorders • Drug effects	Cheyne-Stokes respirations may be normal in the sleeping geriatric patient, and must be interpreted cautiously as a sign of neurologic damage in the absence of other signs and symptoms

• **Cardiovascular function**
 – **Heart rate**
	Look for
	 • Bradycardia
	 • Tachycardia
		Changes in cardiac rate may be due to
		 • Damage to the cardiorespiratory center in the brain stem
		 • Baroreceptor response to changes in intracranial pressure
		   – Bradycardia with increased systolic pressure
		   – Tachycardia with decreased cerebral perfusion pressure (CPP)
		 • Unopposed vagal stimulation
			In the elderly patient, underlying cardiac conduction defects (A-V blocks, bundle branch blocks, sick sinus syndrome) may also be the cause of bradycardia; such defects may also blunt the normal physiologic increase in heart rate with decreased cerebral perfusion
			 Baroreceptor sensitivity may be diminished in the elderly, causing normal tachycardic responses to

Table continued on following page

289

TABLE 6–1 Neuromuscular Assessment Techniques, Tips, Geriatric Considerations *Continued*

CHANGES IN RESPIRATORY PATTERN RELATED TO LEVEL OF BRAIN INJURY

Level	Response	
Cortex:	Cheyne-Stokes respirations	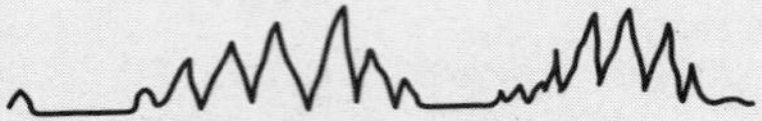
Midbrain:	Central neurogenic hyperventilation	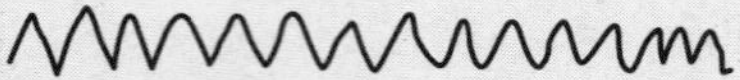
Pons:	Cluster respirations	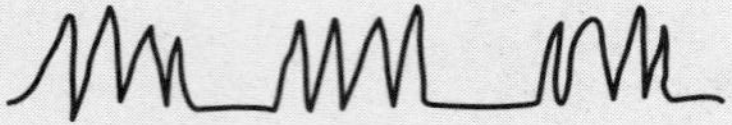
Medulla:	Ataxic or Biot's respirations	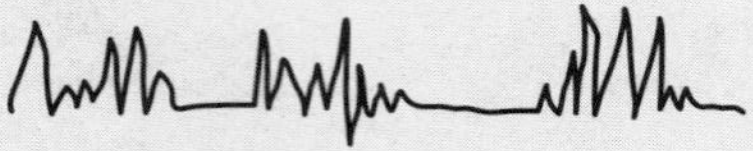

LOSS OF RESPIRATORY MUSCLES BASED ON THE LEVEL OF SPINAL CORD INJURY

Level	Loss
C3–5:	diaphragmatic movement
C5–T1:	pectoralis muscles (chest expansion)
T1–12:	intercostal muscles
T5–12:	abdominal muscles

FIGURE 6–3
Respiratory system responses to central nervous system injuries.

– **Blood pressure**	*Look for* • Hypertension • Hypotension	Changes in blood pressure may be caused by damage to the cardiorespiratory center in the brain stem • Increased systolic blood pressure, widening pulse pressure may be due to increased ICP • Hypotension may be due to decreased peripheral vasoconstriction Vasoinstability is usually present with injury above T6	be diminished; maximal pulse rate also decreases with aging Increased peripheral vascular resistance is a normal change with advancing age Baseline blood pressure and systolic pressure may be higher than expected, especially if hypertension has not been previously diagnosed or treated; this must be distinguished from hypertension associated with neurological disorders
• **Temperature**	*Look for* • Hypothermia or hyperthermia • Changes in core temperature • Changes in temperature, diaphoresis in specific body areas	Changes in temperature may be due to damage to • The temperature regulation center in the brain, which may cause decreased ability of blood vessels to constrict and dilate	Temperature responses may be slower and elevations less dramatic in the older person than in the younger person

Table continued on following page

TABLE 6-1 Neuromuscular Assessment Techniques, Tips, Geriatric Considerations *Continued*

Technique	Performance Tips	Description/Rationale	Geriatric Considerations
		• An area of the spinal cord, which can result in the absence of diaphoresis below the injury level, related to autonomic dysfunction	
• **General behavior**	*Look for* • Uncharacteristic restlessness or calm • Anxiety or confusion • Anger, combativeness, or emotional lability	Changes in behavior can be due to space-occupying lesions, metabolic changes, hypoxemia	Level of consciousness, activity level, and mood may also be affected by depression or underlying dementia
2. Cognitive function: level of consciousness (LOC) • **Arousal** – **To verbal stimuli:** ○ **Eye response** ○ **Verbal response**	*ASSESSMENT TIPS* 1. Begin the assessment as if you were attempting to arouse someone from sleep, first verbally, than	Cognition is the highest level of human function Level of consciousness has two components, which can be evaluated separately:	The elderly have less functional reserve and may develop signs of impaired cognitive function more rapidly than younger persons in the presence of stressors

○ **Motor response**
— **To tactile stimuli:**
  ○ **Eye response**
  ○ **Verbal response**
  ○ **Motor response**

with various levels of touch
2. Gradually increase length of stimulus at each level (see levels below)
3. Proceed through each level of stimuli *until a response is elicited or no response is possible.*
4. At each level look for the following types of response:
   • Eye response
   • Verbal response
   • Motor response
5. It is important to *sustain each stimulus* for 20–30 seconds if necessary to elicit a response; if no response is seen, proceed to the next level of stimulus

1. **Arousal,** or wakefulness
2. **Alertness,** or the awareness of self and the ability to interact purposively with one's surroundings
   Establishing a patient's LOC is fundamental to making decisions about the types of neurological assessments that can be appropriately done and the types of assessment tools that can be used

• It may take many seconds for the brain of the compromised patient to respond to the full level of its potential

When evaluating changes in cognitive function in the elderly patient, take the following into consideration:
• Current disease or injury
• Other conditions in the medical history
  — Concomitant respiratory or cardiovascular problems that may cause cerebral hypoxia
  — Undiagnosed or untreated thyroid conditions
• Fluid or electrolyte imbalance
• Potential adverse effects of current drug therapies on cognitive function (see Geropharmacology in Chapter 3).
• Normal decrease in the number of functioning neurons with age, which can affect the *speed* of impulse transmission and response

Table continued on following page

TABLE 6-1 Neuromuscular Assessment Techniques, Tips, Geriatric Considerations *Continued*

Technique	Performance Tips	Description/Rationale	Geriatric Considerations
	6. Watch while the patient goes through the full range of responses at each level; do not stop until you are certain no further *change* in response to a stimulus will occur	• The final response is the patient's *true* baseline; it is on this basis that succeeding assessments will be evaluated for deterioration or improvement of condition	• Dementia, depression • Sensory deprivations
	7. Assess each stimulus level in the order listed below; do not apply tactile stimuli until after you have attempted verbal stimuli alone; do not apply painful stimuli until you have attempted both verbal and mild tactile stimuli		

Levels of Stimuli

1. Spontaneous response to the environment (light, noise, voices)
2. Response to familiar voices of significant others
3. Response to deliberate verbal stimuli: calling the person's name, beginning with soft, then normal, then loud tone of voice
4. Tactile stimuli, beginning with light touch, then firm touch, then shaking (if not contraindicated)
5. Application of painful stimuli:
   - Centrally to stimulate the brain
   - Peripherally to stimulate the spinal cord

- Levels of stimuli go from higher to lower functional levels
- The *minimal* requirement for full consciousness is intact gray matter of at least one half of the upper brain stem (pontomesencephalic tegmentum) interacting with most or all of one cerebral hemisphere

Assessment of the geriatric patient must take into consideration the normal changes with advancing age and changes produced by disease; limitations that may affect assessment are discussed below

Table continued on following page

TABLE 6-1 Neuromuscular Assessment Techniques, Tips, Geriatric Considerations *Continued*

Technique	Performance Tips	Description/Rationale	Geriatric Considerations
Tactile Stimuli Techniques	Application of the stimuli below are intended to cause pain severe enough to produce a reaction that will help you to clarify the patient's level of consciousness; this will not be enjoyable to you or the patient and may produce bruising; remember, your intention in inflicting pain is to establish a level of arousal; bruising is not your intention but may be an unavoidable result of a good assessment; rotate these techniques, if they are necessary to produce a response, in order to decrease bruising; be sure to explain		

your actions and any skin changes to significant others; document all skin changes as well as patient responses

Central Stimulation
Sternal Rub
1. Grind your knuckle into the midsternal area with sufficient strength to produce an imprint in the patient's soft tissue
2. Sustain the grinding motion for 20–30 seconds, if necessary, to observe the full range of response to persistent stimulation

Trapezius Squeeze
(examiners with long fingernails should take care to avoid damaging the skin)

No response will be elicited from a patient with damage to a sensory or motor pathway at the level of the stimulus

No response will be elicited from a patient with damage to an area of the brain stem through which these sensory and motor pathways travel to and from the cerebral cortex

Table continued on following page

TABLE 6–1 Neuromuscular Assessment Techniques, Tips, Geriatric Considerations *Continued*

Technique	Performance Tips	Description/Rationale	Geriatric Considerations
	1. Pinch about 2 inches (5 cm) of the trapezius muscle with your thumb and two fingers in the angle where the neck and shoulder meet		
	2. Twist the muscle and hold it while you evaluate the full range of the patient's response		
	Supraorbital Pressure (avoid performing this technique in cranial or facial fracture patients or if you have long fingernails)	A nerve runs through this notch; pressure produces sinus pain on the side compressed	
	1. Run finger pad along the orbital rim to a small, midline notch		

2. Apply pressure for 5–10 seconds
3. If no response is elicited on one side, try the other

Peripheral Stimulation: Nail Bed Pressure
1. Place a pencil on base of nail proximal to cuticle
2. With your thumb, roll the pencil up the nail toward the tip with enough force to produce pain
3. Rotate digits with each evaluation of an extremity in order to control bruising

Peripheral stimulation is used to assess the level of response in *unmoving* extremities

Verbal Responses to Stimuli
1. Spontaneous, purposeful response in words or with appropriate head or facial indications of understanding

Verbal response may be limited by
- Injury to oral, neck, or throat structures
- Oral airways, endotracheal tube
- Tracheostomy

Table continued on following page

TABLE 6-1 Neuromuscular Assessment Techniques, Tips, Geriatric Considerations *Continued*

Technique	Performance Tips	Description/Rationale	Geriatric Considerations
	2. Confused verbal response 3. Inappropriate verbal response 4. Incomprehensible verbal response 5. No verbal response	• Preexisting disease affecting speech or cognition.	

	ASSESSMENT TIPS
	1. *Consider characteristics of the individual patient when evaluating responses to verbal stimuli,* such as the ability to
	• Open the eyes
	• See objects in the environment
	• Hear the spoken word (hearing loss may occur with drug therapy, disease, or aging)
		Listed problems will not affect arousal but will require techniques to evaluate cognition that takes these limitations into consideration	Changes with aging that may affect response include
			• *Alterations in vision*
			  – Blurred vision because of pathology or lack of access to usual eyeglasses can cause behaviors that may be mistakenly interpreted as confusion or anxiety by the examiner when they may be due to visual problems
			  – Stroke is a common condition with aging; stroke may

300

- Use language:
  - Comprehend the examiner's language or accent
  - Form words (dysarthria)
  - Comprehend spoken language (receptive aphasia)
  - Verbalize thoughts (expressive aphasia)
  - Move body parts

Also consider
- Possible effects of alcohol, drugs, or therapeutic medications on the ability to respond
- Artificial airways present

affect visual fields (peripheral vision) in many ways (see CN II); this may require the examiner to change position to accommodate possible loss of vision in a specific visual field
- *Alterations in speech* with aging and disease may produce slowed verbal response:
  - Poor articulation may be due to ill-fitting or absent dentures
  - Receptive or expressive aphasia alone will not affect arousal but will require special techniques to evaluate cognition
  - Alzheimer's disease may affect word recognition and response

Table continued on following page

TABLE 6–1 Neuromuscular Assessment Techniques, Tips, Geriatric Considerations *Continued*

Technique	Performance Tips	Description/Rationale	Geriatric Considerations

	2. *Consider characteristics of the individual patient when evaluating response to tactile stimuli:*
	• Loss of sensation in a body part
	• Loss of motor function in a body part
	
	3. *Consider if any eye, verbal, or movement response is deliberate, random, or reflexive*
	• Evaluate the nature of eye contact, with or without accompanying verbal response; is it
	  – Sustained
	  – Random
	  – Absent
		The presence of only reflexive responses is serious in terms of prognosis for survival	• *Alterations in tactile sense with aging and disease may require firmer and more sustained touch to initiate arousal*
			
			The nurse should also be familiar with the patient's medical history, including a history of TIA, CVA, Parkinson's, or other existing disease that might affect verbal or motor response but not be directly related to the current disease process and its extension

- Attempt to distinguish reflexive and deliberate movements
  - Grasping may be reflexive; the ability to *release* a grasp *on command* is deliberate
  - Following a stimulus with the eyes may be reflexive; the ability to *turn away* from a stimulus *on command* is deliberate
- Evaluate the type, speed of initiation, amount, and duration of any eye, verbal, or motor response elicited with stimulation

Table continued on following page

TABLE 6-1 Neuromuscular Assessment Techniques, Tips, Geriatric Considerations *Continued*

Technique	Performance Tips	Description/Rationale	Geriatric Considerations
	• Evaluate the patient's response when the stimulus is terminated (e.g., Is the response sustained or terminated?)		
Motor Responses to Stimuli 1. *Follows commands* • For example, raise two fingers; raise a hand; blink twice • If the patient is able to respond by moving an extremity, this should be followed at some point with an assessment of motor function of all four extremities		*Do not* use the command "squeeze my hand" or "squeeze my fingers," since this is an infantile reflex and may not indicate deliberate action; if it is used, follow it with the request to release the grip, which does require deliberation Verbal or motor response to stimuli may be affected by conditions unrelated to the acute disease state: • Drugs that alter consciousness or produce coma	Geriatric patients may have impaired motor response related to preexisting illnesses such as arthropathies, stroke, or Parkinson's disease; persons with late-stage Alzheimer's disease also have limited abilities to effect a motor response

2. *Localizes response to stimuli*
- Reaches out to stop; attempts to withdraw from the stimulus (the examiner may need to evaluate several areas or extremities if paresis or paralysis is suspected)
- Can also be observed with suctioning, injections, nasogastric tube insertions, etc.

3. *Withdraws from stimuli:* This is not a localized withdrawal; it is a general reaction of the body

- Coexisting diseases that affect the ability to speak or move appropriately

Table continued on following page

TABLE 6-1 Neuromuscular Assessment Techniques, Tips, Geriatric Considerations *Continued*

Technique	Performance Tips	Description/Rationale	Geriatric Considerations
4. *Posturing*		**Posturing:** A pathologic body position or nonverbal response to stimuli	
		Postures are listed from least to most severe re prognosis; the distinction is in upper extremity reaction	
		Postures may be mixed, initially with right and left sides of body reacting differently	
		Cause of Decorticate Posture	
		Lesion of a hemisphere of the cerebral cortex or the corticospinal tracts	
	• Decorticate posture (see Fig. 6–4)		
	– Rigid extension of legs		
	– Internal rotation of legs		
	– *Flexion of elbows,* wrists, fingers, feet (plantar flexion)	***Cause of Decerebrate Posture***	
		Central herniation or lesions of the di- encephalon, upper brain stem (mid-	
	• Decerebrate posture (see Fig. 6–4)		
	– Rigid *extension* of neck, trunk, *arms,* legs		

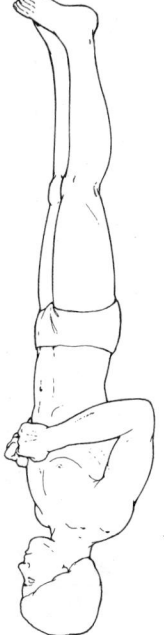

Decorticate posture

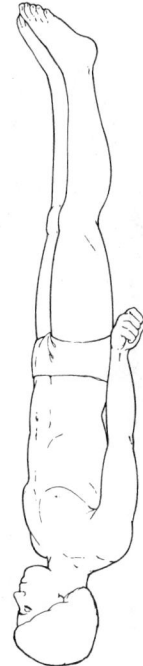

Decerebrate posture

FIGURE 6-4

Characteristics of postures often found in nonresponsive patient. (From Seidel, H. M., Ball, J. W., Dains, J. E., & Benedict, G. W. [1991]. *Mosby's guide to physical examination* [p. 662]. St. Louis: Mosby.)

Table continued on following page

TABLE 6-1 Neuromuscular Assessment Techniques, Tips, Geriatric Considerations *Continued*

Technique	Performance Tips	Description/Rationale	Geriatric Considerations
	– Internal rotation of *arms* and legs – *Flexion* of wrists, fingers, feet, toes (plantar flexed) • Flaccid quadriplegia: Absence of muscle tone and movement in some or all extremities *ASSESSMENT TIPS* 1. Hemiplegia, paraplegia, or quadriplegia must be distinguished from cerebral or spinal shock; this will best be detected by evaluating the motor response of the head as well as of all four extremities for variations in	brain, upper pons) or severe metabolic disorders ***Cause of Flaccid Posture*** *Cerebral shock:* Indicates a nonfunctional brain stem; this may occur with initial injury or may develop before your eyes with succeeding assessments as brain herniation progresses *Spinal shock:* Immediate or delayed response to spinal cord injury that affects motor, sensory, reflex, and sympathetic nervous system function	

reaction to stimulii (see assessment of motor function for additional techniques)

2. Dislocation or fracture of an extremity may cause an extremity not to respond; this must also be distinguished from a plegic response by history or other evaluation (e.g., evidence of deformity from x-ray or scan results)

Best eye, verbal, and motor responses are traditionally recorded using the Glasgow Coma Scale (GCS) or a variant (see Table 6–6, p 371)

If the GCS is used, record *additional notes* about the spe-

The GCS is only a measure of level of consciousness; it *does not* take the place of a complete neurological assessment of the patient

Specific description will allow for accurate and quick recognition of im-

Table continued on following page

TABLE 6-1 Neuromuscular Assessment Techniques, Tips, Geriatric Considerations *Continued*

Technique	Performance Tips	Description/Rationale	Geriatric Considerations
	cific types of stimuli applied to elicit a response, the speed of reactions, stages through which a reaction progresses, and duration of a reaction	provement or deterioration in condition with succeeding assessments	
• Alertness	1. **Alert:** Arousable; responds, appropriately to stimuli 2. **Lethargic:** Arousable but drowsy and falls asleep easily; responds appropriately but slowly to stimuli 3. **Awake:** Arousable: responds to stimuli—may or may not be an appropriate response 4. **Acute confusional state:** Receives information normally, processes it abnormally, responds inappropri-	• Terms used to describe LOC are somewhat subjective, and interpretation may vary with the examiner; definitions presented provide general guidelines • It is *best* to describe the characteristics of a patient's response *specifically* rather than use a label that is not standardized in your facility	In the elderly, confusion may be the result of one or several conditions Consideration must be given to • Adverse drug reactions • Fluid or electrolyte imbalances • Compromised respiratory or cardiovascular function • Inadvertent omission of thyroid hormones for those diagnosed with hypothyroidism or undiagnosed thyroid disease (especially in females) • Infections (e.g., urinary tract, pneumonia)

ately (may be difficult to distinguish from delirium)
5. **Delirium:** Perceives information abnormally, responds inappropriately
6. **Stupor (semicoma):** Briefly arousable with deliberate verbal, tactile, or painful stimuli; responds slowly; response may be appropriate
7. **Coma:** Unable to arouse with stimuli; may respond by posturing (see above)

— **Orientation**
Altered Consciousness
Defer in the patient who does not make a deliberate response to stimuli
Conscious
Evaluate in the patient who makes a deliberate response to stimuli

Awareness of person, place, time, or situation
A patient who is unable to respond verbally may be able to respond
- By deliberate eye movements: side-to-side, up and down, or blinking

Orientations to time and place usually are lost first because they change frequently; person, on the other hand is stable, and situation is somewhat stable; inability to recognize date, time, and place in a critical care area is not, in itself, an abnormal finding

It may be difficult in the elderly person to distinguish among slowed response due to aging, underlying medical conditions, confusion due to sensory deprivation or overload, delirium, depression, or dementia; each of these conditions may affect orientation but

Table continued on following page

TABLE 6-1 Neuromuscular Assessment Techniques, Tips, Geriatric Considerations *Continued*

Technique	Performance Tips	Description/Rationale	Geriatric Considerations
	• By tapping a finger or toes once for "yes" or twice for "no"		not be associated with the acute condition
	Be careful to phrase questions so they can be easily responded to with a "yes" or "no" answer		
	Phrase questions carefully to elicit only one response; avoid "either/or" questions		
	If nonverbal responses are used, clearly define the appropriate response for the patient and practice it prior to asking orientation and memory questions		
	Give the patient time to respond; remember that response time may be slowed with evolving or resolving neurologic deficits		

– Memory

Altered Consciousness
Defer in the patient who does not make a deliberate response to stimuli

Conscious
Evaluate in the patient who makes a deliberate response to stimuli

Ask the patient to recall recent and remote events
Accuracy may need to be verified with significant others
A patient who is unable to respond verbally may be able to respond by
- Deliberate eye movements
- Tapping a finger or toes once for "yes" or twice for "no" (see suggestions under "orientation" above)
Assess new learning by naming three objects (e.g., cat, bell, orange); have the patient repeat the new words immediately; tell the patient that he or she will be asked to recall the words within the next few minutes; evaluate the patient's ability to recall the words

There are three types of memory to be evaluated:
- *Short-term memory:* What happened within the last hours or days (e.g., visitors)
- *Long-term memory:* What happened in the distant past, personally or historically (e.g., past medical history, past presidents)
- *New learning:* e.g, the nurse's name, two to three familiar objects

Persons with Alzheimer's disease or related dementia may be unable to recall recent or remote events; in such cases memory cannot be used as a parameter to evaluate the progression of acute neurologic disorders

Table continued on following page

TABLE 6-1 Neuromuscular Assessment Techniques, Tips, Geriatric Considerations *Continued*

Technique	Performance Tips	Description/Rationale	Geriatric Considerations
	Memory evaluation can be conducted with a translator if necessary		Symptom perception may be altered in the aging patient, who may present with no symptoms or different symptoms than expected (see Chapter 3)
– Symptom analysis			
Altered Consciousness Defer in the patient who does not make a deliberate response to stimuli		In the patient who is not awake or alert, look for changes in usual behavior (e.g., developing restlessness or change in previous level of restlessness) as clues to evolving symptoms	
Conscious Evaluate in the patient who makes a deliberate response to stimuli	*Look for* • Verbal description of symptoms • Intentional indication of distress by nonverbal means when speech is impaired but consciousness is maintained • Changes in usual behavior (thinking, acting) without specific referral to a symptom in the awake but confused patient • Common symptoms of neurologic dysfunction include – Headache		

– Light-headedness
– Vertigo
– Dizziness
– Syncope
– Headache
– Sensory changes
– Weakness
– Altered ability or attempt to move body parts

3. Cranial nerves

Evaluation of cranial nerves will be limited to

- Tests that provide important information on brain stem function in a critically ill person
- Tests that the critically ill person can be reasonably

ASSESSMENT TIPS
1. *Evaluate the symmetry of a response*
- Appropriate responses should be symmetrical
- Describe the nature of each asymmetrical response and whether it was on the right or left side

The 12 pairs of cranial nerves exit at the brain stem; some are sensory, some are motor, and some are mixed nerves; cranial nerves originate as follows:

- CN I, II: Diencephalon
- CN III–IV: Midbrain
- CN V–VIII: Pons
- CN IX–XII: Medulla

Sensory and motor pathways between the peripheral nervous system and

In the geriatric patient there is a normal decrease in the number of functioning neurons with age; this can affect the *speed* of impulse transmission and response during cranial nerve testing

Table continued on following page

TABLE 6–1 Neuromuscular Assessment Techniques, Tips, Geriatric Considerations *Continued*

Technique	Performance Tips	Description/Rationale	Geriatric Considerations
expected to cooperate with or respond to	2. Proximal progression of an abnormal response or progression from unilateral to bilateral indicates decreasing neurological function. 3. Not all cranial nerves can be tested in the unresponsive or uncooperative patient (see left column to identify those tests that can be performed with a patient with altered consciousness [not awake, unaware] and those that can be performed with a patient who is conscious [awake and aware])	the cerebral cortex also pass through the brain stem; loss of brain stem function will affect peripheral responses with or without cerebral cortex damage The level and progression of a lesion can be evaluated by the response of each cranial nerve	

- **Olfactory (CN I)**
- **Optic (CN II)**

Usually deferred by the nurse

Visual Fields

In a conscious patient with suspected loss of visual fields (e.g., CVA or other lesion), it may be helpful to assess for visual field defects

The conscious patient with a visual field defect will be unable to perceive or respond to stimuli presented to the affected field; the practitioner who is unaware of this defect may incorrectly interpret a lack of response to a person or gesture as impaired arousal and alertness rather than impaired vision

Critical care settings do not allow for sophisticated tests for visual field defects; gross

Loss of function of this cranial nerve suggests a lesion or extension in the area of the diencephalon or along the path traveled by this nerve to the sensory visual cortex

Because each eye is innervated by both optic nerves, injury to the right or left optic nerve posterior to the optic chiasm may affect the contralateral (opposite) fields of vision in *both* eyes; injury to the right or left optic nerve anterior to the optic chiasm may produce complete loss of vision on the ipsilateral (same) side (see Table 6–3, p 366)

Altered Consciousness

Defer

Conscious

Visual fields (tests for visual acuity are usually deferred in the critically ill; evaluation of visual fields, however, may provide the nurse with information about the extent of a brain lesion as well as some explanation of the patient's response to visual stimuli)

Table continued on following page

TABLE 6–1 Neuromuscular Assessment Techniques, Tips, Geriatric Considerations *Continued*

Technique	Performance Tips	Description/Rationale	Geriatric Considerations
	evaluation for defects might include the following		
	ASSESSMENT TIPS		
	Lateral temporal loss:		
	Approach the bed from the right or left side and note if the patient responds to your presence		
	All fields		
	1. Test each eye separately; cover the opposite eye		
	2. Have the patient focus on your finger or other object (e.g., penlight, water pitcher); bring your rapidly moving index and middle fingers into each quarter of the visual field for each		

eye; have the patient tell you when he or she is aware of the object; compare this to standard measurements or your own peripheral vision; during the test assure that the patient's gaze does not move from the object on which it should be focused

Altered Consciousness
Fundoscopic examination

Conscious
Fundoscopic examination

Fundoscopic Examination
Provides direct visualization of the retina of the eye, including blood vessels and optic nerve fibers

The optic disc with its physiologic cup is the site at which the retinal nerve fibers unite and exit the eye as the optic nerve
- A deformed disc may indicate demyelination of the nerve
- Papilledema or swelling of the optic disc may indicate increased ICP transmitted to the eye from

A normal fundoscopic examination in the elderly may reveal
- A red reflex that is totally or partially obscured by cataract formation
- Less distinct, paler optic disc margins than in younger adults
- Atherosclerotic changes in vessels, including slight narrowing

Table continued on following page

TABLE 6–1 Neuromuscular Assessment Techniques, Tips, Geriatric Considerations *Continued*

Technique	Performance Tips	Description/Rationale	Geriatric Considerations
	ASSESSMENT TIPS 1. Assure that contact lenses have been removed from the critically ill patient 2. When using the ophthalmoscope, darken the room to enhance pupil dilation 3. If pupils are small, use the smaller diameter white-light aperture instead of the larger white light, which further constricts the pupil 4. Bleeding into the vitreous humor or severe	the subarachnoid space, which extends along the optic nerve path to the occipital lobe • Increased ICP causes ophthalmic vein compression, transudation of fluid into the optic disc, blurred margins and swelling of the disc, and late hemorrhages on the retina	and increased arteriolar light reflex from thickened walls • Increased A-V nicking • Absence of the foveal light reflex in the macula (not visible during routine examination) • Yellow-white drusen bodies in the macular areas

cataracts will preclude retinal examination

5. Examine the patient's right eye with the scope held to your right eye; the left with the scope held to your left eye

6. Stand no more than 10 degrees to the side of the patient, or you will miss the optic disc altogether as you approach the patient

7. Evaluate the red reflex: it should be round and completely red-orange

8. Evaluate the optic disc for
   – Roundness
   – Symmetry
   – Absence of swelling (papilledema)

Table continued on following page

TABLE 6–1 Neuromuscular Assessment Techniques, Tips, Geriatric Considerations *Continued*

Technique	Performance Tips	Description/Rationale	Geriatric Considerations
	9. Evaluate the veins (large red) and arteries (smaller and with a light reflex down the middle) for constriction, bulging, A-V nicking 10. Evaluate the background of the eye for hemorrhage, exudates 11. The macula *will not* be visible unless pupils are dilated		
• Oculomotor (CN III) • Trochlear (CN IV) • Abducens (CN VI)	Loss of function of these three cranial nerves suggests a lesion or extension in the area of the midbrain or along the path traveled by these nerves	Reaction of the pupil to light and accommodation presumes an intact CN II (optic nerve), which discerns light; because of the pattern of innervation of the optic nerve (see	In the aged patient, normal pupil size may be small and light reaction minimal and difficult to discern

to the visual or from the motor cortex

The motor branches of CN III innervate

- Pupil constrictor (parasympathetic) and pupil dilator (sympathetic) muscles of the iris, which cause the pupil to respond to changes in light (pupillary light reaction) perceived by CN II

- Ciliary muscles, which adjust the lens for the distance of an object (accommodation) in the conscious patient with intact CN II

- Most extraocular muscles (medial, superior and inferior recti, and inferior oblique), which move the

Table 6-3, p 366), normal pupillary light response is both direct (the eye stimulated) and consensual (the opposite eye); light responses will vary with lesions at different sites along the route of the optic nerve: retina, optic chiasm, optic tracts, through the thalamus, temporal and parietal lobes, to the visual cortex in the occipital lobe (see Table 6-3, p 366)

Table continued on following page

TABLE 6-1 Neuromuscular Assessment Techniques, Tips, Geriatric Considerations *Continued*

Technique	Performance Tips	Description/Rationale	Geriatric Considerations
	eyes through the six cardinal fields of gaze in the conscious patient • Levator palpebrae and superior tarsal smooth muscles, which keep the eyelid open (prevent ptosis) in the awake patient CN IV and VI assist in extraocular movement: • CN IV: Superior oblique muscle • CN VI: Lateral rectus muscle		
Altered Consciousness Pupil shape Pupil size Pupil equality Pupil reactivity to light (direct)	Before you begin, check for a history of blindness or the presence of a prosthetic eyeball; each will provide an abnormal result during testing	Pupil assessment is one of the most important of the cranial nerve evaluations because it is a reflex and is easily evaluated even in the comatose patient; CN III is located	*Shape:* It is not uncommon in the elderly to find an irregular pupil as the result of previous eye surgery such as an iridectomy

Conscious
Pupil shape
Pupil size
Pupil equality
Pupil reactivity to light (direct and consensual)
Pupil accommodation
Eyelid ptosis
Extraocular movements

Shape: Pupils are normally round
Size: Pupil size varies with amount of light reaching the retina

ASSESSMENT TIP
Evaluate size in ambient (natural) light shining with equal intensity on each eye

Equality: In equal light, pupil sizes should match

ASSESSMENT TIP
Make certain that the light source is of the same intensity for each eye, or the measurement of pupil size will be unequal

Reactivity: can be tested in ambient (natural) light, but more

high in the brain stem and is often affected early in the course of a disease; pupil evaluation may detect subtle changes in condition
Anisocoria is the term used to describe unequal pupils; this occurs normally in 5%–10% of the population
Because CN III passes through the tentorium, pupil changes may be the first sign of hypoxia as well as of increased ICP and herniation as the nerve becomes compressed; pupils will become dilated and fixed ("blown") on the same side as the herniation
Pupil reactivity may be an indication of level and side of herniation:
- *Thalamus:* Small pupils that react to light
- *Midbrain:* Fixed midpoint to dilated pupils with no light reaction

Size, equality, reactivity: Pupil size may diminish with aging, and reactivity may, therefore, be more difficult to evaluate without intense dark-light contrasts
A cataract may affect the pupil in several ways:
- It may appear inordinately large, even appearing to obliterate the iris
- It may give the pupil a light opaque appearance
- It may prevent the affected pupil from reacting to light
Pupil size and reactivity can also be affected by drugs that have a direct or side effect of miosis (pupil constriction) or mydriasis (pupil dilation)
Common drugs administered in critical care settings that may affect pupil size and reactivity:

Table continued on following page

TABLE 6-1 Neuromuscular Assessment Techniques, Tips, Geriatric Considerations *Continued*

Technique	Performance Tips	Description/Rationale	Geriatric Considerations

	intense light (pen or flashlight) should be used if reaction is difficult to see	• *Pons, cerebellum:* Fixed pinpoint with no light reaction
		• *Medulla:* Fixed midpoint to dilated pupils with no light reaction
			• Miotics include
			  – Atropine
			  – Barbiturates
			  – Opiates
			  – Neuromuscular blockers
			  – Medications for glaucoma
			• Mydriatics include amphetamines and other stimulants

	ASSESSMENT TIPS 1. The contrast between dark and light in the testing environment can be enhanced by • Turning off room lights • Closing blinds, drapes tightly • Closing the patient's eyelids for several seconds prior to testing • Having the conscious patient look to a distant object over your shoulder (pupils dilate		

when looking at distant objects) before introducing a light source
2. In the conscious patient, bring the light source in from the side of the patient's head to avoid an accommodation reaction (pupil constriction) from the patient's natural attempt to focus on you or the light (a near object)
3. Record the speed of reaction to light (brisk, sluggish, nonreactive, reactive to light with immediate redilation without removal of light source)
4. In the conscious patient, check for consensual response to light by briefly

Table continued on following page

TABLE 6–1 Neuromuscular Assessment Techniques, Tips, Geriatric Considerations *Continued*

Technique	Performance Tips	Description/Rationale	Geriatric Considerations
	shining the light in one eye and watching for constriction of the pupil of the other eye 5. Record the type and amount of reaction of *each pupil to light* 6. During evaluation of pupils in the patient with altered consciousness, look for complete closure of eyelids following the examination; if the patient is unable to keep eyelids closed, initiate nursing interventions to prevent drying of the corneas		

7. During evaluation of eyes and pupils in the conscious patient, note if any portion of the sclera (white) of the eyes is visible above the iris with eye movement; this is called "lid lag" and indicates exophthalmos, or protruding eyes, which may occur with hyperthyroidism

Altered Consciousness
Defer
Conscious
Extraocular movements

Extraocular Movements
In the awake and alert patient, evaluation of extraocular movements may provide some indication of type and level of injury

Failure of an eye or eyes to move smoothly through the six cardinal fields of gaze indicates damage to the extraocular muscle(s) involved or to the respective cranial nerve that innervates the muscle(s) (see Fig. 6-5)

Table continued on following page

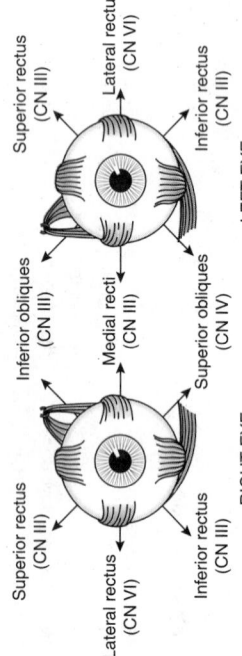

FIGURE 6–5

Eye movements controlled by cranial nerve innervation of extraocular muscles. (Adapted from Swartz, M. H. [1998]. *Textbook of physical diagnosis* [ed. 3, p. 140]. Philadelphia: W. B. Saunders.)

ASSESSMENT TIPS

1. Do not let the patient move the head from midline while following your finger movements

2. Hold your finger or pen-light at least 24 inches from the patient's eyes while performing the test

3. Bring the eyes to the limit of each of the six fields of gaze

4. It is not unusual to observe brief nystagmus at the extremes of lateral gaze in most individuals

5. Normal eye movements are smooth and described as *intact*; any asymmetrical eye movement should be described specifically

Nystagmus is defined as rapid, involuntary eye movements; they can be observed as eyes track the examiners finger

Nystagmus can be caused by vestibular or neural conditions; some nystagmus is hereditary

331

TABLE 6-1 Neuromuscular Assessment Techniques, Tips, Geriatric Considerations *Continued*

Technique	Performance Tips	Description/Rationale	Geriatric Considerations
	6. Abnormal pupil movements can be described by form (horizontal, vertical, rotary, mixed), type (pendular or jerky), direction (uni- or bidirectional), and speed		
• Trigeminal (CN V) • Facial (CN VII)	Testing a sensory branch of CN V requires an intact motor branch of CN VII to evaluate the response		Loss of function of these two cranial nerves suggests a lesion or extension in the area of the pons or along the path traveled by these nerves to the sensory or from the motor area of the frontal lobe of the cerebral cortex (e.g., upper motor neuron palsy or cerebral shock with flaccid paralysis)

Altered Consciousness Facial symmetry at rest and with respiration (VII) Corneal reflex (V) Eyelid closure (VII) **Conscious** Facial symmetry at rest and with movement and respiration (VII) Facial sensation (V) Corneal reflex (V) Eyelid closure against resistance (VII)	In the conscious and unconscious patient, look for facial symmetry at rest and with movement In the conscious patient, one may test for facial sensation (see sensory testing below for technique) and look for facial symmetry at rest and with movement In the unconscious patient, facial sensation may be tested by testing the corneal reflex (CN V) and response evaluated (CN VII) by testing the corneal reflex (V) and looking for upward deviation of the eyes (III) and bilateral blink (VII) as a normal response	Possible signs of facial paralysis include • Facial droop • Eyelid droop • Mouth droop • Loss of movement on one side of the face • Air escaping from one side of the mouth with exhalation • Cheek puffing out on exhalation Facial sensation to light and deep touch may be diminished or lost with • A history of Bell's palsy (CN V) • A history of herpes zoster affecting the facial nerves • Brain stroke If facial sensation is lost because of stroke, the loss will be on the same side as the lesion, and on the opposite side of any extremity paresthesia or paralysis	Parkinson's disease may eventually limit the ability to change facial expression; these patients have a masklike expression Facial asymmetry may also be due to loss of several or all teeth

Table continued on following page

TABLE 6–1 Neuromuscular Assessment Techniques, Tips, Geriatric Considerations *Continued*

Technique	Performance Tips	Description/Rationale	Geriatric Considerations
	Corneal Reflex *ASSESSMENT TIPS* 1. Pull a piece of cotton to form a pointed wisp 2. *Without* touching the eye lashes (gently lift the skin of the upper lid just below the brow, leaving enough slack for the lid to close), touch the cornea (clear covering over the iris and pupil) with the wisp of cotton 3. Watch for upward deviation of the eyes and bilateral lid closure	The response will be diminished or absent in patients wearing contact lenses or in patients who have worn them over a long period of time	Corneal stimulation may need to be more prolonged in the elderly before a response is elicited

Grimacing to Supraorbital Pressure

May also be used to evaluate these cranial nerves:

- Run finger pad along the orbital rim to a small midline notch
- Apply pressure for 5–10 seconds
- Look for facial grimace in response to stimuli
- Test each side separately and note response

A nerve runs through this notch; pressure produces sinus pain on the side compressed

Any grimace will be asymmetrical with acute hemiplegia and absent with midbrain or cortex damage

• **Acoustic (CN VIII)**
Altered Consciousness

Defer or
Oculocephalic reflex
Oculovestibular reflex
(these are special tests and not a routine part of the neuromuscular examination)

Vestibular Response

Oculocephalic reflex (doll's eyes reflex): *This examination can only be performed with a patient with no known pathology of the cervical spine*

This examination can only be accurately performed in the unconscious patient

Lack of contraversive or symmetrical movement or no response to head movement with eyes remaining

Table continued on following page

TABLE 6–1 Neuromuscular Assessment Techniques, Tips, Geriatric Considerations *Continued*

Technique	Performance Tips	Description/Rationale	Geriatric Considerations
		midline is considered indicative of brain-stem damage	
	ASSESSMENT TIPS 1. Hold the head in a neutral position in both your hands 2. Gently hold the eyelids open if necessary 3. Briskly rotate the head side to side or up and down 4. The eyes will normally move opposite to the head movement		
Oculovestibular reflex (ice water calorics)		The test artificially sets up convection currents that circulate fluid in the semilunar canal	
	ASSESSMENT TIPS The nurse may perform or assist according to hospital policy	Vestibular (sensory) nerves are located in the labyrinth of the inner ear and connect with cranial nerves that control extraocular movements	

1. Prior to testing, examine the ears with an otoscope; cerumen occluding the tympanic membrane must be carefully removed for the test to be effective; the test should be deferred if perforation of the tympanic membrane or cerebrospinal fluid is visualized
2. Elevate the head to 30 degrees to position the horizontal semilunar canal vertically
3. Irrigate each ear with 5 ml of ice water
4. Look for normal or abnormal responses; you may need to observe for 20–30 seconds before a

The major ocular sign of vestibular stimulation is nystagmus

Abnormal or no response indicates a supratentorial lesion at some point along this reflex arc

Response may require up to 200 ml of water or be absent in the patient in deep coma, including drug overdose and barbiturate coma

Table continued on following page

TABLE 6-1 Neuromuscular Assessment Techniques, Tips, Geriatric Considerations *Continued*

Technique	Performance Tips	Description/Rationale	Geriatric Considerations
	response occurs (see below)		
	5. Test both ears		
	Result		
	Within normal limits		
	Nystagmus		
	Slow to stimulus side		
	Fast away from stimulus side		
	No net deviation of the eyes		
	Lethargy		
	Slow to stimulus side		
	Less pronounced movement away from stimulus side		

Deviation of eyes to stimulus

Stupor   Deviation of eyes to stimulus

Coma   No movement with stimulus

The individual functions of these nerves need not be isolated; together they innervate the muscles of the palate, pharynx, and larynx

- **Glossopharyngeal (CN IX)**
- **Vagus (CN X)**

Altered Consciousness
Gag reflex
Swallow
Cough

Conscious
Gag reflex
Swallow
Cough
Hoarseness

ASSESSMENT TIPS

1. In the comatose patient, pull down on the chin to open the mouth
2. Stimulate the uvula and watch for it to rise symmetrically; no movement indicates the gag reflex is inadequate to protect from aspiration

Swallow and gag reflexes may be lost with damage to the medullary area of the brain stem or with upper motor neuron damage to the sensory or motor areas of the cerebral cortex

Asymmetrical response suggests damage involving the cranial nerve on the side with limited pharyngeal movement

Coordination of swallowing may be diminished with aging

Table continued on following page

339

TABLE 6-1 Neuromuscular Assessment Techniques, Tips, Geriatric Considerations *Continued*

Technique	Performance Tips	Description/Rationale	Geriatric Considerations
	3. If the uvula rises, stimulate it sufficiently to cause a gag response 4. Do not stimulate enough to produce vomiting, as this may result in aspiration 5. Look for asymmetry of response		
• **Spinal Accessory (CN XI)** *Altered Consciousness* Defer *Conscious* Defer or perform	Strength of sternomastoid and trapezius muscles *ASSESSMENT TIPS* 1. Have patient shrug shoulders while you attempt to hold them in place (trapezius)	Response will be diminished or absent with damage to CN XI or its pathways	Strength against resistance may be diminished because of loss of contractility with normal aging

- **Hypoglossal (CN XII)**

2. Have the patient turn the head right or left while you attempt to hold it in place (sternomastoid)
3. Estimate strength against resistance (see below)

Strength of the tongue muscle against resistance and with formation of words

ASSESSMENT TIPS
1. Have the conscious patient stick out the tongue
2. Have the conscious patient push the tongue against resistance of a tongue blade or the buccal mucosa to measure strength against resistance
3. Observe word formation in the conscious patient

Altered Consciousness
Defer
Conscious
Tongue symmetry, movement, strength
Speech and articulation

Abnormal responses include
- The tongue deviates to the weak side
- Tongue strength is weak on the affected side

In a patient who can speak, word formation requires CN VII, IX, X, XII

In the elderly patient the tongue may normally have a slight tremor with the effort of pushing against resistance
Excessive tremor or weakness should be considered abnormal
If a patient has difficulty forming words (dysarthria) consider
- Cerebral vascular accident
- Previous oral injuries or surgeries

Table continued on following page

TABLE 6–1 Neuromuscular Assessment Techniques, Tips, Geriatric Considerations *Continued*

Technique	Performance Tips	Description/Rationale	Geriatric Considerations
		Labial sounds (me, be) = VII Guttural sounds = IX, X Hoarseness = X Nasal speech = X Lingual sounds (la) = XII Word recognition = cerebral cortex	• Loss of teeth • Absent dentures
4. Sensory function (somatic): **Light touch, pressure, vibratory sense** *Altered Consciousness* See central and peripheral stimulation to assess arousal, above *Conscious* Light touch Pain Vibratory sense	Testing of the sensory branches of the cranial nerves has already been accomplished above; sensory testing here is of the trunk and extremities Sensation can be lost because of damage to • A specific peripheral nerve • A segment of the spinal	Somatic sensory stimuli enter the central nervous system through the dorsal or posterior root Two major tracts carry sensory (afferent) nerve fibers to the sensory cortex: 1. *The spinothalamic tracts* • Located in the anterolateral aspects of the white matter of the	There is a normal decrease in the number of functioning neurons with age, which can affect the *speed* of impulse transmission to the sensory cortex and subsequent response Light touch may need to be administered with slightly more intensity with aging patients

cord containing a spinal nerve root that innervates a specific band of dermis (dermatome)
- A segment of the spinal cord above the peripheral nerve or dermatome affected
- Damage to the brain stem, through which sensory (afferent) stimuli travel to the sensory cortex
- Damage to the sensory cortex of the parietal lobe

Loss of sensation may occur even in the presence of normal motor function

Loss of sensation may prevent motor response to a stimulus even with an intact motor pathway

spinal cord, they carry sensations of touch, pain, and temperature
- Fibers cross to the opposite side of the cord within 1–2 segments of their entry
- Produce contralateral sensory loss of touch, pain, and temperature sensation below the level of a lesion

2. The posterior (dorsal) columns
- Located in the posterior aspects of the white matter of the spinal cord
- Carry sensations of proprioception, pressure, and vibration
- Fibers cross to the opposite side of the body at the medulla
- Produce ipsilateral (same-side) loss of proprioception, pressure and vibration below the level of the lesion

Responses to deep pain and temperature may be diminished in the elderly

Common problems in older persons that may affect sensory function include
- Peripheral neuropathies such as might be caused by diabetes, alcoholism, nutritional deficiencies
- Stroke
- Herpes zoster (shingles)

Elderly patients may tire easily with extensive sensory testing; this may result in inaccurate evaluation; to prevent this, do the following:
- Perform sensory testing early in the examination
- Perform sensory testing as a separate examination when the patient is not fatigued

Table continued on following page

TABLE 6–1 Neuromuscular Assessment Techniques, Tips, Geriatric Considerations *Continued*

Technique	Performance Tips	Description/Rationale	Geriatric Considerations
	ASSESSMENT TIPS 1. The patient's eyes should be closed during testing 2. Compare sensations on contralateral body parts 3. Test for light touch with a wisp of cotton whisked lightly over a small patch of skin • Avoid callused areas • If extremities are cold, testing will not be accurate 4. Test for pain sensation with a large-bore sterile needle or a clean safety pin		• Do not perform sensory testing in a noisy or otherwise distracting environment where other sensations compete for the patient's attention

- Avoid puncturing the skin
- Discard the needle or pin immediately after use to prevent inadvertent transmission of blood-borne infections from accidental skin puncture

5. Test vibratory sense by setting a low-frequency tuning fork (128 Hz, 256 Hz) in motion and placing it on a bony prominence of each upper extremity (wrist, elbow) and lower extremity (metatarsal, ankle, knee); ask the patient to close his or her eyes and tell you if he or she can feel the vibration

Table continued on following page

TABLE 6-1 Neuromuscular Assessment Techniques, Tips, Geriatric Considerations *Continued*

Technique	Performance Tips	Description/Rationale	Geriatric Considerations
	and to tell you when it stops; stop the vibration by touching the tines 6. Clearly describe or map areas of sensory loss 7. Compare the area of sensory loss with a dermatome chart (see Fig. 6–2) or known innervation patterns of specific peripheral nerves		
5. Motor function (somatic)	Testing of the motor branches of the cranial nerves has already been accomplished above; motor testing here is of the trunk and extremities Movement can be lost because of damage to	Somatic motor stimuli exit the central nervous system through the ventral or anterior root of the spinal cord. The major tracts carry motor (efferent) impulses from the motor cortex in the posterior frontal and anterior parietal lobes to the effector organs	There is a normal decrease in the number of functioning neurons with age, which can affect the *speed* of impulse transmission and response

- The motor cortex of the frontal and parietal lobes
- The brain stem, through which motor (efferent) stimuli travel from the motor cortex
- An upper motor neuron (UMN)
- A segment of the spinal cord above the peripheral nerve or myotome affected
- A specific peripheral motor nerve
- A segment of the spinal cord containing a spinal nerve root that innervates a specific band of muscle (myotome); a neuron at this level is called a lower motor neuron (LMN)

The corticospinal tracts
- Are located in the posterolateral area of the spinal cord
- Conduct impulses to effect voluntary movement
- Cross in the brain stem at approximately the level of the medulla
- Synapse in the anterior gray matter before leaving the cord

Table continued on following page

347

TABLE 6–1 Neuromuscular Assessment Techniques, Tips, Geriatric Considerations *Continued*

Technique	Performance Tips	Description/Rationale	Geriatric Considerations
	Loss of voluntary movement may occur even with an intact sensory pathway		
	Paralytic drugs will prevent response even in the presence of intact motor pathways		
• **General**	Evaluate for fractures or dislocations	Above this synapse motor neurons are termed *upper motor neurons* (UMN), and below they are termed *lower motor neurons* (LMN)	
	Look for muscle atrophy or hypertrophy	Injuries to these neurons have differing clinical signs (see Clinical Findings in Motor Neuron Damage below)	
	Look for spontaneous extremity movement		
	Evaluate extremity movement in response to stimuli (see above)		
	Look for asymmetry in deliberate or reflexive extremity movement		

• Tone

Altered Consciousness

Passive range of motion

Limb-drop tests

Conscious

Passive range of motion

Limb-drop tests

Active range of motion

ASSESSMENT TIPS
1. When moving a joint through its range of motion, support the areas distal and, where appropriate, proximal to each joint and protect the patient from injury and protect the patient from pain
2. Observe muscles for obvious atrophy
3. Palpate muscles for tone, bulk, and pain

Tone is initially evaluated by passively moving the extremities

Tone is loosely defined as subtle muscular resistance to passive movement

Tone is largely regulated by stimulation of LMNs, by receptors in muscles and skin

Causes of spasticity usually originate in lesions of the pyramidal tract

Causes of rigidity usually originate in lesions of the extrapyramidal tracts

Causes of flaccidity usually originate in lesions of LMNs or impulses arriving via the dorsal roots

Flaccid paralysis also occurs with spinal shock and is accompanied by loss of sensation and reflexes, bradycardia and hypotension, and may last for 7–10 days after injury

Parkinson's disease is accompanied by increased muscle tone, causing a characteristic rigidity with passive or active range of motion; this produces a cogwheel or ratchetlike movement when joints are ranged

Arthritic changes can limit range of motion with grating of the articular surfaces of joints

Limited use of muscles will produce muscle atrophy; asymmetric muscle mass can be a clue to chronic disability (greater than a few weeks)

Patients with advanced Alzheimer's disease may display fluctuating resistance to joint movement (Gegenhalten)

Table continued on following page

TABLE 6–1 Neuromuscular Assessment Techniques, Tips, Geriatric Considerations *Continued*

Technique	Performance Tips	Description/Rationale	Geriatric Considerations
	4. Observe muscles for fasciculations 5. Observe head and extremities for tremors; describe tremors (see Table 6–2, p 365)	The normal finding is subtle resistance to movement Abnormal findings include • Spasticity: increased muscle resistance to brisk movement of a joint, which quickly fades away • Rigidity: increased muscle resistance to passive movement of a joint that is sustained throughout the range	

- Flaccidity: absence of resistance to passive movement

Evaluate for flaccid paralysis in a limb without tone; this can be done with the following techniques

In deep coma with flaccid paralysis these tests are invalid, as all extremities will be atonic

Wrist-Drop Test

ASSESSMENT TIPS
1. Grasp both forearms above the wrist
2. Hold the forearms vertical
3. A hemiplegic wrist will drop at right angles
4. A nonhemiplegic wrist will remain somewhat vertical

Table continued on following page

TABLE 6–1 Neuromuscular Assessment Techniques, Tips, Geriatric Considerations *Continued*

Technique	Performance Tips	Description/Rationale		Geriatric Considerations

Clinical Findings in Motor Neuron Damage

		UMN	LMN
Paralysis		Spastic	Flaccid
Muscle atrophy		Minimal	Severe
Fasciculations		Absent	Present
Reflex activity		Hyper	Hypo
Babinski's reflex		May be absent	Absent

Arm-Drop Test

ASSESSMENT TIPS
1. Grasp both forearms
2. Raise forearms vertically
3. Release both arms simultaneously
4. A hemiplegic arm drops limply
5. A nonhemiplegic arm drops more slowly

Leg-Drop Test

ASSESSMENT TIPS
1. Flex the patient's knees and support them on one forearm
2. Grasp one ankle at a time and extend it

Injury to the spinal cord will be reflected in diminished or absent motor activity of muscle groups innervated by nerves at and below the level of injury; normal motor function by spinal cord segment is illustrated in Table 6–4, page 368

	3. Release the lower leg 4. A hemiplegic leg drops limply and loudly to the bed 5. A nonhemiplegic leg drops more slowly and softly	
• **Strength**		
Altered Consciousness		
Defer	Strength is evaluated by having the patient push or pull against resistance; patients may also grasp or pinch the examiner's fingers; as far as possible, upper and lower extremities should be tested separately and results compared; strength is graded with one of two scales	
Conscious		
Strength against resistance		Grade strength against resistance in the conscious patient carefully, looking for subtle changes (e.g., 5/5 to 4/5 or 100% to 75%)
Pronator drift		It may be normal for the healthy older person to have strength against resistance of 4/5 because of loss of muscle contractility with normal aging

Table continued on following page

353

TABLE 6-1 Neuromuscular Assessment Techniques, Tips, Geriatric Considerations *Continued*

Technique	Performance Tips		Description/Rationale	Geriatric Considerations
	5-Point Scale	% Scale		
	0/5	0%	No voluntary movement of an extremity	
	1/5	10%	Contraction of extremity muscles without movement of the extremity	
	2/5	25%	Movement of an extremity side-to-side but not against gravity	
	3/5	50%	Movement of an extremity against gravity but with out resistance applied	
	4/5	75%	Movement of an extremity against gravity and against mild resistance applied by the examiner	
	5/5	100%	Movement of an extremity against gravity and against strong resistance applied by the examiner	

	Pronator Drift Test	This test detects subtle loss of muscle strength in the cooperative patient
	ASSESSMENT TIPS 1. Have the conscious patient hold both arms outstretched with palms up 2. Have patient close eyes 3. Watch for lowering of an arm or drift of a wrist toward palm-down	
6. Reflex Activity • **Deep tendon reflexes** (also called muscle-stretch reflexes, or MSRs)		Loss of a muscle-stretch reflex indicates that a component of a reflex arc is damaged
	ASSESSMENT TIPS The likelihood of eliciting a deep tendon reflex may be increased with the following techniques:	MSRs are elicited by stimulation of sensory receptors deep in the skin, which stimulate an immediate motor response (reflex arc)
Altered Consciousness MSRs ***Conscious*** MSRs		There is a normal decrease in the number of functioning neurons with age, which can affect the *speed* of impulse transmission and response

Table continued on following page

TABLE 6-1 Neuromuscular Assessment Techniques, Tips, Geriatric Considerations *Continued*

Technique	Performance Tips	Description/Rationale	Geriatric Considerations
	1. Do *not* announce to a conscious patient your intent to test reflexes; the patient will tense 2. Identify the location of each tendon to be struck 3. Hold the extremity so that the tendon is slightly stretched (intermediate between full extension and full flexion) 4. Hold the portion of the extremity expected to react loosely and clearly within your line of sight; do not stand where you might get hit by a hypertonic response	The response is elicited without the stimulus traveling up the central nervous system to the brain; it does, however, require some intact cortical function MSRs will be absent at or above the level of damage with LMN disease (see Table 6–5, p 368) MSRs may be hyperactive in acute UMN disease MSRs may be normal, diminished, or increased in cerebral shock In spinal shock, reflexes will be lost below the level of injury and will usually return in an inferior to superior direction MSRs should be interpreted with caution without a previous baseline Hyperreflexia can also be caused	Reflex response may be less brisk in the elderly person (1+); reinforcement may be required in the alert patient to achieve accurate results The Achilles, or ankle-jerk, reflex is often absent in the elderly

5. Strike the tendon once (or your finger for the biceps reflex) lightly and briskly. The hammer should swing loosely and quickly glancing off the target tendon; use whichever side of the reflex hammer will give you the best strike

6. If no response is elicited, try again after repositioning the extremity slightly; after 2–3 tries the reflex is likely obliterated; go on to another reflex and return to the one not elicited later in the examination

7. In the conscious patient use reinforcement (distraction) when a reflex

by electrolyte imbalance or medications

Clonus is a sustained hyperreflexia usually indicative of UMN (pyramidal tract) disease

Table continued on following page

TABLE 6-1 Neuromuscular Assessment Techniques, Tips, Geriatric Considerations *Continued*

Technique	Performance Tips	Description/Rationale	Geriatric Considerations
	will not respond; this is a voluntary isometric contraction of another muscle group by the patient (such as clenching the teeth, making a fist) while the reflex is being tested		
	8. Compare sides immediately for symmetry of reaction		
	9. No reaction is graded as 0: minimal reaction as 1+; normal brisk reaction as 2+; very brisk as 3+; and hyperreflexia as 4+		
	In addition to the traditional MSRs the examiner might try the following		

Jaw Reflex

ASSESSMENT TIPS

1. Lay the index finger horizontally across the relaxed lower jaw below the lower lip
2. Strike your index finger with the reflex hammer
3. The jaw should move to close the mouth

- **Superficial (pathologic) reflexes**

Superficial reflexes elicit muscle response by stimulation of receptors on the surface of the skin

A pathologic response indicates the presence of a UMN lesion or brain herniation

Pathologic response will be absent in acute spinal or cerebral shock

Table continued on following page

TABLE 6–1 Neuromuscular Assessment Techniques, Tips, Geriatric Considerations *Continued*

Technique	Performance Tips	Description/Rationale	Geriatric Considerations
Altered Consciousness Plantar reflex Selected additional reflexes ***Conscious*** Plantar reflex	*ASSESSMENT TIPS* To elicit a response to plantar stimulation, 1. *Lightly* drag a pointed object such as the handle of a reflex hammer up the lateral side of the sole of *each* foot and across the ball of the foot in one continuous motion 2. Apply only enough pressure for stimulus to be felt; heavy pressure may cause reflex withdrawal of the foot from the stimulus 3. Accurate assessment cannot be done if feet are cold		In some cases the plantar reflex will be absent in the elderly If present, the normal plantar reflex may be difficult to identify in the elderly; this may be due to • Arthropathy of the tarsal and metatarsal joints • Bunion deformities that limit natural movement of the great toe • Peripheral neuropathy

4. Do not be distracted by the patient's pulling away or withdrawal of the foot and leg from the stimulus; this in itself *is not* an abnormal response
5. Look at the movement of the great toe to evaluate the reflex

The *normal response* in adults and children above the age of 2–3 years is flexion of the great toe and often the other toes of the stimulated foot
The *abnormal response* in adults and children above the age of 2–3 years is dorsiflexion of the great toe, with or without flaring of the other toes on the stimulated foot (see Fig. 6–6)

Table continued on following page

TABLE 6-1 Neuromuscular Assessment Techniques, Tips, Geriatric Considerations *Continued*

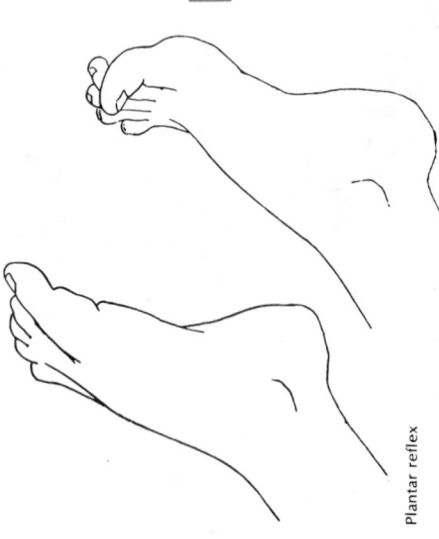

Plantar reflex

Babinski reflex

FIGURE 6-6

The normal (plantar reflex) and abnormal (Babinski's reflex) response of an adult to stimulation of the plantar reflex. (From Price, S. A., & Wilson, L. M. [1992]. *Pathophysiology: Clinical concepts of disease processes* [4th ed., p. 759]. New York: McGraw–Hill.)

The normal response is described as a
- Positive plantar reflex, or a Negative Babinski reflex

The abnormal response is described as a
- Negative plantar reflex, or a Positive Babinski reflex

Selected Special Reflexes: Frontal Release Signs

ASSESSMENT TIPS

1. *Snout reflex*
   - Stimulate the circumoral area by tapping lightly with a finger or reflex hammer
   - Puckering and protrusion of the lips is an abnormal response
2. *Sucking reflex*

These pathological reflexes reflect damage to the frontal lobe of the brain

These reflexes may be seen in persons with degenerative brain disease such as Alzheimer's disease

Table continued on following page

TABLE 6–1 Neuromuscular Assessment Techniques, Tips, Geriatric Considerations *Continued*

Technique	Performance Tips	Description/Rationale	Geriatric Considerations
	• Stimulate the lips by gently placing a finger on the lip at midline • Sucking movements are an abnormal response 3. *Glabellar reflex* • Repeatedly tap the forehead with a finger, midline, just above the nose • Repeated eye blinking is an abnormal response 4. *Grasp reflex* • Touch the palm of a hand with the fingers (must have motor function) • A continuous grasping reaction is an abnormal response		

TABLE 6-2 Comparison of Common Types of Tremors

Tremor Type	Oscillation Characteristics	Relation to Movement	Factors that Accentuate Tremor	Factors that Suppress Tremor
Postural (physiologic)	Fine amplitude—usually invisible to naked eye	Occur with movement or in fixed position	Anxiety Caffeine Hyperthyroidism Lithium Tricyclics	
Essential (familial/senile)	Larger amplitude (visible)—frequently slower than physiologic, but faster than Parkinson's	Absent at rest; accentuated by voluntary tasks requiring precision	Fatigue Emotional factors Phenothiazines Halperidol Alcohol	Alcohol Propranolol
Cerebellar disease	Large, irregular, slow oscillations of progressively increased amplitude as person brings limb closer to target	Occur with movement; not present while limb at rest		
Parkinson's disease	Slow oscillations of relaxed, supported limb	Occur with limb at rest; diminish on voluntary movement	Phenothiazines Halperidol	Sleep Voluntary movement L-dopa anticholinergics

Developed from *Primary Care Medicine* (2nd ed., pp. 733–735) by A. Goroll, L. May, and A. Muller, 1987. Philadelphia: J.B. Lippincott.

TABLE 6-3 **Visual Field Defects Produced by Selected Lesions in the Visual Pathways**

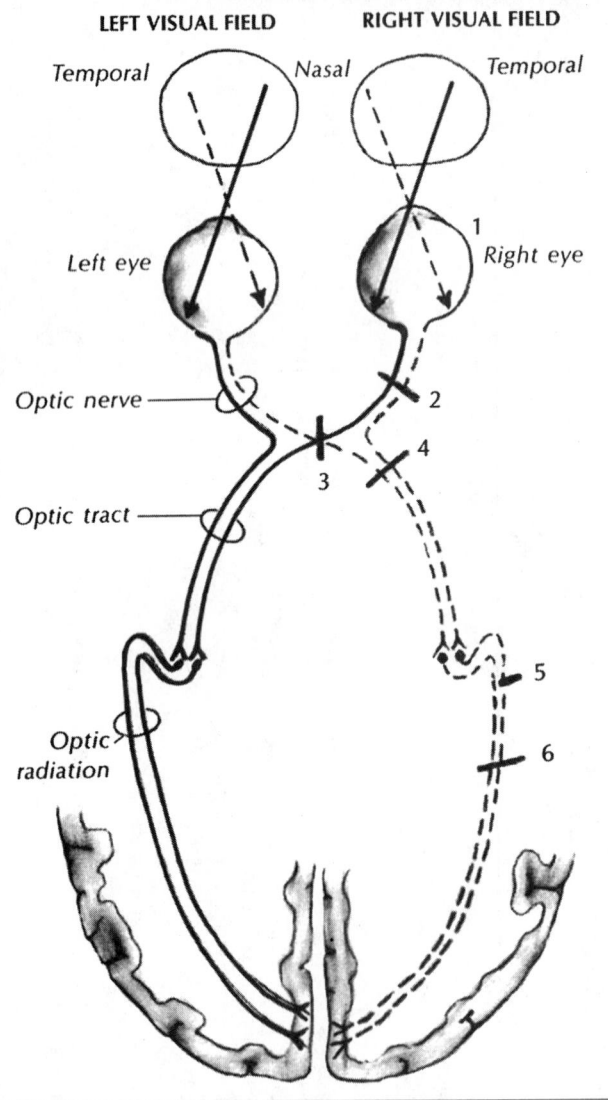

LEFT VISUAL FIELD   RIGHT VISUAL FIELD

Temporal   Nasal   Temporal

Left eye   1   Right eye

Optic nerve   2

3   4

Optic tract

5

Optic radiation   6

Blind right eye *(right optic nerve)*
A lesion of the optic nerve, and of course of the eye itself, produces unilateral blindness

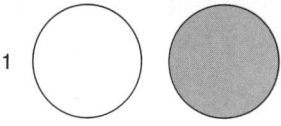

Bitemporal hemianopsia *(optic chiasm)*
A lesion at the optic chiasm may involve only the fibers that are crossing over to the opposite side. Since these fibers originate in the nasal half of each retina, visual loss involves the temporal half of each field.

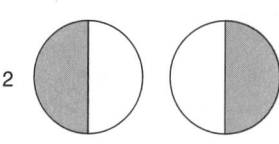

Left homonymous hemianopsia
(right optic tract)
A lesion of the optic tract interrupts fibers originating on the same side of both eyes. Visual loss in the eyes is therefore similar (homonymous) and involves half of each field (hemianopsia).

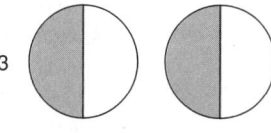

Homonymous left upper quadrantic defect *(optic radiation, partial)*
A partial lesion of the optic radiation may involve only a portion of the nerve fibers, producing, for example, a homonymous quadrantic defect.

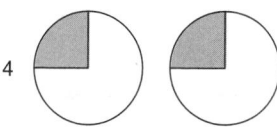

Left homonymous hemianopsia
(right optic radiation)
A complete interruption of fibers in the optic radiation produces a visual defect similar to that produced by a lesion of the optic tract.

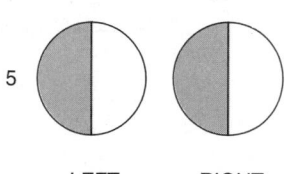

LEFT   RIGHT

367

TABLE 6-4 Motor Function According to Cord Segments

Area of Body	Action Tested	Cord Segment
Shoulder	Flexion, extension, or rotation of neck	C1–C4
Arm	Adduction of arm	C5–C8, T1
	Abduction of arm	C4–C6
	Flexion of forearm	C5–C6
	Extension of forearm	C6–C8
	Supination of forearm	C5–C7
	Pronation of forearm	C6–C7
Hand	Extension of hand	C6–C8
	Flexion of hand	C7–C8, T1
Finger	Abduction of thumb	C7–C8, T1
	Adduction of thumb	C8, T1
	Abduction of little finger	C8, T1
	Opposition of thumb	C8, T1
Hip	Flexion of hip	L1–L3
	Extension of leg	L2–L4
	Flexion of leg	L4–L5, S1–S2
	Adduction of thigh	L2–L4
	Abduction of thigh	L4–L5, S1–S2
	Medial rotation of thigh	L4–L5, S1
	Lateral rotation of thigh	L4–L5, S1–S2
	Flexion of thigh	L4–L5
Foot	Dorsiflexion of foot	L4–L5, S1
	Plantar flexion of foot	L5, S1–S2
Toe	Extension of great toe	L4–L5, S1
	Flexion of great toe	L5, S1–S2
	Spreading of toes	S1–S2

From Swartz, M. H. (1998). *Textbook of physical diagnosis: History and examination* (3rd ed., p. 547). Philadelphia: W. B. Saunders.

TABLE 6-5 Spinal Cord Levels for Five Common Muscle-Stretch Reflexes (MSRs)

Reflex	Expected Response	Cord Level
Biceps reflex	Flexion of forearm	C5–C6
Triceps reflex	Extension of forearm	C7–C8
Brachioradialis reflex	Flexion, supination of forearm	C5–C6
Quadriceps reflex	Extension of lower leg	L2–L4
Achilles reflex	Plantar flexion of foot	L5–S2

NEUROMUSCULAR DISORDERS

Neuromuscular disorders may affect mental status (level of arousal, speech, and behavior), movement, sensation, the ability to maintain respiration, reflexes, and vital signs. Life-threatening deterioration may occur rapidly with the disruption of consciousness and ventilation.

Many neuromuscular disorders also lead to multisystem dysfunction, because they may affect central nervous system and endocrine regulation of numerous body systems. Motor and sensory deficits may lead to immobility, affecting other systems. Neurogenic shock, adult respiratory distress syndrome (ARDS), pneumonia, pulmonary embolism, diabetes insipidus (DI), syndrome of inappropriate antidiuretic hormone (SIADH), and hyperglycemic, hyperosmolar, nonketotic coma (HHNK) are some of the complications of neuromuscular disorders.

Neuromuscular disorders may be divided into two categories. The first includes disorders that may affect both consciousness and ventilation. The second includes disorders that may affect ventilation but may not affect the level of consciousness.

Neuromuscular Disorders Affecting Consciousness and Ventilation

With certain neuromuscular disorders, altered levels of consciousness may result in the loss of the voluntary ability to protect the airway. Secondary effects of the disorder may increase intracranial pressure (see Chapter 14) and cause cerebral ischemia, cerebral edema, and brain herniation.

Brain Herniation Syndromes

Pathophysiology

Brain herniation may occur when changes in cerebral compliance cause an increase in intracranial pressure beyond compensatory levels (see Chapter 14 for related information on intracranial pressure [ICP], cerebral compliance, and cerebral perfusion pressure [CPP]). Brain tissue protrudes or is pushed through openings or linings of the intracranial cavity. Brain herniation syndromes may be classified as cingulate, or lateral; central downward, or transtentorial; uncal; downward cerebellar, or tonsillar; or upward cerebellar.

Assessment

Clinical manifestations of brain herniation syndromes reflect the location of herniation and the order of central nervous system (CNS) involvement (see Clinical Findings 6–1). Progressive changes in the level of consciousness (LOC), motor function, plantar reflex, respiratory patterns, eye responses, and vital signs indicate deterioration (see Clinical Findings 6–1).

Level of Consciousness (LOC)

The reticular activating system (RAS) is responsible for maintaining consciousness. The RAS originates in the brain stem and relays messages from the spinal cord to the thalamus and cerebrum to control arousal and wakefulness. Because of its widespread influence, *a change in the level of consciousness is often the first indication of deteriorating brain function.*

In critical care settings, the Glasgow Coma Scale (GCS) is commonly used to give an accurate reflection of the level of consciousness, as well as a prediction of outcome for brain-injured patients (see Table 6–6). The critically ill adult who is hearing impaired, unable to speak English, has an endotracheal tube or tracheostomy, has an eye injury or a limb fracture, is paralyzed or has a neuromuscular deficit associated with an underlying neuromuscular disorder, is intoxicated with drugs or alcohol, or who is uncooperative may need special consideration to avoid an unreliable score.

Motor Function

The critically ill adult should be assessed for voluntary versus involuntary movement, changes in muscle strength and tone, and symmetry of responses (see Table 6–1 for related information on the evaluation of motor function). In general, weakness, paralysis, and abnormal posturing progressing from one side of the body to both (bilateral involvement) may be indications of deteriorating brain function.

Plantar Reflex (Babinski's Sign)

A positive Babinski reflex (see Fig. 6–6) is usually an indication of deterioration in brain function in the critically ill adult at risk for herniation (see Table 6–1 for related information on the evaluation of superficial reflexes).

TABLE 6–6 A Typical Glasgow Coma Scale

Parameter Assessed	Reaction	Score
Eye opening	Spontaneous	4
	To voice	3
	To pain	2
	None	1
	Closed by swelling	C
Verbal response	Oriented	5
	Confused	4
	Inappropriate words	3
	Incomprehensible sounds	2
	None	1
	Endotracheal tube or tracheostomy	T
Motor response	Obeys commands	6
	Localized pain (purposeful movement, i.e., pushes stimulus away)	5
	Withdraws from pain (moves away from stimulus)	4
	Flexion response (decorticate)	3
	Extension response (decerebrate)	2
	None (flaccid)	1
	Paralysis	P
	BEST POSSIBLE SCORE	15

Respiratory Pattern

Changes in respiratory patterns may be used to assess the progression through the loss of consciousness and deterioration of brain function, as well as to assess the return of reversible loss of function (see Table 6–1 and Fig. 6–3 for related information on the evaluation of respiratory patterns).

Eye Responses

In the critically ill adult with an impaired level of consciousness, the lack of response to head movement with the eyes remaining midline (doll's eyes) and an abnormal or absent response to activation of the oculovestibular reflex (ice-water calorics) may be an indication that brain deterioration has progressed to the brain stem (see Table 6–1 for related information on the evaluation of cranial nerves and the oculocephalic and oculovestibular reflexes).

Vital Signs

Blood pressure, pulse, and respirations are controlled by structures in the medulla and brain stem. Changes in these parameters usually occur late in the process of herniation and should not be relied upon to protect the patient from harm.

POINTS TO REMEMBER

▶ Brain herniation may rapidly progress to brain-stem ischemia and death.

▶ The major difference between central and uncal herniation is the initial pupil changes in uncal herniation. In uncal herniation, associated changes in the level of consciousness and motor function can occur almost simultaneously with ipsilateral pupil dilation.

▶ Because clinical manifestations of brain herniation may be detected before irreversible damage occurs, a thorough nursing history (see Tables 1–1 and 6–1 and Clinical Findings 6–1) is crucial to identifying patients at risk.

▶ In addition to the initial and baseline assessments (see Table 2–1), a focused neuromuscular assessment (see Tables 2–1 and 6–1), as well as a focused assessment of the underlying pathology should be completed as often as the patient's condition dictates to detect or anticipate and prevent the progression of deterioration.

▶ Ongoing assessment incorporates the evaluation of responses to diagnostic procedures and therapeutic interventions aimed at the reduction of increased intracranial pressure; it includes collaboration with other members of the health team to prevent irreversible neurologic decompensation.

Clinical Findings 6–1   *Location and Progression of Brain Herniation Syndromes*

I. CINGULATE (LATERAL) HERNIATION

A lesion in one cerebral hemisphere causes lateral displacement across the midline of the intracranial cavity under the falx cerebri and may lead to compression of the internal cerebral vein and ipsilateral anterior cerebral artery.

A. Predisposing factors
1. Head trauma (subdural or epidural hematoma, intracranial hemorrhage)
2. Cerebral aneurysm
3. Tumor
4. Cerebral edema related to infection or metabolic and electrolyte disturbances

B. Progression of herniation and physical assessment findings: Midline shift
1. May be asymptomatic.
2. Compression of blood vessels may contribute to cerebral ischemia and increased intracranial pressure (see Chapter 14 for related information on ICP).
3. May progress to transtentorial herniation.

II. CENTRAL DOWNWARD (TRANSTENTORIAL) HERNIATION

Downward displacement of the cerebral hemispheres pushes the diencephalon and midbrain through the tentorial notch, compressing branches of the basilar artery and causing deterioration of the brain stem.

A. Predisposing factors: Same as lateral herniation

B. Progression of herniation and physical assessment findings
1. Diencephalon
   - *LOC*
     - Difficulty concentrating
     - Memory lapses
     - Lethargy
     - Decreased purposeful movement
     - Stupor
     - Coma
     - Decorticate posturing (see Fig. 6–4)
   - *Motor function:* Ipsilateral weakness or paralysis
   - *Plantar reflex:* Positive Babinski's response (see Fig. 6–6)
   - *Respiratory pattern:* Cheyne-Stokes respirations or normal pattern with yawns, sighs, or pauses
   - *Eye responses:* Small (1–3 mm), equal, and reactive pupils
   - *Vital signs:* Increasing blood pressure
2. Midbrain
   - *LOC:* Decerebrate posturing
   - *Motor function:* Bilateral weakness or paralysis
   - *Respiratory pattern:* Central neurogenic hyperventilation
   - *Eye responses:* Fixed, dilated (3–5 mm) pupils
   - *Vital signs:* Temperature fluctuations

3. Pons
   - *Eye responses:* Absent oculocephalic and oculovestibular reflexes
   - *Respiratory pattern:* Cluster respirations (slow to absent)
4. Medulla
   - *Motor function:* Absent motor responses
   - *Respiratory pattern:* Ataxic respirations
   - *Eye responses:* Dilated pupils
   - *Vital signs*
     - Variable pulse rate
     - Hypotension
5. Cervical spinal cord
   - *Reflexes*
     - Absent Babinski's response
     - Absent deep tendon reflexes
   - *Respiratory pattern:* Respiratory arrest

III. UNCAL HERNIATION

An expanding mass in the temporal lobe or middle fossa pushes the uncus toward or over the edge of the tentorium, compressing the oculomotor nerve, midbrain, and brainstem.

A. Predisposing factors
1. Temporal lobe fracture (epidural hematoma)
2. Unilateral cerebral tumor

B. Progression of herniation and physical assessment findings
1. Compression of CN III, same side as mass (early third nerve stage)
   - *Eye responses:* Same-side dilation (ipsilateral) of pupil (sluggish or no reaction)
2. Irreversible damage to CN III (late third nerve sign); dysfunction of midbrain (RAS and motor tracts involved)
   - *LOC*
     - Restlessness
     - Confusion
     - Stuporous
     - Opposite side extension posturing
   - *Motor function:* Same-side weakness, paralysis
   - *Eye responses:* Same-side fixed and dilated pupil
3. Infarction of midbrain (irreversible damage to midbrain and upper pons)
   - *LOC:* Bilateral extension posturing
   - *Respiratory pattern:* Central neurogenic hyperventilation
   - *Eye responses:* Bilateral fixed and dilated pupils

4. Pons, medulla, and cervical spinal cord: Progression same as downward central herniation

IV. DOWNWARD CEREBELLAR (TONSILAR) HERNIATION

Rapid descent of the contents of the posterior fossa into the foramen magnum and onto the medulla.

A. Predisposing factors: Basilar skull fracture

B. Progression of herniation and physical assessment findings
1. Dysfunction of lower pons, medulla
   - *LOC:* Rapid deterioration in LOC
   - *Motor response:* Acute, flaccid quadriplegia
2. Infarction of medulla: Cardiopulmonary arrest

V. UPWARD CEREBELLAR HERNIATION

Contents of the posterior fossa are pushed upward, compressing the midbrain.

A. Predisposing factors
1. Occipital skull fracture (epidural or subdural bleeding)
2. Rapidly expanding cerebellar abscess or tumor

B. Progression of herniation and physical assessment findings: Midbrain
1. *Respiratory pattern:* Ataxic respirations or apnea may be the first sign (cerebellum compresses the structures regulating respiration in the pons and the medulla)
2. *Eye responses*
   - Pupils constricted and nonreactive (the parasympathetic fibers of CN III are compressed)
   - Rapidly expanding masses result in decompensation and progression of herniation as above.

Seizures and Status Epilepticus

Pathophysiology

Episodes of excessive discharge of cerebral neurons may cause seizure activity, resulting in motor or sensory dysfunction, behavioral alterations, or loss of consciousness. Anything that disturbs the environment of cerebral neurons may cause a seizure.

Seizures may be classified as partial (focal), or generalized. Partial seizures may be further classified as simple (no loss of consciousness), or complex (loss of consciousness). Generalized seizures are associated with impairment of consciousness and may be further classified as absence (petit mal), myoclonic, clonic, tonic, tonic-clonic (grand mal), or atonic seizures.

Epilepsy is a chronic seizure disorder of primary (idiopathic) or secondary (acquired) origin. Status epilepticus refers to continuous and prolonged seizure activity, with or without loss of consciousness, and without recovery between attacks.

Assessment

Seizure activity may include a pre-ictal (aura), ictal (seizure activity), and post-ictal (recovery period) phase. Clinical manifestations in each phase may vary with the type and extent of seizure activity (see Clinical Findings 6–2).

Seizure activity should be assessed through each phase (from onset to termination) with emphasis on the evaluation of the level of consciousness and motor activity. In general, be aware of the following:

- Partial seizures have a local onset and may evolve to generalized tonic-clonic seizures (bilaterally symmetrical).
- Petit mal seizures may be characterized by a brief loss of consciousness or decreased awareness.
- Myoclonic seizures may be characterized by a momentary loss of consciousness and single uncontrollable short, abrupt muscle contraction of one or more extremities.
- Clonic seizures may be characterized by loss of consciousness and repetitive jerking motions.
- Tonic seizure activity may be characterized by loss of consciousness and excessive muscle contraction (muscles become stiff and rigid).
- Grand mal seizure activity may be characterized by loss of consciousness and muscle rigidity followed by clonic jerking (convulsions).
- Atonic seizures may be characterized by a loss of consciousness and muscle tone (drop attacks).

POINTS TO REMEMBER

▶ In the absence of emergency intervention, grand mal status epilepticus may cause prolonged apnea, cerebral hypoxia, severe neurological deficits, and death.

▶ Because seizure activity is a manifestation of central nervous system irritability associated with a variety of underlying disorders, a thorough nursing history (see Tables 1–1 and 6–1 and Clinical Findings 6–2) is crucial to identify patients at risk (the most common cause of status epilepticus is the discontinuance or insufficient administration of anticonvulsant medication).

▶ Because seizure activity may increase cerebral oxygen consumption, metabolic demands, and intracranial pressure, and compromise an already deteriorating status for many critically ill adults, in addition to the initial and baseline assessments (see Table 2–1) and a focused assessment of the underlying disorder, a focused neuromuscular assessment (see Tables 2–1 and 6–1) should be completed as often as the patient's condition dictates to detect or anticipate and prevent seizure activity, status epilepticus, and complications such as hypoglycemia, hyperthermia, hypoxemia, increased intracranial pressure, and hypotension.

▶ The critically ill adult on controlled ventilation and paralytic drugs may not demonstrate a motor response. The patient should be assessed for sudden increases in ICP accompanied by pupil dilation (see Figs. 14–7 and 14–8 and Table 14–4).

▶ Ongoing assessment incorporates the evaluation of responses to diagnostic procedures and therapeutic interventions aimed at identifying the type of seizure and protecting the patient from harm; it includes collaboration with other members of the health team to gain and maintain control of the seizure activity.

Clinical Findings 6–2 *Seizure Activity*

I. HISTORY

A. Predisposing factors

1. Head trauma
2. Intracranial aneurysm
3. Subarachnoid hemorrhage
4. Cerebrovascular accident (CVA)
5. Brain tumor
6. Drug or alcohol abuse
7. Infection
8. Encephalitis

    9. Meningitis

   10. Fever

   11. Electrolyte imbalances such as hypocalcemia and hyponatremia

   12. Endocrine disorders such as hyperosmolar nonketotic hyperglycemia

   13. Hypoglycemia

   14. Hypoxia

   15. Hypercapnia

   16. Excessive environmental stimuli such as sensory overload and sleep deprivation

   17. Life-threatening dysrhythmias

   18. Discontinuance of, or insufficient, anticonvulsant medication

B. Subjective findings: An aura (Complaints of headache, dizziness, numbness or other sensations of feeling or movement may precede the ictal phase)

II. LABORATORY AND BEDSIDE MONITORING FINDINGS

A. Computed tomography (CT) scan or magnetic resonance imaging (MRI): May be used to assess intracranial abnormalities and lesions of the skull and meninges

B. Electroencephalogram (EEG)
1. May assist in determining the type of seizure
2. May isolate the focus of the seizure through detection of abnormal neuron activity

C. Cerebrospinal fluid (CSF) analysis (see Chapter 13 for related information on CSF): Changes in color, cell count, and pressure may assist in diagnosing the cause of the seizure

D. Arterial blood gas studies (see Chapter 13 for related information on arterial blood gas studies): May reveal hypoxemia or hypercapnia as an underlying cause of seizure activity

E. Other laboratory studies: Electrolytes, glucose, BUN, creatinine, complete blood count (CBC), antiepileptic drug (AED) concentrations, and toxicology screens may be completed to identify correctable causes of seizure activity such as electrolyte and metabolic imbalances, or to identify other underlying disease processes (see Chapter 13 for related information on metabolic and acid-base disorders)

F. ECG
1. Bradycardia or tachycardia may be associated with seizure activity
2. Dysrhythmias may be related to electrolyte or acid-base imbalances

G. Hemodynamic parameters: Increased blood pressure may be associated with seizure activity

H. ICP (see Chapter 14 and Figs. 14–7 and 14–8 for related information): Abrupt and sustained increases in intracranial pressure may be associated with seizure activity

III. PHYSICAL ASSESSMENT FINDINGS

A. General observations (inspection)
 1. Increased salivation, diaphoresis, and incontinence of stool or urine may accompany generalized seizures
 2. May be periods of apnea or hyperventilation during seizure activity (ictal phase)

B. LOC: An impaired level of consciousness is associated with partial complex and generalized seizures related to the spread or occurrence of abnormal neuron discharge throughout the cerebral hemispheres

C. Behavior
 1. Inappropriate behavior, confusion, and memory loss may be associated with temporal lobe seizures
 2. Confusion or psychological impairment may be associated with frontal lobe seizures
 3. Confusion, disorientation, and memory loss may occur during the post-ictal phase

D. Speech: Speech difficulty or aphasia may be associated with temporal or frontal lobe seizures

E. Motor function
 1. Automatisms such as lip-smacking, chewing, and rubbing may be associated with temporal lobe seizures
 2. Kicking or thrashing may be associated with frontal lobe seizures
 3. Drop attacks may be associated with frontal lobe seizures
 4. Unilateral extremity involvement may be associated with partial seizures (may be unilateral residual weakness in post-ictal phase)
 5. Bilateral extremity involvement may be associated with generalized seizures

F. Sensation: Tingling sensations or loss of body awareness may be associated with parietal lobe seizures

G. Cranial nerves (eye responses)
 1. Dilated and nonreactive pupils may be associated with generalized seizures
 2. Staring may be associated with petit mal, temporal lobe, or frontal lobe seizures

3. Blurred vision, nystagmus, visual hallucinations, or blinking may be associated with occipital lobe seizures
4. Deviation of the eyes and head to the contralateral side may be associated with frontal lobe seizures

Acute Head Injury

Pathophysiology

The term *head injury* refers to any injury involving the scalp, skull, or brain tissue. Head injuries may be classified as open or closed:

- Open head trauma may result from a skull fracture with a laceration of the scalp, allowing exposure of the contents to the environment or from a penetrating injury (missile or impalement).
- Closed head trauma may result from an accelerated force (the head is struck by a rapidly moving blunt object) or decelerated force (the head hits a hard surface).

Primary and Secondary Injury

Primary injury refers to brain damage resulting from the direct impact of the injury. Primary injury may involve

- The site of impact (coup)
- The side opposite to the site of impact (contrecoup, or rebound injury)
- Diffuse axonal injury (DAI) to the white matter, resulting from the twisting and shearing of brain tissue during rotation of the head

Primary injuries include lacerations, skull fractures, concussions, and contusions. Primary injuries may lead to hematoma formation and secondary injuries such as hypoxia, hypotension, cerebral ischemia, cerebral edema, increased intracranial pressure (see Chapter 14), or brain herniation (see Clinical Findings 6–1).

Skull Fractures

Skull fractures may be categorized as linear, comminuted, depressed, compound, or basilar:

- Linear fractures involve a simple break in the bone (however, a fracture over the temporal bone may tear the dura or meningeal artery and cause an acute epidural hematoma).

- Comminuted fractures involve a break in the bone with fragments.
- Depressed fractures are characterized by the displacement of bone inward into the brain.
- Compound fractures may involve linear, comminuted, or depressed fractures that communicate with a scalp laceration, a sinus, or the middle ear cavity.
- Basilar skull fractures are often compound linear fractures extending to the base of the skull and involving the anterior, middle, or posterior fossa. (Basilar skull fractures often tear the dura and allow the leakage of cerebral spinal fluid and the creation of a pathway for intracranial infection.)

Concussion

A concussion refers to a transient period of unconsciousness caused by jarring of the head due to blunt trauma.

Contusion

A contusion involves bruising and tearing of the brain tissue, and may lead to capillary hemorrhage and edema. DAI involves widespread stretching and shearing of brain tissue and nerve fibers, and may lead to severe brain swelling.

Hematoma

Hematomas may be epidural, subdural, or intracerebral.

- Epidural hematomas may be acute or chronic:
  - An acute epidural hematoma involves bleeding into the potential space between the skull and the dura, and is often associated with temporal or parietal skull fractures and laceration of the meningeal artery.
  - A chronic epidural hematoma is less common. The dura mater is torn over the sagittal or transverse sinus, resulting in a slow venous bleed with symptoms not appearing for several days.
- A subdural hematoma is a collection of blood, usually venous, in the space between the dura and the arachnoid layers. A subdural hematoma may be acute or chronic:
  - An acute subdural hematoma is often associated with massive cerebral or brain-stem contusions and lacerations.
  - A chronic subdural hematoma accumulates over several weeks, and a vascular membrane may form a wall around the

hematoma. The expanding mass may lead to localized manifestations or signs of increased intracranial pressure.

- An intracerebral hematoma involves bleeding into the brain parenchyma and may be associated with contusions, lacerations, penetrating injuries, or hemorrhagic stroke. The expanding mass may cause secondary injuries, including hypoxia, hypotension, compression of brain tissue, or cerebral edema.

Assessment

Clinical manifestations vary with the type, extent, and mechanism of head injury (see Clinical Findings 6–3).

POINTS TO REMEMBER

▶ A thorough nursing history (see Tables 1–1 and 6–1, and Clinical Findings 6–3), including details of the accident or injury and the patient's immediate response, is crucial to assist in identification of the type and extent of head injury.

▶ In addition to the initial and baseline assessments (see Table 2–1), as well as focused assessments of all the systems involved with associated injuries (head injuries are often associated with cervical spine injury [see Clinical Findings 6–7] or multiple trauma [see Clinical Findings 12–2], a focused neuromuscular assessment [see Tables 2–1 and 6–1]), should be completed as often as the patient's condition dictates to detect or anticipate and prevent complications such as hypoxia, hypotension, intracranial hypertension (see Chapter 14), brain herniation (see Clinical Findings 6–1), infection (aspiration or pneumonia; see Clinical Findings 4–3 and 4–4), neurogenic pulmonary edema (hypothalamic activation of descending fibers of the sympathetic nervous system or the release of vasoactive catecholamines may cause vasoconstriction of the pulmonary circulation, leading to hypoperfusion, hypoxemia, and the initiation of the chain of events described for ARDS; see Clinical Findings 4–1), seizures (see Clinical Findings 6–2), diabetes insipidus (see Clinical Findings 9–3), syndrome of inappropriate secretion of antidiuretic hormone (see Clinical Findings 9–3), gastrointestinal ulceration and hemorrhage (parasympathetic stimulation may lead to increased secretion of hydrochloric acid, while sympathetic stimulation may shunt blood away from the gastric mucosa and lead to ischemia; see Clinical Findings 7–1), or neurogenic or hypovolemic shock (see Clinical Findings 12–3).

▶ Ongoing assessment incorporates the evaluation of responses to diagnostic procedures and therapeutic interventions aimed at the reduction of cerebral edema and intracranial hypertension; it includes collaboration with other members of the health team to maintain cerebral perfusion pressure and prevent neurologic deterioration and further injury.

Clinical Findings 6–3   *Acute Head Injury*

I. HISTORY

A. Predisposing factors

1. Motor vehicle accidents
2. Motorcycle accidents
3. Falls
4. Assaults
5. Penetrating injuries (bullets and other foreign objects that may pierce the head)

B. Subjective findings

1. Headache, dizziness, nervousness, and irritability may be associated with concussion
2. Salty taste may be associated with rhinorrhea and drainage of CSF into the throat (basilar skull fracture)

II. LABORATORY AND BEDSIDE MONITORING FINDINGS

A. Skull x-ray: May reveal skull or facial fracture

B. CT scan: May reveal contusions, hematomas, hemorrhages, edema

C. MRI

1. May reveal air in sinuses or intracranial air suggestive of a basilar skull fracture
2. Differentiates between gray and white matter and may reveal small hemorrhages associated with diffuse axonal injury

D. Arterial blood gas studies (see Chapter 13 for related information on arterial blood gas studies): Hypoxemia, hypercapnia, or acid-base imbalances may be present related to respiratory insufficiency

E. Other laboratory studies

1. Elevated WBC count may be present, related to infection (see Table 13–9)

    2. Alterations in hemoglobin, hematocrit, and coagulation profiles may be present, related to bleeding (see Table 13–8)

    3. Alterations in sodium, potassium, chloride, glucose, and serum osmolality may be present, related to dehydration, diuretic therapy, or complications such as DI and SIADH (see Table 13–5 and Clinical Findings 9–3)

F. ECG: Tachycardia-bradycardia dysrhythmias may be present, related to intracranial injury and alterations in intracranial pressure

G. Hemodynamic parameters

    1. Increased systolic pressure may be present, related to increased ICP (Systolic pressure increases to maintain cerebral perfusion pressure in the presence of increased intracranial pressure)

    2. Hypotension may be related to hypovolemia

    3. Widened pulse pressure may reflect severe deterioration (increased systolic pressure, widened pulse pressure, and bradycardia)

H. Intracranial pressure and cerebral perfusion pressure (CPP) (see Chapter 14 and Figs. 14–7 and 14–8 for related information)

    1. An increased ICP may be related to space-occupying lesions, hematomas, concussions, hemorrhage, diffuse tissue injury, or cerebral edema

    2. A decreased CPP may be related to an increased ICP or a decrease in the mean arterial pressure (MAP)

III. Physical Assessment Findings

A. General observations (inspection and palpation)

    1. Scalp lacerations, bumps, bruising, and areas of tenderness may be present, related to the site of impact

    2. Bloody or CSF drainage from the ears, nose, or mouth may be present, related to dural tears

    3. Findings associated with basilar skull fractures may include tinnitus (ringing, cracking, or buzzing in the ears), hearing difficulties, facial nerve palsy, and

      • *Anterior fossa*
        – Rhinorrhea (CSF and blood draining from the nose)
        – Raccoon's eyes (bilateral periorbital ecchymosis from bleeding into the paranasal sinuses)

      • *Middle fossa*
        – Otorrhea (CSF and blood draining form the middle ear)
        – Battle's sign (ecchymosis over the mastoid bone)

    4. Partial or generalized seizures may be present related to the area and extent of brain injury (see Clinical Findings 6–2)

B. LOC: Alterations in the level of consciousness may vary with the type and extent of injury.

1. Immediate loss of consciousness of short duration and with no residual effects may be related to a concussion
2. Altered levels of consciousness and neurological deficits may be related to a severe contusion
3. Immediate and prolonged loss of consciousness may be related to DAI
4. Immediate loss of consciousness followed by a lucid interval and then progressive deterioration in neurological status may be related to an epidural hematoma (immediate surgical intervention may be necessary to prevent uncal herniation)
5. Restlessness, confusion, agitation, or slowed cognition followed by a deterioration in the LOC may be related to a subdural hematoma (immediate surgical intervention may be necessary to prevent central downward herniation)
6. Rapid deterioration of LOC may be related to an intracerebral hematoma (see Tables 6–1 and 6–6 for related information on assessment of LOC and Chapter 14 and Clinical Findings 6–2 for related information on increased intracranial pressure and brain herniation syndromes)

C. Cranial nerves

1. Speech may be slurred, confused, repetitive, or absent related to the type and extent of injury
2. Swallow, cough, and gag reflexes may be impaired, related to direct injury to the brain stem, edema, or herniation
3. Variations in the size, shape, and reaction of pupils as well as ocular movements may be related to the type of injury, increases in ICP, or herniation

(see Table 6–1 for related information on evaluation of cranial nerve function and Chapter 14 and Clinical Findings 6–1 for related information on pupil changes associated with increased ICP and brain herniation syndromes)

D. Motor and sensory function: Deficits in movement and sensation may include hemiplegia and hemiparesis related to the area of injury, increased ICP, or brain herniation

(see Table 6–1 for related information on evaluation of motor and sensory function and Chapter 14 and Clinical Findings 6–1 for related information on changes associated with increased ICP and brain herniation)

E. Reflexes

1. Positive Babinski's reflex may be related to increased ICP or herniation
2. Deep tendon reflexes will be absent with brain death

(see Table 6–1 and Fig. 6–3 for related information on evaluation of reflexes and Chapter 14 and Clinical Findings 6–1 for changes associated with increased ICP and brain herniation syndromes)

F. Vital signs

1. Change in pattern and rate of respiration may be related to increased ICP or herniation (see Table 6–1 for related information on evaluation of respiratory patterns and Chapter 14 and Clinical Findings 6–1 for related information on changes associated with increased ICP and brain herniation syndromes)
2. Loss of temperature control (hypothermia or hyperthermia) may be related to involvement of the hypothalamus

Subarachnoid Hemorrhage

Pathophysiology

The most common cause of a subarachnoid hemorrhage (SAH) is a ruptured intracranial aneurysm. Other causes of SAH include arteriovenous malformations, head injury, and bleeding from a cerebral tumor.

With intracranial aneurysm, a weakened segment in the arterial wall (often a saccular or berry aneurysm in the circle of Willis) bulges out and ruptures. Blood flows into the subarachnoid space and may initiate an inflammatory reaction in the neural and meningeal tissues, coat nerve roots, impair CSF absorption and circulation, and lead to a secondary hydrocephalus. The blood may also flow into the brain parenchyma and increase intracranial pressure.

Rebleeding and Vasospasm

Complications of a ruptured aneurysm include rebleeding and cerebral vasospasm. Rebleeding may occur between the third and eleventh day (peak incidence about the seventh day) as the original clot is absorbed.

Vasospasm may occur 4 to 12 days (peak 7 to 10 days) after SAH. The exact cause of vasospasm has not been clearly delineated, but spasm of the vessel may be related to vasoactive substances such as serotonin, prostaglandin, and histamine, which are released at the time of rupture. These substances are thought to increase the flux of calcium into the vascular smooth muscle and may alter muscle cell contraction, resulting in cerebral ischemia or infarction.

Assessment

Clinical manifestations may be associated with SAH (see Clinical Findings 6-4). Clinical manifestations may also be associated with re-bleeding and vasospasm.

Clinical manifestations related to rebleeding may include sudden onset of or increased headache accompanied by nausea and vomiting, fluctuating levels of consciousness with motor and sensory deficits, increased blood pressure, and alterations in respiratory rate and patterns.

Clinical manifestations of vasospasm may be related to the cerebral artery involved and the area of cerebral ischemia. In general, manifestations may include increase in headache, alterations in the level of consciousness, inappropriate behavior, speech impairment, visual deficits, focal motor paresis, seizures, and increased blood pressure.

POINTS TO REMEMBER

▶ Because the critically ill adult with SAH related to a ruptured intracranial aneurysm is at risk for rebleeding or vasospasm, a thorough nursing history (see Tables 1–1 and 6–1 and Clinical Findings 6–4) is crucial to identify precipitating factors such as hypertension.

▶ Because SAH may lead to hydrocephalus, cerebral ischemia, or infarction, in addition to the initial and baseline assessments (see Table 2–1), a focused neuromuscular assessment (see Tables 2–1 and 6–1) should be completed as often as the patient's condition dictates to detect or anticipate and prevent such complications.

▶ Ongoing assessment incorporates the evaluation of responses to diagnostic procedures and therapeutic interventions aimed at the reduction of cerebral edema and ischemia; it includes collaboration with other members of the health team to restore cerebral perfusion and prevent further injury.

Clinical Findings 6–4   *Subarachnoid Hemorrhage*

I. HISTORY

A. Predisposing factors

1. Congenital malformations
2. Atherosclerosis
3. Hypertension

4. Head trauma
5. Middle age
6. Female sex

B. Subjective findings
1. Explosive headache, which may be associated with nausea and vomiting related to a sudden increase in ICP
2. Nuchal rigidity, photophobia, and blurred vision related to meningeal irritation and inflammation

II. LABORATORY AND BEDSIDE MONITORING FINDINGS

A. CT scan: May reveal presence of blood in the subarachnoid space or presence of hydrocephalus
B. Cerebral angiography: May visualize presence and location of aneurysm
C. Cerebrospinal fluid (CSF) analysis (see Chapter 13 for related information on CSF); CSF may be bloody grossly with an increased number of red blood cells, elevated protein levels, and increased pressure, related to the subarachnoid hemorrhage
D. Other laboratory studies: Elevated WBC count may be related to meningeal irritation (see Table 13–9 for related information on WBC count)
E. ECG: Tachycardia may be present, related to increased ICP and decreased CPP
F. Hemodynamic parameters: Hypertension may be present, related to increased ICP
G. ICP and CPP
1. Increased ICP may be related to subarachnoid hematoma or edema
2. Decreased CPP may be related to vasospasm or increased ICP
(See Chapter 14 for related information on ICP, cerebral compliance, and CPP)

III. PHYSICAL ASSESSMENT FINDINGS

A. General observations (inspection): Partial or generalized seizures may occur (often at the time of rupture or with a rebleed) related to ischemia, edema, or increased intracranial pressure (see Clinical Findings 6–2 for related information on seizures)
B. LOC: Transient or sustained loss of consciousness may be related to cerebral ischemia, infarction, edema, increased intracranial pressure, hydrocephalus, or meningeal irritation (see Tables 6–1 and 6–6 for related information on evaluation of LOC, and see Chapter 14 for related information on increased intracranial pressure)
C. Behavior: Irritability or restlessness may be related to meningeal irritation or increased intracranial pressure

D. Cranial nerves

1. Speech deficits or aphasia may be present, related to edema, ischemia, or increased intracranial pressure
2. Visual disturbances, papilledema, and alterations in pupil response may be present, related to edema, ischemia, or increased intracranial pressure (see Table 6–1 for related information on cranial nerve function, and see Chapter 14 for related information on increased intracranial pressure)

E. Motor and sensory function

1. Kernig's sign (inability to extend the leg when lying with the thigh flexed on the abdomen) may be present, related to meningeal irritation
2. Brudzinski's sign (when lying in the supine position, flexion of the neck produces flexion of the knees and hips) may be present, related to meningeal irritation
3. Numbness, hemiparesis, or hemiplegia may be related to cerebral ischemia, edema, or increased intracranial pressure (see Table 6–1 for related information on the evaluation of motor and sensory function, and see Chapter 14 for related information on increased intracranial pressure)

F. Reflexes: Positive Babinski's sign may be present, related to increased intracranial pressure (see Table 6–1 for related information on the evaluation of reflexes)

G. Vital signs

1. Alterations in respiratory rate and pattern may be related to increased intracranial pressure (see Table 6–1 and Fig. 6–3 for related information on respiratory patterns)
2. Increased temperature may be present, related to meningeal irritation or inflammation

Cerebrovascular Accident (CVA)

Pathophysiology

A CVA (stroke) results from a sudden interruption of blood supply to the brain tissue. The brain tissue is deprived of oxygen and neurological deficits may occur as a result of cerebral ischemia, infarction, or edema.

Strokes may be classified as thrombotic, embolic, hemorrhagic, or ischemic:

- A thrombotic stroke is associated with thrombus formation, which may obstruct one or more of the arteries supplying the brain (most common cause of CVA).
- An embolic stroke is caused by an embolus formed outside the cerebral circulation (usually the heart) that enters the carotid system and often lodges in the left middle cerebral artery.
- A hemorrhagic stroke is associated with rupture of a cerebral blood vessel with bleeding or pressure extending into the brain tissue.
- An ischemic stroke is associated with decreased blood flow to the brain.

Assessment

Clinical manifestations vary with the type of stroke and the location and extent of the injury (see Clinical Findings 6–5). Alterations in memory, thought, speech, visual fields, movement, and sensation may be temporary or permanent and may reflect left or right cerebral hemisphere involvement (see Fig. 6–1).

Thrombotic and embolic strokes may cause loss of consciousness with occlusion of the main stem of the middle cerebral artery or damage to an entire cerebral hemisphere. Hemorrhagic strokes may cause loss of consciousness from direct effects on the RAS or from brain swelling and increased intracranial pressure.

Brain-stem strokes may impair cranial nerve function and airway protection (the vertebral and basilar arteries supply the cerebellum, brain stem, and spinal cord). "Locked-in" syndrome is a brain-stem stroke that impairs all cranial nerve function but spares the RAS. The patient may be fully alert but has no speech or movement except for the eyes.

POINTS TO REMEMBER

▶ The critically ill adult may present with a severe hemorrhagic stroke and loss of consciousness. Assessment is similar to the patient with increased intracranial pressure or a brain herniation syndrome (see Chapter 14 and Clinical Findings 6–1).

▶ Because the critically ill adult is susceptible to the development of a stroke and may also present with an unrelated condition but have neurologic deficits related to a previous stroke, a thorough nursing history (see Tables 1–1 and 6–1 and Clinical Findings 6–5) is crucial to identify patients at risk or who may have residual deficits.

▶ Because complications of a stroke include pneumonia (see Clinical Findings 4–4), pulmonary embolism (see Clinical Findings 4–7), and heart disease, in addition to the initial and baseline assessments (see Table 2–1), focused neuromuscular, respiratory, and cardiovascular assessments (see Tables 2–1, 6–1, 4–1, and 5–1), should be completed as often as the patient's condition dictates to detect or anticipate and prevent further neurological injury and such complications.

▶ Ongoing assessment incorporates the evaluation of responses to diagnostic procedures and therapeutic interventions aimed at establishing the cause of the stroke and the restoration of cerebral blood flow; it includes collaboration with other members of the health team to prevent further injury and ischemia.

Clinical Findings 6–5   *Cerebrovascular Accident (CVA)*

I. HISTORY AND PREDISPOSING FACTORS

A. Thrombotic CVA

1. Atherosclerosis
2. Hypertension
3. Hyperlipidemia
4. History of transient ischemic attacks (TIAs)
5. Diabetes mellitus
6. Hypercoagulability
7. Smoking
8. Obesity

B. Embolic CVA

1. Atrial fibrillation
2. Infective endocarditis
3. Cardiomyopathy
4. Mitral valve prolapse
5. Prosthetic heart valves
6. Atrial myxoma
7. Myocardial infarction
8. Hypercoagulable states
9. Oral contraceptives
10. Fat emboli (trauma or long bone fracture)
11. Tumor emboli

C. Hemorrhagic CVA

1. Hypertension
2. Congenital arteriovenous malformation
3. Anticoagulant therapy
4. Bleeding disorders

D. Ischemic CVA

1. Hypotension
2. Dehydration

II. LABORATORY AND BEDSIDE MONITORING FINDINGS

A. CT scan: May distinguish between hemorrhage and infarction

B. Cerebral angiography: May visualize cerebral vessels, aneurysms, and AV malformations

C. Arterial blood gas studies (see Chapter 13 for related information on arterial blood gas studies and acid-base disorders): Hypoxemia, hypo- or hypercapnia, or acid-base imbalances may be present, related to respiratory insufficiency

D. CSF analysis (see Chapter 13 for related information on CSF analysis)

1. A normal pressure and clear fluid may be associated with thrombosis and embolism
2. An elevated pressure and bloody fluid may be associated with subarachnoid and intracerebral hemorrhage

E. Other laboratory studies

1. Elevated cholesterol or triglycerides or both may be present with atherosclerosis (see Table 13–2 for related information on cholesterol and triglycerides)
2. Elevated serum glucose may be present with diabetes mellitus (see Table 13–7 for related information on blood glucose)
3. Elevated WBC count may be present, related to inflammation (see Table 13–9 for related information on WBC count)
4. Decreased hemoglobin may be present, related to hemorrhage or underlying disorder (see Table 13–8 for related information on hemoglobin)

F. ECG: Tachycardia may be present related to hypoxemia or increased ICP and decreased CPP

G. Hemodynamic parameters

1. Hypertension may be present, associated with hemorrhagic stroke
2. Hypertension may be present, related to increased ICP

III. Physical Assessment and Findings

A. Findings associated with the artery involved

1. Confusion, memory loss, personality changes, incontinence, contralateral motor and sensory loss, and alterations in eye tracking may be associated with involvement of the anterior cerebral artery (supplies medial, frontal, and parietal lobes)

2. Widespread damage, including contralateral motor and sensory loss, functional deficits (see left and right hemisphere below), blindness or ipsilateral visual blurring may be associated with involvement of the internal carotid artery (supplies cerebral hemisphere)

3. A loss of consciousness with contralateral motor and sensory loss (arm more affected than the leg), contralateral visual field loss, aphasia if dominant hemisphere affected, spatial-perceptual deficits in nondominant hemisphere, or vasomotor paresis may be associated with involvement of the middle cerebral artery (supplies the lateral surface of the four cerebral lobes)

4. Contralateral sensory loss, homonymous hemianopsia, color blindness, depth-of-field perception, perseverative behavior, memory loss, oculomotor nerve palsy, nystagmus, conjugate gaze deficits, and pupil abnormalities may be associated with involvement of the posterior cerebral artery (supplies the occipital lobe, medial and inferior surface of the temporal lobe, midbrain, and posterior diencephalon)

B. General observations (assessment of the responsive patient focuses on identification of motor and sensory deficits; see Table 6–1 and Fig. 6–2 for related information on evaluation of motor and sensory function)

1. *Left hemisphere involvement*
   - Behavior
     – Emotional lability (cry and laugh)
     – Perseveration (repetitive behaviors that are often verbal)
     – Apraxia (unable to plan action)
   - Speech
     – Expressive aphasia (loss of ability to verbalize)
     – Receptive aphasia (loss of ability to understand)
   - Motor and sensory function: Right hemiparesis and or hemiplegia (affected extremities may be flaccid at first and then spastic)

2. *Right hemisphere involvement*

- Behavior: Perseveration (repetitive behaviors may be motor and verbal)
- Speech: Dysarthria (slurred speech)
- Motor and sensory function
  - Left hemiparesis or hemiplegia
  - Left hemisensory perceptual deficits
  - Denial of paralysis of left side of body
  - Apraxia (inability to perform planned motor acts)

Bacterial Meningitis

Pathophysiology

Bacteria may invade the meninges and subarachnoid space surrounding the brain and spinal cord and cause acute inflammation. A purulent exudate develops, which may cover the base of the brain and extend into the cranial and spinal nerves. Brain swelling may cause increased intracranial pressure. Increased pressure on cerebral vessels may lead to areas of necrosis. Cranial nerve damage may be life-threatening if airway protection is compromised.

Assessment

The clinical manifestations of meningitis initially result from irritation of the meninges (see Clinical Findings 6–6). Manifestations of increased intracranial pressure (see Chapter 14) may follow.

POINTS TO REMEMBER

▶ Because the critically ill adult may present with bacterial meningitis and is also susceptible to the development of bacterial meningitis, a thorough nursing history (see Tables 1–1 and 6–1 and Clinical Findings 6–6) is crucial to identify the causative pathology or patients at risk.

▶ Because the accumulation of exudate may cause an obstructive hydrocephalus, which may contribute to increased intracranial pressure and the potential for herniation, and vascular changes may lead to venous and arterial thrombosis and contribute to decreased cerebral blood flow, in addition to the initial and baseline assessments (see Table 2–1), a focused neuromuscular assessment (see Tables 2–1 and 6–1) should be completed as often as the patient's condition dictates to detect or anticipate and prevent such complications.

▶ Ongoing assessment incorporates the evaluation of responses to diagnostic procedures and therapeutic interventions aimed at early detection of the infecting agent and prevention of the spread of infection; it includes collaboration with other members of the health team to increase cerebral perfusion pressure and prevent further injury.

Clinical Findings 6–6   *Bacterial Meningitis*

I. HISTORY

A. Predisposing factors

1. Common pathogenic bacteria include *Streptococcus pneumoniae, Neisseria meningitidis* (meningococcus), and *Haemophilus influenzae*
2. Less common pathogenic bacteria include *Staphylococcus aureus* and gram-negative bacteria such as *Klebsiella, Pseudomonas,* and *Escherichia coli*
3. Head injuries (compound skull fractures and penetrating trauma)
4. Neurosurgical procedures
5. Lumbar puncture
6. Otitis media
7. Sinusitis
8. Pneumonia
9. Immunodeficiency states

B. Subjective findings

1. Severe headache, which may be accompanied by nausea and vomiting
2. Neck, shoulder, and back pain, or stiffness related to meningeal irritation

II. LABORATORY AND BEDSIDE MONITORING TECHNIQUES

A. Skull x-ray: May reveal infected sinuses

B. CSF analysis (see Chapter 13 for related information on CSF)

1. Elevated pressure (>175 mm H_2O)
2. Purulent and turbid fluid related to infectious process
3. Elevated protein levels related to increased protein volume associated with bacteria and increased WBCs (100–500 mg/dl)
4. Elevated leukocytes (particularly polymorphonuclear neutrophils) related to infectious process (10,000–30,000/mm³)
5. Decreased glucose level related to consumption of glucose by bacteria (<40 mg/dl)

C. Other laboratory studies: Cultures of CSF, blood, or sputum may reveal the causative organism

III. PHYSICAL ASSESSMENT FINDINGS

A. General observations (inspection)
   1. Skin rash or petechiae related to meningococcal organism
   2. Seizures related to meningeal irritation (see Clinical Findings 6–2 for related information on seizures)

B. LOC: Loss of consciousness may be present, related to increased ICP (see Chapter 14 for related information on increased ICP)

C. Behavior: Irritability, confusion, restlessness, agitation, or delirium may be present, related to meningeal irritation or deteriorating LOC

D. Cranial nerves
   1. Photophobia may be present, related to meningeal irritation
   2. Nystagmus may be present, related to meningeal irritation
   3. Aphasia may be present, related to meningeal irritation

E. Motor and sensory function
   1. Kernig's sign may be present, related to meningeal irritation (see Clinical Findings 6-4 for related information on Kernig's sign)
   2. Brudzinski's sign may be present related to meningeal irritation (see Clinical Findings 6–4 for related information on Brudzinski's sign)

F. Vital signs: Fever, tachycardia, or tachypnea may be present, related to the infectious process

Neuromuscular Disorders That May Affect Ventilation But Not the Level of Consciousness

Certain neuromuscular disorders involve the loss of respiratory muscle function or sensory and motor reflexes that protect the airway, which may result in ineffective breathing patterns and airway clearance. Immobility may predispose the patient to atelectasis or pneumonia, resulting in impaired gas exchange. Assessment focuses on identifying motor and sensory limitations and the prevention of life-threatening complications such as respiratory failure.

Spinal Cord Injury

Pathophysiology

Damage to the spinal cord may result from mechanical injury to the spinal cord nerve tissue as well as hemodynamic changes that may cause ischemia, vasospasm, and hypoxia. In addition, concussion may cause shaking of the cord with a transient loss of function (usually resolves within 48 hours), and contusion may cause hemorrhage, edema, and possible necrosis.

Mechanism of Injury

Mechanisms of spinal cord injury include hyperextension (may cause a fracture of the posterior elements of the spine and ligament), hyperflexion (may cause tearing of the posterior ligaments and unstable or dislocated vertebra), rotation (an involuntary twisting of the body), and compression (may cause a burst fracture or a simple compression fracture). A penetrating injury may also result in transection of the cord.

Complete and Incomplete Injury

Spinal cord injury may affect the cervical, thoracic, or lumbar area. The injury may be complete or incomplete.

Complete Injury. Complete transection of the cord results in a total loss of motor and sensory function below the level of the lesion. Motor and autonomic output from the cerebral hemispheres and brain stem are unable to reach the periphery beyond the injured area (descending tracts). Sensory and reflex input from the unaffected cord beyond the level of the injury are unable to reach the brain (ascending tracts).

Incomplete Injury. Incomplete transection of the cord leaves some tracts intact and results in a varying degree of loss of motor and sensory function below the level of the lesion. Incomplete lesions include central cord syndrome, anterior cord syndrome, and Brown-Sequard syndrome.

Central Cord Syndrome. Central cord syndrome is usually associated with a hyperextension injury that results in compression of the central portion of the spinal cord or interruption of blood flow via the anterior spinal arteries:

- Damage may be caused by microscopic hemorrhages and edema in the central gray matter of the cord.
- Motor weakness is more marked in the upper extremities than in the lower extremities.
- Sensory impairment varies but may be more pronounced in the upper extremities.
- Bladder dysfunction is common.

Anterior Cord Syndrome. Anterior cord syndrome is usually associated with a flexion injury that results in compression or interruption of the anterior spinal artery which supplies blood to the anterior two thirds of the cord:

- Damage may be caused by herniated discs, bony fragments, or thrombotic occlusion of the anterior spinal artery.
- There is complete motor paralysis with loss of pain, deep touch, and temperature sensations below the level of the lesion.
- Sensations of light touch, motion, position, and vibration are preserved (posterior cord tract remains intact).

Brown-Sequard Syndrome. Brown-Sequard syndrome is usually associated with a penetrating injury that results in a transverse hemisection of the spinal cord:

- There is ipsilateral motor paralysis and loss of light touch, position, vibration, and motion sensations (corticospinal tracts) below the level of the lesion.
- There is contralateral loss of pain and temperature sensations (spinothalamic tracts) below the level of the lesion.

Assessment

Clinical manifestations of spinal cord injury vary with the level of injury and the type of injury (see Fig. 6–7 and Clinical Findings 6–7). In addition, to motor and sensory losses, respiratory and cardiovascular function, temperature regulation, gastrointestinal motility, elimination, and skin integrity may be affected.

POINTS TO REMEMBER

▶ A thorough nursing history (see Tables 1–1 and 6–1 and Clinical Findings 6–7), including details of the accident or injury and the patient's immediate response, is crucial to assist in identifying the type and extent of spinal cord injury.

▶ Because edema and intracord hemorrhage may extend damage up or down the cord during the first few hours after injury, and spinal cord injury may affect multiple systems, in addition to the initial and baseline assessments (see Table 2–1), focused respiratory, cardiovascular, neuromuscular, gastrointestinal, genitourinary, and integumentary assessments (see Tables 2–1, 4–1, 5–1, 6–1, 7–1, 8–1, and 11–1) should be completed as often as

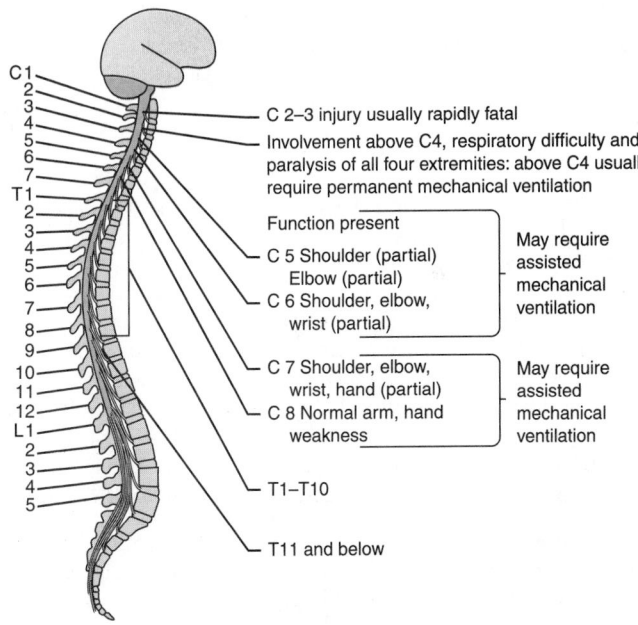

FIGURE 6–7

Level of spinal cord injury and function preserved. (Adapted from Brunner, L. S., & Suddarth, D. S. [1988]. *Textbook of Medical-Surgical Nursing* [6th ed., p. 1505]. Philadelphia: J. B. Lippincott.)

the patient's condition dictates to establish a baseline of normals from whence alterations may be detected, and to detect or anticipate deterioration in respiratory, cardiovascular, and neuromuscular status and prevent complications such as spinal shock (see below), autonomic dysreflexia (see below), pulmonary embolism (see below and Clinical Findings 4–7), pneumonia (see below and Clinical Findings 4–4), and stress ulcer (see below).

Spinal Shock

The critically ill adult with spinal cord injury may present with spinal shock or is at risk for the development of spinal shock. Spinal shock is related to the abrupt cessation of descending impulses, which results in flaccid paralysis and the loss of autonomic and somatic reflex activity below the level of the injury. Spinal shock is more severe in cervical and high thoracic injuries as cord transection above T5 interrupts sympathetic nervous system influence (see Clinical Findings 12–3 for related information on neurogenic shock). Multisystem effects may include

- Bradycardia and dysrhythmias related to unopposed vagal stimulation in the heart
- Hypotension related to the loss of peripheral vasoconstriction
- Decreased gastrointestinal mobility and paralytic ileus related to loss of sympathetic innervation
- Atonic bladder (urinary retention) related to the imbalance between sympathetic and parasympathetic stimulation
- Impaired temperature regulation related to loss of the ability to constrict skin vessels and conserve heat in cool environments, and dilate skin vessels and sweat to lose heat in hyperthermic environments (the patient takes on the temperature of the environment)

Spinal shock may last for days, weeks, or sometimes months. The appearance of spastic paralysis and the return of reflexes signifies that spinal shock is ending. The anal reflex may be tested as one of the earliest to return (insertion of a gloved finger into the rectum will produce contraction of the anal sphincter).

Autonomic Dysreflexia

The critically ill adult with spinal cord injury is at risk for the development of autonomic dysreflexia. Autonomic dysreflexia is a potentially life-threatening situation that can occur in patients with lesions above T6 once spinal shock has subsided. A distended bladder, full rectum, or activation of the skin or pain receptors below the level of the lesion may stimulate the sensory receptors and trigger a reflex arteriolar spasm that increases the blood pressure.

- Uncontrolled blood pressure may result in a stroke (see Clinical Findings 6–5), myocardial infarction (see Clinical Findings 5–3), or seizure (see Clinical Findings 6–2).
- Bradycardia may occur as baroreceptors sense the hypertension and stimulate the parasympathetic nervous system.
- Throbbing headache, nausea, blurred vision, flushing of the face and neck, nasal congestion, and sweating above the level of the lesion may accompany the hypertension and bradycardia.

Pulmonary Embolism

The critically ill adult with spinal cord injury is at risk for the development of a pulmonary embolism (see Clinical Findings 4–7) related to deep vein thrombosis.

- Hypotension and bradycardia result in decreased blood flow.
- Loss of muscle tone contributes to decreased venous return and venous pooling in the pelvis and lower extremities.

Pneumonia

The critically ill adult with spinal cord injury is at risk for the development of pneumonia (see Clinical Findings 4–4) related to atelectasis (see Clinical Findings 4–3) or aspiration.

- Loss of respiratory muscle function may contribute to atelectasis and the retention of secretions.
- Aspiration of stomach contents may contribute to infection.

Stress Ulcer

The critically ill adult with spinal cord injury is at risk for the development of a stress ulcer (see Clinical Findings 7–1) related to an increased production of gastric acid, decreased blood flow to the stomach, paralytic ileus, or the increased production of adrenocorticotropic hormone (ACTH).

Summary

Ongoing assessment incorporates the evaluation of responses to diagnostic procedures and therapeutic interventions aimed at the evaluation of cord instability or damage and the prevention of further injury; it includes collaboration with other members of the health team to increase cord tissue perfusion, prevent life-threatening complications, and optimize recovery.

Clinical Findings 6–7   *Spinal Cord Injury*

I. HISTORY

A. Predisposing factors
1. Males 15–25 years of age
2. Motorcycle and motor vehicle accidents
3. Falls (elderly more at risk)

    4. Violence (stab and gunshot wounds)

    5. Sports injuries

    6. Drugs or alcohol may be contributing factors

B. Subjective findings

    1. Pain over any area of the spinal column

    2. Inability to move extremities

    3. Decreased sensation in the trunk or extremities

II. Laboratory and Bedside Monitoring Findings

A. Spinal x-rays: May reveal presence of a fracture, dislocation, or subluxation (partial or incomplete dislocation)

B. CT scan: May reveal areas of bone injury and cord compression not seen on x-ray

C. Pulmonary function studies (see Table 13–1 for related information on pulmonary function studies)

    1. Decreased vital capacity and tidal volume may be related to loss of respiratory muscle function

    2. Fractures above C4 result in loss of phrenic nerve function to the diaphragm, and permanent mechanical ventilation is usually required

    3. Patients with fractures of C4–C6 may have diaphragmatic function but will have loss of intercostal muscle function and may require assisted ventilation

    4. Patients with fractures of C7 and C8 have diaphragmatic function, but loss of intercostal function may require assisted ventilation (see Fig. 6–7)

D. Arterial blood gas studies

    1. Pao_2 <80 mm Hg may indicate hypoxemia related to hypoventilation

    2. $Paco_2$ >45 mm Hg may indicate hypercapnia related to hypoventilation

E. ECG

    1. Bradycardia may be associated with acute cervical and high thoracic injuries, related to the loss of sympathetic influence on the heart

    2. Dysrhythmias may be associated with acute cervical and high thoracic injuries, related to vagal (parasympathetic) influence, hypothermia, or hypoxia

F. Hemodynamic parameters

    1. Hypotension may be associated with acute cervical or high thoracic injuries related to disconnection of the sympathetic fibers as they exit the spinal cord in the thoracolumbar area (sympathetic influence maintains vasomotor tone; loss of sympathetic activity leads to vasodilation and decreased venous return, resulting in hypotension)

    2. Decreased cardiac output may be related to decreased systemic vascular resistance

III. PHYSICAL ASSESSMENT FINDINGS

A. General observations (inspection)

1. Ineffective rate and depth of respirations may be associated with high cervical and thoracic injuries, related to the loss of diaphragmatic or intercostal muscle function (see Table 6–1 and Fig. 6–3 for related information on the evaluation of respiratory muscle function)
2. Abdominal distention may be related to paralytic ileus and decreased gastrointestinal motility associated with injuries above the lumbar area (abdominal distention may compromise respiratory function and contribute to hypoventilation and hypoxemia as well as increase the risk for vomiting and aspiration)

B. Palpation

1. *Skin*
   - May be cool with hypothermia (common in critical care areas because of air conditioning) related to injuries above T6 and loss of thermoregulation
   - May be warm with hyperthermia related to injuries above T6 and loss of thermoregulation
   - Diaphoresis may be absent below the level of the lesion, related to autonomic dysfunction
2. *Chest wall and thorax:* Chest expansion may be decreased, related to loss of respiratory muscle function
3. *Peripheral pulses:* May be slow or irregular, related to bradycardia and dysrhythmias

C. Percussion: Abdomen may be dull to percussion with injuries above the sacral area, related to retained feces or urine

D. Auscultation

1. *Breath sounds:* May be decreased or absent, related to respiratory muscle insufficiency and decreased chest expansion, or areas of atelectasis
2. *Adventitious sounds:* Crackles or wheezes may be present, related to retained secretions associated with ineffective airway clearance, aspiration, or immobility (atelectasis or pneumonia) or pulmonary edema associated with overzealous fluid administration
3. *Heart sounds:* May be slow or irregular, related to bradycardia or dysrhythmias
4. *Bowel sounds:* May be diminished or absent, related to decreased gastrointestinal mobility

E. Motor and sensory function (in general, cervical injuries may result in quadriplegia, and thoracic and lumbar injuries may result in paraplegia)

1. C3, C4, and C5: May be able to move head and shrug shoulders
2. C6: May have gross arm movement and be able to use thumb and move head and shoulders
3. C7 and C8: May be able to flex elbow, use first, second, third, or fourth digits, roll over, sit up
4. T1 to L1 or L2: May have arm function with no leg function
5. Below L2: May have mixed motor and sensory loss, dependent on intact nerve fibers

(the patient should be able to assist with the assessment unless the level of consciousness is impaired because of an accompanying head injury or sedation. See Tables 6–1 and 6–4 and Figs. 6–2 and 6–7 for related information on the evaluation of motor and sensory function)

F. Reflexes (see Tables 6–1 and 6–5 for related information on the evaluation of reflex activity): The presence of deep tendon and superficial reflexes will vary with complete or incomplete injury and the presence of spinal shock

Myasthenia Gravis

Pathophysiology

Myasthenia gravis is an autoimmune disease affecting neuromuscular transmission. The destruction of receptor sites for acetylcholine (neurotransmitter) diminishes transmission of the nerve impulse across the myoneural junction to the muscle. Voluntary muscles become weak with exercise and improve with rest.

Assessment

Clinical manifestations of myasthenia gravis vary with remission and exacerbation (see Clinical Findings 6–8). In myasthenia crisis, severe weakness may affect the respiratory muscles and cause respiratory insufficiency (extreme dyspnea). Additional manifestations may include difficulty speaking and swallowing, tachycardia, increased blood pressure, anxiety, increased bronchial secretions, and weakness of the extremities.

POINTS TO REMEMBER

▶ The critically ill adult with myasthenia gravis may present with, or develop, myasthenia crisis associated with an exacerbation of the disease process or undermedication.

▶ The critically ill adult with myasthenia gravis may present with, or develop, cholinergic crisis associated with overmedication or after a thymectomy:

  – Too much acetylcholine at the myoneural junction may cause a clinical presentation similar to myasthenia crisis.

  – The Tensilon (edrophonium chloride) test may be used to differentiate myasthenia crisis from cholinergic crisis: If the patient's symptoms improve after the administration of Tensilon, the crisis is myasthenic. Cholinergic crisis will worsen.

▶ A thorough nursing history (see Tables 1–1 and 6–1 and Clinical Findings 6–8) is crucial to identify patients at risk for myasthenia crisis or cholinergic crisis.

▶ In addition to the initial and baseline assessments (see Table 2–1), focused neuromuscular and respiratory assessments (see Tables 2–1, 4–1, and 6–1) should be completed as often as the patient's condition dictates to detect or anticipate and prevent complications such as choking, aspiration, and pneumonia.

▶ Ongoing assessment incorporates the evaluation of diagnostic procedures and therapeutic interventions aimed at the detection or prevention of myasthenia and cholinergic crises (these are medical emergencies and may require immediate intervention, such as endotracheal intubation and mechanical ventilation to support respiration); it includes collaboration with other members of the health team to optimize ventilation and decrease respiratory muscle fatigue.

Clinical Findings 6–8   *Myasthenia Gravis*

I. History

A. Predisposing factors

  1. Thymoma (tumor of the thymus gland)
  2. Thymic hyperplasia
  3. Respiratory infection
  4. Surgery
  5. Trauma
  6. ACTH therapy
  7. Inadequate anticholinesterase medication
  8. Excess anticholinesterase medication

9. Menstrual cycle
10. Pregnancy (especially the first trimester)
11. Anxiety
12. Fatigue
13. Alcohol
14. Medications that may increase muscle weakness or precipitate crisis include quinine, quinidine, procainamide, propranolol, phenothiazines, barbiturates, tranquilizers, narcotics, aminoglycoside antibiotics

B. Subjective findings

1. Extreme weakness and fatigue related to weakness of skeletal muscles
2. Double vision related to weakness of ocular muscles
3. Difficulty speaking and swallowing related to weakness of laryngeal and pharyngeal muscles (increased risk of aspiration)
4. Extreme anxiety associated with crisis
5. Dyspnea related to respiratory muscle fatigue

II. LABORATORY AND BEDSIDE MONITORING FINDINGS

A. CT scan: May reveal the presence of a thymoma

B. Pulmonary function studies (see Table 13–1 for related information on pulmonary function studies): Decreases in tidal volume, vital capacity, and inspiratory force may be present, related to respiratory muscle fatigue and decreased lung expansion

C. Arterial blood gas studies (see Chapter 13 for related information on arterial blood gas studies)

1. Pao_2 <80 mm Hg may indicate hypoxemia related to hypoventilation
2. $Paco_2$ >45 mm Hg may indicate hypercapnia related to hypoventilation

D. Electromyelogram (EMG): May reveal decreased muscle action potential

E. ECG: Tachycardia or dysrhythmias may be present, related to anxiety or hypoxia (crisis)

III. PHYSICAL ASSESSMENT FINDINGS

A. General observations (inspection)

1. Ptosis (drooping of the eyelid) may be present, related to weakness of the ocular muscles
2. Loss of facial expression may be present, related to weakness of the facial muscles
3. Tachypnea may be present, related to anxiety or the need to move more oxygen and maintain CO_2 levels (crisis)
4. Decreased respiratory excursion may be present, related to weakness of respiratory muscles

B. Palpation: *Chest wall and thorax.* Chest expansion may be decreased associated with weakness of the respiratory muscles

C. Auscultation
1. *Abnormal breath sounds:* Diminished or absent breath sounds may be present, related to respiratory muscle insufficiency and decreased lung expansion or areas of atelectasis
2. *Adventitious sounds:* Crackles or wheezes may be present, related to retained secretions associated with ineffective airway clearance or immobility, or increased secretions associated with crisis

D. Motor function: Strength of voluntary muscles may be decreased (sensation and reflexes remain intact)

Guillain-Barré Syndrome (GBS)

Pathophysiology

Guillain-Barré syndrome is an acute inflammatory disease that affects the peripheral nervous system, including cranial and spinal nerves. The cause of GBS is unknown, but it is thought that an autoimmune reaction causes lymphocytes to attack the myelin sheath surrounding the axon of the neuron, causing demyelination. As the axon becomes damaged, the muscles innervated by the affected nerves become weak and atrophy. If there is no cell death, regeneration of the nerve takes place, and recovery is usually complete. Extensive demyelination and axon destruction may result in permanent neurologic deficits.

Assessment

Clinical manifestations may vary with the progression and extent of nerve involvement (see Clinical Findings 6–9). In general, the syndrome is characterized by progressive ascending and symmetrical weakness, and motor paralysis (function returns in descending order). Sensory deficits and diminished or absent reflexes are common.

The syndrome may become life-threatening with the involvement of the diaphragm and the potential for respiratory failure. As well, the autonomic nervous system may be affected resulting in disturbances such as sinus tachycardia (heralding sign), orthostatic hypotension, episodes of hypertension, the syndrome of inappropriate ADH secretion (SIADH), diaphoresis, facial flushing, bowel and bladder incontinence, and abnormal vagal responses, including bradycardia, heart block or asystole.

POINTS TO REMEMBER

▶ The critically ill adult with GBS may be totally paralyzed and unable to speak, swallow, breathe, or blink but is usually fully conscious and able to hear.

▶ A thorough nursing history (see Tables 1–1 and 6–1 and Clinical Findings 6–9) is crucial to identify the causative factor.

▶ Because GBS may affect multiple systems, in addition to the initial and baseline assessments (see Table 2–1), focused assessments of the neuromuscular, respiratory, cardiovascular, gastrointestinal, genitourinary, and integumentary systems (see Tables 2–1, 6–1, 4–1, 5–1, 7–1, 8–1, and 11–1) should be completed as often as the patient's condition dictates to detect or anticipate and prevent complications such as respiratory failure, infection, atelectasis (see Clinical Findings 4–3), aspiration, pneumonia (see Clinical Findings 4–4), deep vein thrombosis, pulmonary embolism (see Clinical Findings 4–7), SIADH (see Clinical Findings 9–3), and urinary retention.

▶ Ongoing assessment incorporates the evaluation of responses to diagnostic procedures and therapeutic interventions aimed at the detection of muscle weakness and the prevention of potentially fatal complications associated with progressive nerve involvement and related neuromuscular deficits; it includes collaboration with other members of the health team to support respiration and optimize recovery.

Clinical Findings 6–9   *Guillain-Barré Syndrome*

I. History

A. Predisposing factors
1. Viral infections (usually respiratory or gastrointestinal)
2. Viral immunizations
3. Immunocompromised states such as AIDS, organ transplantation, pregnancy, malignant neoplasms (chemotherapy)

B. Subjective findings
1. Paresthesia (tingling or numbness) and weakness of the lower extremities
2. Pain, aching, burning, or cramping of the affected areas

II. LABORATORY AND BEDSIDE MONITORING FINDINGS

A. Pulmonary function studies (see Table 13–1 for related information on pulmonary function studies): Decreased tidal volume (<5 ml/kg), decreased vital capacity <12 to 15 ml/kg), and negative inspiratory force (<20 cm H_2O) may be present, related to respiratory muscle weakness (may indicate the onset of respiratory failure and the need for mechanical ventilatory support)

B. Arterial blood gas studies (see Chapter 13 for related information on arterial blood gas studies)

1. Pao_2 <80 mm Hg may indicate hypoxemia related to hypoventilation
2. $Paco_2$ >45 mm Hg may indicate hypercapnia related to hypoventilation

C. CSF analysis (see Chapter 13 for related information on CSF): Elevated protein count (may be normal initially and then peak 4 to 6 weeks after the onset of symptoms)

D. Other laboratory studies: Hyponatremia may be present, related to SIADH (see Table 13–5 for related information on electrolyte imbalances)

E. Nerve conduction studies: Decreased velocity of nerve impulse conduction

F. ECG

1. Tachycardia may be present, related to autonomic nervous system dysfunction
2. Bradycardia, heart blocks, or asystole may occur, related to involvement of the vagus nerve (see Table 14–3 for related information on dysrhythmias)

G. Hemodynamic parameters: Orthostatic hypotension or hypertension may occur, related to autonomic nervous system involvement

III. PHYSICAL ASSESSMENT FINDINGS

A. General observations (inspection)

1. Facial weakness, inability to blink, diplopia, or difficulty in chewing, speaking, or swallowing may be present, related to involvement of cranial nerves III, IV, V, VI, VII, IX, X, XI, and XII (see Table 6–1 for related information on evaluation of the cranial nerves)
2. Decreased or paradoxical chest excursion may be present, related to involvement of the diaphragm or respiratory muscles
3. Abdominal distention may be present, related to urinary retention

B. Palpation: Decreased chest expansion may be present, related to involvement of the respiratory muscles

C. Auscultation

1. *Abnormal breath sounds:* Diminished breath sounds may be present, related to decreased chest expansion or areas of atelectasis

2. *Adventitious breath sounds:* Crackles or wheezes may be present, related to ineffective airway clearance and retained secretions

D. Motor and sensory function

1. Decreased strength against resistance beginning in the lower extremities and progressing to paralysis involving the trunk, upper extremities, and facial muscles, related to peripheral and cranial nerve involvement

2. Decrease in position or vibratory sense related to nerve involvement (see Table 6–1 and Fig. 6–2 for related information on the evaluation of motor and sensory function)

E. Reflexes: Diminished or absent deep tendon reflexes may be present, related to nerve involvement (see Table 6–1 for related information on the evaluation of reflexes)

7

Gastrointestinal Assessment

FUNCTION OF THE GASTROINTESTINAL SYSTEM

The purpose of the gastrointestinal (GI) system is to provide nutrients and drugs to the body. It is essentially an air- and fluid-filled muscular tube through which foods, liquids, and oral medications are transported and prepared for ultimate delivery to cells. It involves the processes of **ingestion, digestion, and absorption** of nutrients as well as **elimination** of solid waste products of the process. The rapid turnover of epithelial cells lining the GI tract makes it sensitive to the effects of chemotherapy and radiotherapy.

Usual entry of nutrients and drugs into the body requires the ability to chew and swallow. Digestion begins in the **mouth** with the process of mastication and secretion of the enzyme ptyalin by salivary glands to begin the digestion of starches. Once a bolus reaches the **esophagus,** it is transported by gravity and the process of peristalsis through the lower esophageal sphincter (LES) to the stomach.

The **gastric mucosa** secretes the hormone gastrin into the blood stream, which stimulates production of hydrochloric acid and pepsin in the stomach for protein digestion. It also stimulates secretion of intrinsic factors needed for absorption of vitamin B_{12} in the distal small intestine, as well as hepatic and pancreatic digestive enzymes, and insulin. Peak gastric activity occurs approximately two hours after eating. Gastric secretions can also be stimulated by caffeine, nicotine, alcohol, nonsteroidal anti-inflammatory drugs (NSAIDs), long-term steroid use, and stress.

Chyme passes through the pyloric sphincter into the **duodenum**, where digestion of fats occurs principally through the emulsifying action of bile produced in the **liver** and stored in the **gallbladder**, and by pancreatic lipase produced by the acinar cells of the pancreas. The **pancreas** also secretes proteolytic enzymes, including trypsin, as well as pancreatic amylase for further digestion of starches. Cells of the pancreatic duct secrete bicarbonate, which is added to pancreatic juice and helps neutralize the acidity of the food bolus as it leaves the stomach. In addition to producing bile the liver is involved in the metabolism and synthesis of carbohydrates, fats, and proteins delivered to it from the intestines via the portal vein, in the storage of vitamins and minerals, and in detoxification of drugs and other substances harmful to the body.

The functional units of the **small intestine** are villi, which secrete enzymes (maltase, sucrase, lactase, lipase, and several proteolytic enzymes) to complete the digestive process, hormones to stimulate the gallbladder and pancreas, and mucus to protect the small intestine. The **duodenum** is the site for absorption of calcium, iron, and most water- and fat-soluble vitamins. The distal portion of the small intestine (**ileum**) provides for absorption of sugars, fats, amino acids, water, and vitamin B_{12} as well as reabsorption of bile.

Preparation of solid waste from the digestive process is accomplished in the **large intestine** after passage of GI contents through the ileocecal valve. It provides a final opportunity for absorption of water and nutrients. Here with the aid of intestinal bacteria, vitamin K and B vitamins are synthesized, and conjugated bilirubin in bile is reduced to fecal urobilinogen, which gives stool its brown color. Water and mucus are added, and feces are stored for elimination, which occurs within approximately 24 hours of ingestion. Elimination is accomplished through voluntary contraction of the external **anal sphincter** in response to a sensation of rectal fullness produced by fecal distention of the rectum.

Parasympathetic fibers (vagus) inhibit and **sympathetic** (splanchnic) nerve fibers stimulate gastrointestinal motility. Major blood supply to the area is through the **celiac and mesenteric arteries**. The **peritoneum** is the protective serous membrane lining the abdominal cavity. Because it is contiguous with the outer surface of most gastrointestinal organs, damage to them may cause inflammation of the peritoneum or fluid accumulation in the peritoneal cavity.

Gastrointestinal function can be compromised by disruption of normal motility, by secretory dysfunction, by mechanical obstruction, by disease states, or by drugs, chemicals, or organisms that affect the gastrointestinal system. This may result in maldigestion, malabsorption, and fluid, electrolyte, vitamin, or other nutrient imbalances. Because of the close proximity of the upper respiratory and upper gastrointestinal systems, respiratory obstruction and aspiration can easily occur.

If nutrients are delivered to the gastrointestinal system artificially (e.g., enteral tubes), digestive processes begin at the point at which the nutrients come in contact with the digestive enzymes and gastrointestinal mucosa. Nutrients delivered intravenously are supplied in elemental forms that can be immediately used by the body or can be further metabolized with passage through the portal circulation of the liver.

Changes with Aging

Changes in the gastrointestinal system with aging are usually minor. Of themselves, such changes have little effect on function. In the presence of systemic disease these changes may severely compromise the elderly patient. Poor nutritional status is a significant predictor of morbidity and mortality in this age group.

Taste sensation, especially for sweet and salty flavors, may diminish with age and affect appetite and food preferences. **Teeth** may be less effective in mastication, and mandibular bone may become osteoporotic. **Pharyngeal muscles** may become weak and less coordinated during the swallowing process, and esophageal contractions may be less coordinated (presbyesophagus). Such changes are more likely related to neurologic or vascular disease than to normal aging. While not a normal change, many elderly experience **gastroesophageal reflux** disease (GERD) due to incompetence of the lower esophageal sphincter. This may result in complaints of heartburn and an increased incidence of esophagitis.

There is a **decreased gastric acid secretion** in the stomach, which may be associated with *Helicobacter pylori* infection, **decreased mucus production,** and **slowed gastric emptying.** Such changes may delay absorption of acid-soluble drugs or prolong their exposure to gastric mucosa, resulting in gastric irritation.

In the small intestine motility may be increased, and enzymes and **absorptive activities decreased. Lactose intolerance** may result from a decrease in the production of lactase. Water, electrolytes, vitamin D, calcium, and iron absorption may be decreased with age. Conversely, other fat-soluble vitamins (A, E, K) may be more readily absorbed.

In the large intestine, mucus production is decreased, **transit time slowed,** and **peristaltic contractions** may be weakened. **Diverticular pockets** form that have the potential to become inflamed and infected. The rectal and anal walls become less motile and less elastic, and the **stimulus to defecate** may be more subtle and more easily disregarded. Constipation, however, is more likely due to changes in routine, activity, diet, and fluid intake.

Hepatocytes decrease in number, resulting in smaller liver size. Hepatic blood flow decreases, as does synthesis of proteins and possibly albumin. These changes may adversely affect a drug's volume of distribution and clearance (see Chapter 3). The **acinar glands** diminish, which may affect secretion of certain digestive enzymes. The **gallbladder** more easily forms gallstones.

Because of **the decrease in total body water** with aging, the older person is more quickly affected by rapid loss of body fluids through vomiting and diarrhea. Water deprivation may more rapidly produce dehydration and elevation of blood chemistry values due to poor dilution. Pain in gastrointestinal organs may be poorly localized, absent, minimal, or atypical. The nurse must be alert to potential problems affecting the GI system through thorough baseline, initial, focused, and ongoing assessments.

Examples of Drugs That Affect Gastrointestinal Function

Drug Classification	Potential Adverse Effects on Gastrointestinal Function
Antacids	Altered absorption of vitamins, minerals; diarrhea (magnesium), constipation (aluminum, calcium)
Antiarrhythmics, antihypertensives, antihypotensives	Constipation (calcium channel blockers), nausea and vomiting (dobutamine, bretylium), diarrhea (quinidine).
Antibiotics	Diarrhea, vitamin and mineral deficiencies
Anticholinergics: tricyclic antidepressants, anti-psychotics (e.g., lithium), antihistamines, antiparkinsonians	Dry mouth, constipation, intestinal obstruction, worsening GERD
Anticoagulants	Gastrointestinal hemorrhage
Antidiarrheals	Bloating, constipation
Antineoplastics	Anorexia, gastrointestinal bleeding
Corticosteroids	Gastritis, peptic ulceration, calcium deficiency (long-term therapy)
Digitalis glycosides	Anorexia, nausea, vomiting, diarrhea
Diuretics	Dehydration, electrolyte imbalances (potassium, magnesium, zinc), constipation
H_2 receptor agonists	Anorexia
Hyperlipemics	Altered absorption of nutrients, constipation (bile-acid resins), gallstones (fibrates, estrogen)
Laxatives	Diarrhea, abdominal pain and cramping, electrolyte imbalances, vitamin deficiency, dehydration
Narcotics	Constipation, nausea, intestinal obstruction
Nonsteroidal anti-inflammatory drugs	Gastrointestinal bleeding, ulceration, perforation, hepatitis, diarrhea

Common Causes of Abdominal Pain

Epigastric Pain
Angina
Esophageal rupture
Stomach disorders: pyloric obstruction, gastritis, gastroenteritis, peptic ulcer, perforation
Liver tumors, enlargement, vascular congestion
Acute pancreatitis
Acute gallbladder disease
Appendicitis
Small bowel obstruction
Mesenteric artery or vein occlusion, ischemia

Umbilical Pain
Small bowel obstruction
Mesenteric artery or vein occlusion
Appendicitis
Gastroenteritis
Abdominal aortic aneurysm
Trapped umbilical hernia

Hypogastric Pain
Colon disorders: colitis, obstruction, fecal impaction
Acute prostatitis
Acute urinary tract disorders: urinary retention, infection, calculi
Colon: diverticulitis, obstruction, perforation
Gynecologic disorders

Generalized Abdominal Pain
Perforation, rupture of an abdominal organ
Bowel strangulation, infarction, necrosis
Peritonitis
Ruptured tubal pregnancy, ovarian cyst

Hypochondrial Pain
Lower lobe pneumonia
Subphrenic abscess
Costochondritis
Splenic disorders (left)
Peptic ulcer (rare), gastric dilatation (left)
Hepatic disease
Gallbladder disease (right)
Acute pancreatitis (left)
Colon: splenic flexure disease, diverticulitis (left)
Renal abscess, infarction

Iliac Pain
Gastroenteritis
Appendicitis (right)
Diverticulitis (left)
Colitis (left)
Ureteral colic
Ovarian, tubal disease
Renal disease

Back Pain
Pleuritis
Aortic aneurysm
Renal disease

Developed from Wiener, S. L. (1993). *Differential diagnosis of acute pain by body region.* New York: McGraw-Hill.

TABLE 7-1 Gastrointestinal Assessment Techniques, Tips, Geriatric Considerations

Technique	Performance Tips	Description/Rationale	Geriatric Considerations
Pertinent History			
1. Related medical history	Review the patient's known medical history for **actual or potential disease states** that may affect gastrointestinal function	These may include diseases or surgeries that involve • Gastrointestinal organs • Vascular supply to GI organs • Neurologic innervation of GI organs • Nutritional disorders • Lifestyle behaviors: alcohol, drugs, tobacco, stress	While the gastrointestinal tract undergoes minimal changes with aging, underlying disease states may affect ingestion, digestion, absorption, and elimination of nutrients and drugs
2. Related drug history	Review the patient's recent past and current **drug therapy** for medications that may • Increase GI symptoms • Mask GI symptoms • Affect nutritional status	Drugs taken prior to admission or administered in the critical care setting may have adverse effects on gastrointestinal function (see p. 415)	The elderly may develop gastrointestinal symptoms related to drug therapy due to • Polypharmacy • Increased potential for drug interactions • Increased drug sensitivity

Table continued on following page

TABLE 7–1 Gastrointestinal Assessment Techniques, Tips, Geriatric Considerations *Continued*

Technique	Performance Tips	Description/Rationale	Geriatric Considerations
	ASSESSMENT TIPS 1. Attempt to correlate a new symptom with a recently administered drug or changed dose 2. Attempt to correlate improvement of a symptom with discontinuance of a drug or with a changed dose		• Incorrect dosing • Altered absorption • Dehydration • Immobility
3. Common complaints and observations that indicate the need for a focused assessment of the gastrointestinal system	*Look for* • Dry mouth • Difficulty swallowing • Drooling • Nausea or retching • Eructation (belching, burping) • Coughing • Emesis, hematemesis	Common causes of abdominal pain (see p. 416)	Conditions of the gastrointestinal tract commonly experienced by the elderly include • Gastroesophageal reflux disease (GERD) • Vitamin B_{12} and iron deficiency anemias

	• Heartburn, chest pain • Upper or lower abdominal pain • Gastric and abdominal distention • Gastric and abdominal cramping • Flatus • Constipation • Diarrhea	• Diverticulosis • Diarrhea • Constipation and laxative dependence
4. Cultural and psychosocial considerations related to GI functions	*Look for* • Stoicism, denial • Moaning, crying • Food rituals and preferences	
	Many individuals find it difficult to discuss bowel elimination Many individuals find it embarrassing to eliminate solid waste in the close confines of a hospital room, cubicle Disregarding the urge to defecate retains stool in the colon for longer periods, allowing for continuing water absorption and constipation or impaction	These behaviors can contribute to constipation and bowel obstruction, especially in the elderly patient

Table continued on following page

TABLE 7-1 Gastrointestinal Assessment Techniques, Tips, Geriatric Considerations *Continued*

Technique	Performance Tips	Description/Rationale	Geriatric Considerations
Physical Examination: Inspection			
1. General observations • Nonverbal behaviors	*Look for* • Changes in activity level • Changes in facial expression • Changes in mental status	May be caused by • Abdominal pain (see below) • Fluid and electrolyte imbalance • Active GI bleeding with resultant anemia, hypotension	The older person is more quickly affected by fluid deprivation or overload than a younger person because of changes with aging as well as disease Dehydration can be caused by fluid restriction (voluntary or iatrogenic), functional impairment, cognitive impairment, or medications
2. Integument	*ASSESSMENT TIP* Use natural light, if possible. Incandescent and fluorescent lighting may alter skin colors		

- Skin color

Look for
- Paleness
- Palmar erythema
- Jaundice

ASSESSMENT TIPS
1. True jaundice includes yellow color of eye sclerae, whereas elevated serum carotene does not discolor sclerae
2. The underside of the tongue may yellow early in the process
3. In dark-skinned patients jaundice may be evaluated by inspecting the hard palate, which will appear yellowed or green brown

Pale skin may be result of malnutrition and anemias

Red palms are common in late cirrhosis

Jaundice is the result of increased circulating bile pigment (hyperbilirubinemia); it can result from
- Overproduction of bilirubin in hemolytic disease
- Hepatocellular disease: hepatitis, cirrhosis, malignancy, drugs
- Liver or gallbladder obstructions

The frail elder confined to bed will usually be pale; loss of subcutaneous fat and muscle atrophy increase the prominence of superficial blood vessels, giving the skin a bluish hue; this may also indicate nutritional deficiencies

Table continued on following page

TABLE 7-1 Gastrointestinal Assessment Techniques, Tips, Geriatric Considerations *Continued*

Technique	Performance Tips	Description/Rationale	Geriatric Considerations
• Pruritus		Generalized itching of skin may be caused by • Dry skin • Skin lesions, inflammations, infections • Hepatic disease • Renal disease • GI malignancies • Lymphomas	
• Hydration	*Look for* • Skin texture • Skin turgor	Dryness suggests dehydration Skin turgor can be assessed by pinching up the skin over the forehead, sternum, or inner thigh; hydrated skin should snap back briskly; dehydrated skin will tent In the well-hydrated patient, mucous membranes are moist and glistening; in dehydration, membranes are dry and dull	Dry skin may be normal with aging Loss of skin elasticity with aging can also cause skin to tent and must be cautiously interpreted as dehydration in the absence of other signs and symptoms The elderly patient may have little or no fever with infection
	• Mucous membranes: – Mouth – Conjunctivae		

| • Nutrition | • Skin temperature, moisture
• Peripheral edema
Look for signs of undernourishment:
• Dry, flaky skin
• Thin, dry hair
• Generalized muscle atrophy
• Temporal muscle wasting
• Small muscle wasting in hands
• Sunken eyes | Fever may be a response to infection or dehydration
Malnutrition (over- or under-nourishment) can adversely affect patient outcomes; it must be identified and treatment begun as soon as possible
Maintenance of adequate nutrition and hydration can contribute to positive outcomes in critically ill patients
Generalized symmetrical loss of muscle mass suggests undernourishment
Extremity wasting with trunkal obesity may be due to long-term steroid therapy
Extremity wasting with abdominal distention may suggest starvation, malignancy, or liver disease
Physical findings that suggest malnourishment are most definitively evaluated through biochemical and hematological analyses | Physical signs of malnutrition may be difficult to distinguish from changes with aging in the very old or frail elderly; after age 70 most elderly will have a mild decline in weight
The frail elderly who have a history of prolonged physical inactivity will also present with generalized muscle atrophy
The frail elderly may also experience loss of appetite as a consequence of chronic disease, drugs, dietary restrictions, alterations in function, mental status, economics, or depression and loss of social networks |

Table continued on following page

TABLE 7-1 Gastrointestinal Assessment Techniques, Tips, Geriatric Considerations *Continued*

Technique	Performance Tips	Description/Rationale	Geriatric Considerations
3. Breath odors	*Look for* • Fruity odor of diabetic ketoacidosis • Alcohol • Tobacco • Food odors • Vomitus • Ammonia odor of uremia • Musty odor of liver disease (fetor hepaticus) • Fetid odor of dental, respiratory infection	Halitosis may provide indication of recent activities, lifestyle behaviors, and systemic disease; this may be especially important information in the nonresponsive patient	The elderly patient may present with poor dental hygiene; this may be due to physical, cognitive, or emotional limitations associated with age or disease; it may also suggest, in certain circumstances, caregiver neglect
4. Nose, mouth, and throat	*Look for* • Nasal obstruction • Tongue size, contour, coating • Dry mouth • Copious or thick mucus • Drooling • Cough: dry, loose	It is important to perform a thorough examination of the mouth and throat of each patient to assess for • Airway obstruction by the tongue, food, secretions, tonsils, masses, dentures, foreign objects • Accurate placement of feeding or	In the elderly person the oral examination will commonly reveal • Discolored teeth from prolonged exposure to staining pigments (cigarettes, coffee, etc.) • Worn chewing surfaces (attrition)

- Eructation
- Retching
- Vomiting, vomitus
- Hemoptysis, hematemesis
- Cerebrospinal fluid in ears, nose, mouth

ASSESSMENT TIPS

1. Evaluation of the nose, mouth, and throat are critical in *every* gastrointestinal assessment because of the close proximity of the upper gastrointestinal and upper respiratory systems
2. Inspect and palpate the oral cavity (see Fig. 7–1) using a good light source and a tongue depressor or gauze pad and gloved fingers to move the tongue

- suction tubes and artificial airways
- Secretions, vomitus that cannot be cleared by the patient and may be aspirated into the respiratory tree
- Loose teeth that may be dislodged during oral procedures such as suctioning, intubation, anesthesia delivery
- Dry mucous membranes (xerostomia) that cause discomfort and increased susceptibility to inflammation and oral infection
- Infections of the teeth, gums, oral mucosa, or tongue that may indicate underlying disease (e.g., AIDS, cancer, diabetes), drug side effect, or neglect
- Ability to clear secretions, foreign materials with an intact cough and gag reflex

- Lost or loose teeth due to periodontitis or osteoporotic changes in the jaw bones
- Dentures or bridges
- Gum recession and gum-line caries
- Xerostomia due to diminished secretions of salivary glands, diseases such as diabetes, medication side effects, dehydration, electrolyte imbalances
- Plaque, food particles which may suggest neglect or inability to attend to oral hygiene
- Dysphagia due to poor coordination of the phases of swallowing with aging; severe dysphagia always indicates disease of the involved musculature or nervous system innervation

Table continued on following page

425

TABLE 7-1 Gastrointestinal Assessment Techniques, Tips, Geriatric Considerations *Continued*

Technique	Performance Tips	Description/Rationale	Geriatric Considerations

Hard palate
Soft palate
Uvula
Posterior pillar
Anterior pillar
Tonsils
Tongue

Incisors
Canine
Premolars
Molars

Molars
Premolars
Canine
Incisors

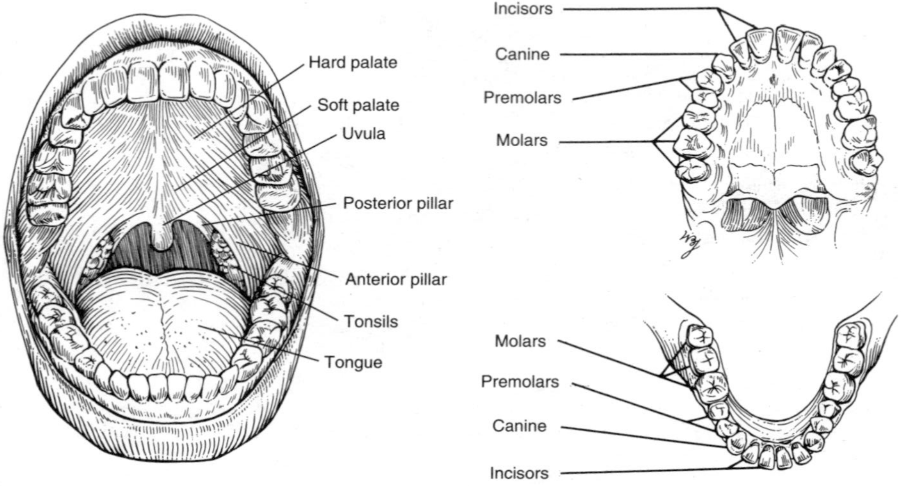

FIGURE 7-1

Structures of the oral cavity. (Adapted from Swartz, M. H. [1998]. *Textbook of physical diagnosis* [3rd ed., pp. 221, 223]. Philadelphia: W. B. Saunders.)

	Look for	Clinical significance	Geriatric considerations
and retract the oral and buccal mucosae; a gauze pad and gloved fingers provide more definitive information on oral contours, textures, and masses 3. Always perform a thorough mouth examination when the enteral tubes are in place to evaluate placement and possible naso-oropharyngeal or upper respiratory obstruction		• Undiagnosed pathologies such as leukoplakia, erythroplakia, tongue or pharyngeal masses most prevalent in middle-aged and elderly persons with a history of significant cigarette and alcohol use • Hematemesis due to upper gastrointestinal bleeding from a pre-existing peptic ulcer or a stress gastritis, which commonly develops during critical illness • Hemoptysis due to airway irritation or lung pathology • Deviation of the tongue or slackness of the cheek with brain stroke	• Gastroesophageal reflux disease (GERD) with esophagitis due to reflux of gastric acid through an incompetent lower esophageal sphincter is a common cause of heartburn in the elderly
5. Cough, gag, swallow reflex	Cough, gag, swallow reflexes (CN IX, X, XII; see Chapter 6) Look for • Guarding, gagging, coughing when the back of the throat	Absence of these reflexes increases the possibility of aspiration and precludes oral feeding Swallowing difficulties may be due to	The elderly patient may be at greater risk for aspiration because of normal changes with aging: • Pharyngeal muscles may be-

Table continued on following page

427

TABLE 7-1 Gastrointestinal Assessment Techniques, Tips, Geriatric Considerations Continued

Technique	Performance Tips	Description/Rationale	Geriatric Considerations
	is stimulated with a tongue blade or suction catheter • Voluntary transfer of solids, liquids, or saliva to the oropharynx • Spontaneous swallowing when liquids or saliva move to the oropharynx	• Decreased level of consciousness • Oral obstruction • Neurological disorders such as brain stroke or Parkinson's disease • Degenerative disorders of the neuromuscular system	come weak and less coordinated with aging • Esophageal contractions may be less coordinated with aging
6. Abdomen	*ASSESSMENT TIPS* 1. Stand on the patient's right side 2. The patient must be in a supine position for accurate assessment with arms at sides and knees sufficiently flexed to	Results will be inaccurate if abdominal contents are displaced during assessment; when full supine position is not possible, interpret abnormal results cautiously	

relax abdominal muscles; it may be necessary to place a small pillow or blanket under the knees to do this	
3. **Visualize abdominal organs** during the examination	Visualizing organs will help you to clarify your findings
4. Describe location of findings in terms of the four abdominal quadrants or nine regions (see Fig. 7–2)	Accurate description allows your results to be reproduced by others
5. Inspection and auscultation of the abdomen should be performed **before percussion and palpation**	Percussion and palpation manipulate abdominal contents; this can change the baseline bowel sound, usually causing hyperactivity, or possibly hypoactivity
6. **Assess painful areas last**	Once pain is elicited, the patient will resist further evaluation

Table continued on following page

TABLE 7-1 Gastrointestinal Assessment Techniques, Tips, Geriatric Considerations *Continued*

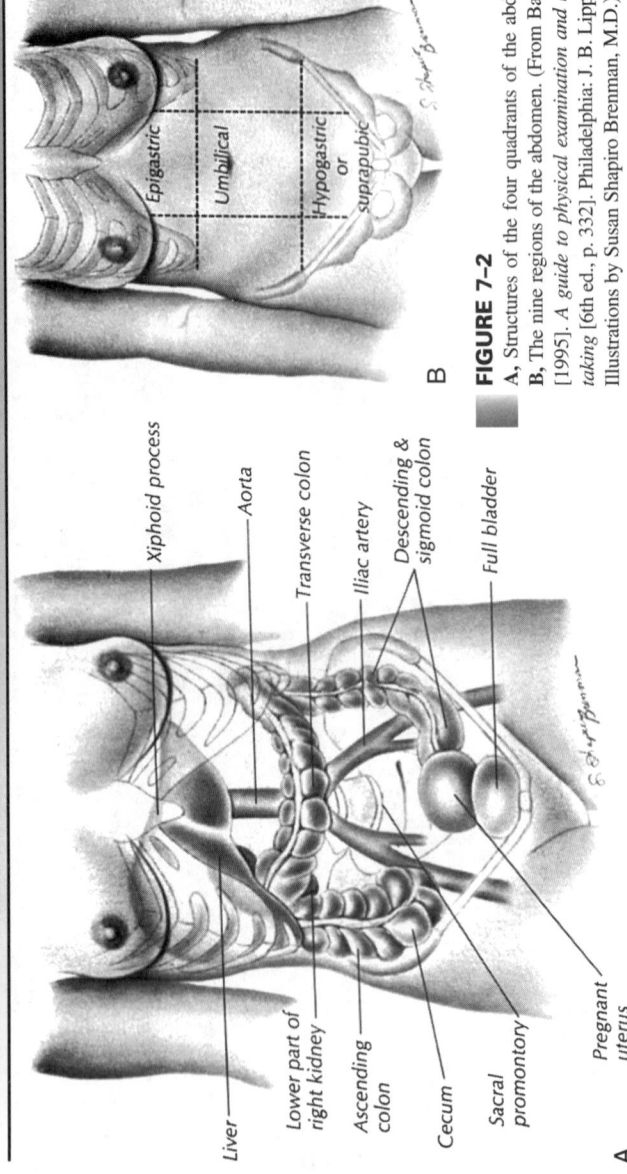

FIGURE 7-2

A, Structures of the four quadrants of the abdomen. **B,** The nine regions of the abdomen. (From Bates, B. [1995]. *A guide to physical examination and history taking* [6th ed., p. 332]. Philadelphia: J. B. Lippincott. Illustrations by Susan Shapiro Brenman, M.D.)

	7. Inspect the abdomen while you are auscultating	This will save time and increase the efficiency of your examination
	8. Make certain you have good light reflecting across the abdomen during inspection to better assess movements	Proper lighting will allow the examiner to see abdominal contours and sometimes, peristaltic movements
	9. Warm the stethoscope in your hand or by rubbing it	Cold implements on the abdomen may cause involuntary tensing of abdominal muscles on contact, which may alter results of the assessment
	10. Always perform a thorough abdominal examination when enteral tubes are in place	Abdominal distention in the presence of an enteral tube may indicate obstruction of a suction tube or slowed gastric emptying with a feeding tube; either can lead to regurgitation and aspiration
• General observations	*Look for*	
	• **Body movement in the presence of abdominal pain**	Restlessness: colicky pain, obstruction
		Flexed knee position: renal, urethral lithiasis
		Stillness with flexed knees: peritonitis
		Pain of gastrointestinal origin may be poorly localized, absent, minimal or atypical in presentation in the geriatric patient

Table continued on following page

TABLE 7-1 Gastrointestinal Assessment Techniques, Tips, Geriatric Considerations *Continued*

Technique	Performance Tips	Description/Rationale	Geriatric Considerations
	• **Breathing pattern**	Left knee to thigh: diverticulitis Right knee to thigh: appendicitis This is a respiratory assessment, but can be reevaluated during the abdominal examination Abdominal breathing is common for males or patients with chronic obstructive pulmonary disease (COPD) who must use abdominal muscles as accessory muscles of exhalation	Abdominal breathing is a common pattern in aging as the chest becomes less compliant and the lungs lose elastic recoil
• Inspection	• Symmetry *ASSESSMENT TIP* Do not palpate any area of asymmetry until after the abdomen has been auscultated.	Asymmetry suggests the presence of an abdominal pathology that can be defined more specifically later in the examination	In the cachectic patient some asymmetry may be explained by the clearer outline of asymmetrical abdominal organs

	• Contour
	  – Flat, rounded
	  – Scaphoid: concave contour
		Contour of the well-conditioned person
		Indicates low body mass, usually related to disease or malnutrition	

- Protuberant: attempt to assess cause

Possible causes:
Obesity: abdomen is soft or consistent with underlying musculature
Aerophagia: abdomen may be firm due to air swallowing. It may occur following CPR, with displaced artificial airway, or during positive pressure ventilation
Distention with everted umbilicus may indicate ascites due to liver disease, portal hypertension, congestive heart failure (CHF), peritonitis, hernia, or neoplasia. Skin is taut and shiny

Distention may be enhanced by delayed gastric emptying with aging

- **Scars:** Will confirm or identify previous abdominal surgeries (Fig. 7-3)
- **Striae:** Ruptured elastic fibers resulting from rapid and prolonged stretching

Previous surgeries may produce adhesions that can cause discomfort or obstruction

Common causes
Obesity, pregnancy (pink, blue, silver)
Long-term adrenocorticosteroid exposure (purple-blue) from Cushing's syndrome or long-term corticosteroid use causes fragility of skin components

Table continued on following page

433

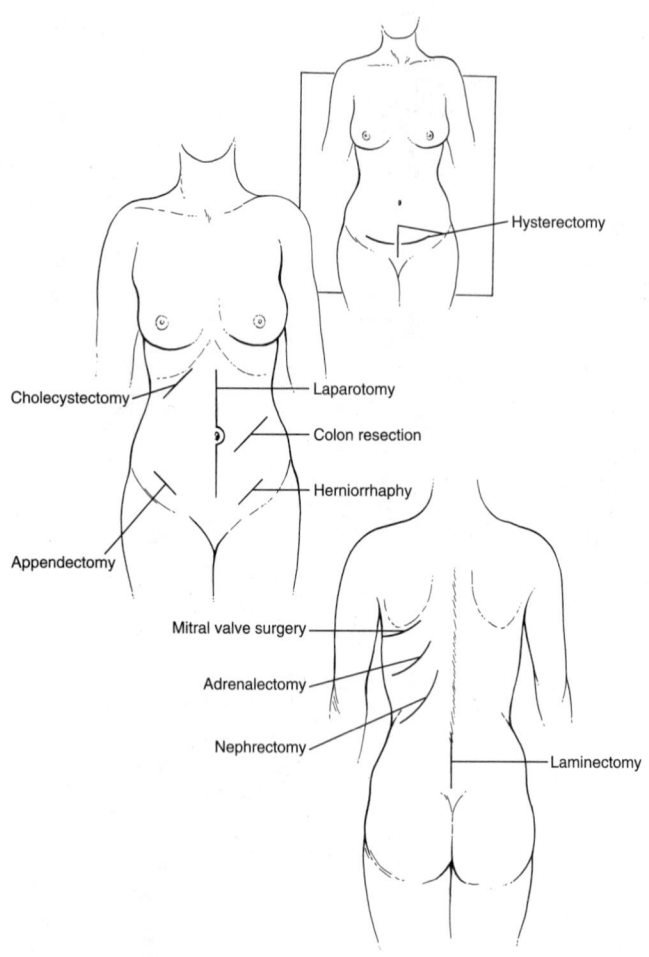

FIGURE 7–3
Locations of common surgical scars. (From Swartz, M. H. [1998]. *Textbook of physical diagnosis* [3rd ed., p. 338]. Philadelphia: W. B. Saunders.)

TABLE 7-1 Gastrointestinal Assessment Techniques, Tips, Geriatric Considerations *Continued*

• **Venous patterning**	Spider angiomas on chest or abdomen may indicate liver disease, pregnancy, collagen disease	
	Prominent, dilated superficial veins (caput medusae) on a distended abdomen are seen in liver disease with portal hypertension	
	Ecchymoses on abdomen, flanks (Grey Turner's sign) may be present in severe intra-abdominal bleeding	
	A blue umbilical area (Cullen's sign) may indicate possible hemoperitoneum	
• **Pulsations**		
— Midepigastric	Midepigastric pulsations of the abdominal aorta can be seen in thin people and with hypertension, aortic insufficiency, and thyrotoxicosis	Pulsations may be more easily visible in the elderly patient due to decreased abdominal muscle mass and tone and decreased connective tissue
	Pulsations of the abdominal aorta should be no wider than an inch and consistent with cardiac sounds; a	

Table continued on following page

435

TABLE 7-1 Gastrointestinal Assessment Techniques, Tips, Geriatric Considerations *Continued*

Technique	Performance Tips	Description/Rationale	Geriatric Considerations
– Peristaltic		wide area of pulsation may indicate an abdominal aortic aneurysm and may be accompanied by a bruit, heard on auscultation	
		Oblique peristaltic movements may be seen in thin persons or patients with enteritis; peristalsis may also be visible above an area of impending or actual bowel obstruction, usually accompanied by colicky pain and borborygmi (see below)	
• Obvious masses		Masses are usually visible only in the thin person	Masses may be more easily visible in the elderly patient due to decreased abdominal muscle mass and tone, and decreased connective tissue
	ASSESSMENT TIP At this point in the examination, do not palpate any suspected mass; manipulation of abdominal contents may alter bowel sounds	A hernia is a protrusion of abdominal contents through weakened abdominal musculature; it may only be seen with increased intra-abdominal pressure such as with a cough or ascites; it should be soft, nontender, reducible	

Look for
- Hernias
- Abdominal aorta (midline, epigastric area)
- Enlarged liver (right and possible left upper quadrant) or spleen (left upper to lower quadrant); these are rare findings
- Distended colon (any quadrant, especially left lower)
- Distended bladder (suprapubic)

- *Umbilical:* Protuberant umbilicus
- *Incisional:* In the area of a scar
- *Inguinal:* In the groin area, above the inguinal ligament or in the ipsilateral scrotal sac
- *Femoral:* Medial aspect of the thigh

Any suspected hernia should be reducible (see below); a strangulated hernia constitutes a surgical emergency

Auscultation
1. Bowel sounds

ASSESSMENT TIPS
1. Warm the stethoscope before placing on the abdomen
2. Begin assessment in the **right lower quadrant (RLQ)**

Cold equipment may cause discomfort and abdominal guarding

Normal bowel sounds are easily transmitted, but in the critically ill patient, bowel sounds may be diminished and difficult to hear; in the

Table continued on following page

TABLE 7-1 Gastrointestinal Assessment Techniques, Tips, Geriatric Considerations *Continued*

Technique	Performance Tips	Description/Rationale	Geriatric Considerations
	3. In critical care settings listen for bowel sounds in **all four abdominal quadrants**	area of the ileocecal valve in the RLQ, bowel sounds are normally audible; listening throughout the abdomen may pinpoint an area of obstruction	
	4. Bowel sounds are high-pitched and can usually be heard with the diaphragm of the stethoscope		
	5. Lay the stethoscope *gently* on the abdomen; do not apply pressure	Heavy pressure on the abdomen changes the rate of movement of air and fluids and alters normal bowel sounds for some period of time	
	6. If bowel sounds are not readily heard, pull up a chair, sit, and **listen for at least 2–5 minutes before declaring sounds absent**	A decision that bowel sounds are absent will have treatment consequences for the patient	

Listen for

- Tinkling, gurgling sounds at the approximate rate of 5–30 per minute
- Diminished bowel sounds
- Hyperactive bowel sounds
- Borborygmi

Hyperperistalsis (borborygmi) occurs with hunger, enteritis, or early intestinal obstruction

Diminished or absent bowel sounds occur with paralytic ileus, abdominal surgery, or peritonitis

2. Abdominal bruits

ASSESSMENT TIPS

1. Listen first with the **diaphragm** pressed firmly on the abdomen
2. Soft, low-pitched murmurs may only be heard with the **bell** held lightly to the abdomen
3. Attempt to **differentiate** an **abdominal** bruit in the aortic area from a **cardiac murmur** transmitted to the abdomen

A bruit is produced by turbulent blood flow through a large artery; this may be caused by arterial stenosis or aortic dissection; while abdominal bruits represent cardiovascular problems (see Chapter 4), they may only be discovered during auscultation of the abdomen

Bruits may be difficult to detect through an obese or distended abdomen

Auscultation over the source of the murmur will usually produce a

Table continued on following page

TABLE 7–1 Gastrointestinal Assessment Techniques, Tips, Geriatric Considerations *Continued*

Technique	Performance Tips	Description/Rationale	Geriatric Considerations
	Listen in the following areas (Fig. 7–4): • Aortic • Renal • Iliac • Femoral	louder sound than over a transmitted area, except when a cardiac murmur is very loud (grade IV–VI) and the patient very thin	
3. Venous hums	*ASSESSMENT TIP* Use the stethoscope bell *Listen in the following regions:* • Periumbilical • Epigastric	This is a soft, continuous, machinery sound produced by collateral circulation between systemic and portal circulatory systems in the presence of liver disease	
4. Friction rubs	*Listen in the following areas:* • Hepatic (right, left upper quadrants) • Splenic (left upper quadrant)	This is a grating sound with respiratory movement produced by inflammation of the peritoneal surface of the liver or spleen; a friction rub heard over the liver or spleen is *rare* and usually heard at or above the border of the organ	

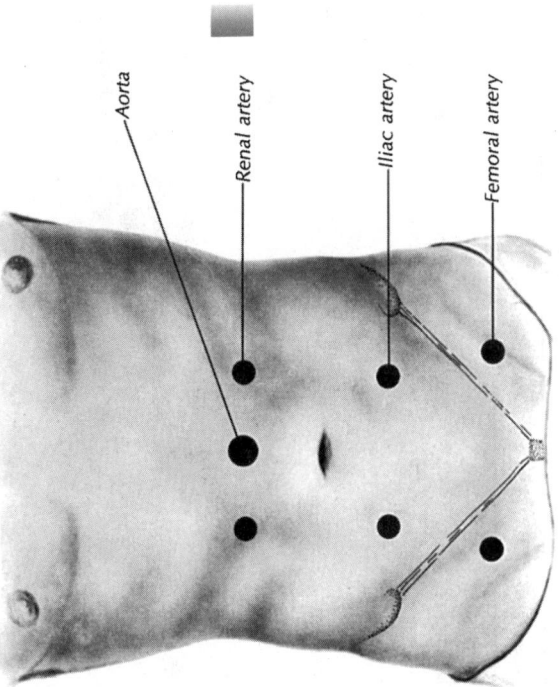

FIGURE 7-4

Sites for auscultation of renal, iliac, and femoral arteries. (From Bates, B. [1995]. *Textbook of physical diagnosis* [6th ed., p. 338]. Philadelphia: J. B. Lippincott. Illustration by Susan Shapiro Brenman, M.D.)

Aorta

Renal artery

Iliac artery

Femoral artery

Table continued on following page

TABLE 7-1 Gastrointestinal Assessment Techniques, Tips, Geriatric Considerations *Continued*

Technique	Performance Tips	Description/Rationale	Geriatric Considerations
Percussion **1. General**	*ASSESSMENT TIPS* 1. Percussion can provide important information about abdominal symptoms and evolving pathologies 2. Percussion needs to be practiced for proficiency 3. **Defer** abdominal percussion if you suspect appendicitis, pancreatic pseudocyst, or aortic aneurysm; also defer percussion with recent abdominal organ transplant or polycystic kidneys	The normal abdominal percussion note is tympany; this is a hollow, drum-like sound produced by abdominal gas bubbles that rise toward the ventral surface of the stomach and intestines when the patient is in the supine position A dull percussion note is heard over nonhollow organs (liver, spleen), fluid-filled organs (full bladder), or hollow organs filled with solid material (stool-filled colon)	

		A resonant percussion note is heard over lung tissue
		The obese abdomen may produce a dull percussion note throughout because of the thickness of the adipose layer
	4. Percuss the entire abdomen systematically, listening for unexpected percussion notes	
	5. See Chapter 4 for technique	
	6. Coordinate percussion results with those of palpation	
2. Masses		Masses will have a dull percussion note
3. Shifting dullness		Significant amounts of ascitic fluid in the peritoneal cavity will produce a dull percussion note
		Since fluid seeks the lower level in a cavity because it is heavier than air (gas), this dull percussion note will shift as the patient is repositioned to a side-lying position (Fig. 7–5)

Table continued on following page

TABLE 7–1 Gastrointestinal Assessment Techniques, Tips, Geriatric Considerations *Continued*

Technique	Performance Tips	Description/Rationale	Geriatric Considerations

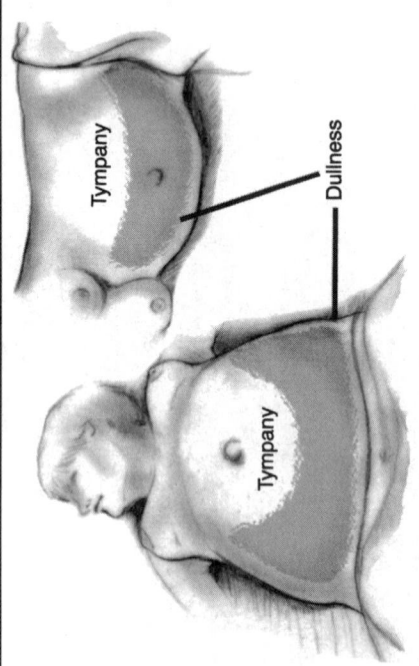

FIGURE 7–5

Location of tympany when percussing for the shifting dullness of ascites. (From Delp, M. H., & Manning, R. T. [1981]. Major's physical diagnosis: An introduction to the clinical process [9th ed., p. 326]. Philadelphia: W. B. Saunders.)

4. Liver, spleen

ASSESSMENT TIPS

1. **Percussion** of specific organs **is not routinely performed** by the critical care nurse

2. Use percussion to further **evaluate and describe abdominal masses or tenderness**

3. With hypatomegaly, general percussion of the upper abdomen may reveal dullness over the lower border of the liver below the costal margins

4. A simple method to assess splenomegaly involves percussing in the last full intercostal space (9th) at the left anterior

While nurses do not routinely percuss for specific organs, in certain situations it may reveal an evolving pathology

Percussion over the liver produces a dull note; dullness at the lower costal margins in the upper abdominal quadrants is also produced by percussion of ribs or by percussion over a transverse colon containing feces

The spleen is situated under the left costal margin below the diaphragm and behind the stomach (Fig. 7–6); enlargement may be due to cirrhosis, cytopenic diseases, inflammatory diseases, or abdominal trauma

In the elderly patient the normal liver decreases in size; the borders are within or at the costal margin and are not easily percussed

Table continued on following page

445

TABLE 7-1 Gastrointestinal Assessment Techniques, Tips, Geriatric Considerations *Continued*

Technique	Performance Tips	Description/Rationale	Geriatric Considerations

10th rib

Midaxillary line

Spleen

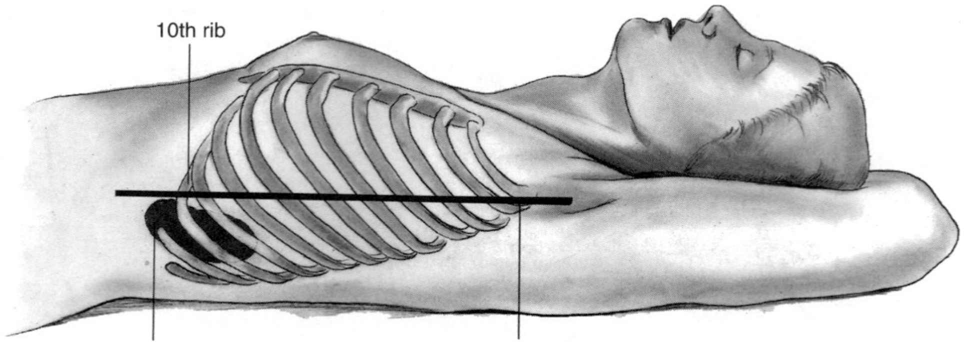

FIGURE 7-6

Location of the spleen. (From Jarvis, C. [1996]. *Physical examination and health assessment* [3rd ed., p. 601]. Philadelphia: W. B. Saunders.)

axillary line during normal breathing and with deep inspiration; both notes should be tympanic; dullness on inspiration suggests splenomegaly; this examination can only be done with a cooperative patient

Enlargement progresses down the left quadrants of the abdomen as an area of dullness; dullness in these areas may also be due to a full descending colon

Palpation: General, Light

ASSESSMENT TIPS
1. **Defer** abdominal palpation if you suspect appendicitis, pancreatic pseudocyst, or aortic aneurysm; also defer palpation with recent abdominal organ transplant or polycystic kidneys

Light and especially deep palpation may rupture an inflamed organ, dissect an aneurysm, dislodge a cyst, or damage a transplant

Table continued on following page

TABLE 7-1 Gastrointestinal Assessment Techniques, Tips, Geriatric Considerations *Continued*

Technique	Performance Tips	Description/Rationale	Geriatric Considerations
	2. **Warm your hands** before touching the abdomen	Cold hands may cause abdominal guarding, making accurate assessment difficult	
	3. **Palpate with the pads of the fingers** of the dominant hand, or place the nondominant hand on top of this hand to exert sufficient pressure to compress the abdomen about 1–2 cm	Finger pads are sensitive to changing contours and masses	
	4. **Develop a systematic pattern of palpation** that covers all four quadrants	Without a system, areas of tenderness or pathology may be missed	
	5. **Palpate areas of known tenderness or pain last**	Once pain has been initiated, the awake patient will be unwilling to continue the examination and incur more discomfort	

6. **Watch the face** of the conscious and unconscious patient while palpating for nonverbal signs of discomfort

7. **Coordinate palpation results with percussion findings**

Feel for

• **Consistency**

The healthy abdomen is soft and compliant

In patients with well-developed abdominal musculature, the consistency is firm

In the very thin person, a bony mass may be felt in the midline of the lower quadrants; this is the concave sacral promontory of the spine but may be misinterpreted as a lower abdominal mass

Table continued on following page

TABLE 7-1 Gastrointestinal Assessment Techniques, Tips, Geriatric Considerations *Continued*

Technique	Performance Tips	Description/Rationale	Geriatric Considerations
		The protuberant abdomen may be rigid in the presence of ascites or hemoperitoneum	Masses may be more easily palpable in the elderly patient due to decreased abdominal muscle mass and tone, and decreased connective tissue
• **Masses**	*ASSESSMENT TIPS* 1. Have a cooperative patient, if able, raise his or her head off the pillow, superficial masses will become more prominent; deeper masses will disappear beneath abdominal musculature 2. Have the alert patient take a deep breath or cough, or inspect the abdomen during a sponta-	Masses that may be normally palpable include • Hernias • Aorta (midline, epigastric area) • *Enlarged* liver (right and possible left upper quadrant) • *Enlarged* spleen (left upper to lower quadrant) • Fecal material (any quadrant, especially left lower) • Distended bladder (suprapubic area) Other masses may indicate neoplasia or other pathology	

neous deep breath or cough; this may enhance abdominal contours and help identify asymmetry and masses

• **Ascites**

ASSESSMENT TIPS

1. If ascites are suspected, **measure abdominal girth** at the largest diameter of the abdomen

2. Before removing the tape measure, **mark the abdomen** on each side of the tape near the midline and at the flanks so that successive measurements will be consistent among examiners

Ascites is an accumulation of fluid within the abdominal cavity. It may occur with
• Portal or venous hypertension in liver disease
• Hypoalbuminemia
• Inflammatory processes of the peritoneum that increase peritoneal capillary permeability
• Cardiac conditions such as advanced CHF or constrictive pericarditis

Table continued on following page

TABLE 7-1 Gastrointestinal Assessment Techniques, Tips, Geriatric Considerations *Continued*

Technique	Performance Tips	Description/Rationale	Geriatric Considerations
	3. Note increase or decrease in girth with each measurement		
• **Tenderness**		Some abdominal areas are normally mildly tender to palpation, including the proximal abdominal aorta and the sigmoid colon	
		These areas can be palpated routinely	
		Other painful areas should be palpated at the end of the examination	
• **Guarding**		Guarding is involuntary muscle contraction over an area of tenderness	
		Rebound tenderness occurs as fingertip pressure is quickly released following compression of a tender area; it is caused by an inflamed peritoneum; it can also often be elicited in the abdominal quadrant contralateral to the area of pathology	

- **Liver, spleen borders**

ASSESSMENT TIPS
1. Palpation of specific organs is **not routinely performed** by the critical care nurse
2. With hepatomegaly, general palpation of the upper abdomen may reveal the lower border of the liver below the costal margins; with severe enlargement, it may be visible; with sclerosis, it will be firm to the touch; with inflammation, it will be tender

During routine palpation the inferior border of an enlarged or sclerosed liver may be palpated at or below the costal margins

In the elderly patient the normal liver decreases in size; the borders are within or at the costal margin and are not usually palpable.

Table continued on following page

TABLE 7–1 Gastrointestinal Assessment Techniques, Tips, Geriatric Considerations *Continued*

Technique	Performance Tips	Description/Rationale	Geriatric Considerations
Rectal/Anal Area			
1. Stool characteristics	Absence of stool or constipation	Healthy adults have a stool every 1–4 days Illness may cause alteration in the usual pattern of elimination; constipation may be due to • Disruption of usual toileting routine • Changes in activity • Changes in diet • Medication side effects (e.g., anticholinergics, calcium channel blockers, narcotics) • Enteral or parenteral nutrition • Tumor, stricture, adhesion, volvulus or other obstruction • Electrolyte imbalances (e.g., hypercalcemia, hypokalemia) • Endocrine disorders (e.g.,	The geriatric patient may also present with laxative overuse; this often leads to an atonic colon and laxative dependence; in the absence of an accurate history of laxative use, constipation and impaction may be the first signs of the problem; if an elderly patient has unexplained diarrhea in small amounts, the first assessment should be for fecal impaction

| Consistency of stool | hypothyroidism, diabetic autonomic neuropathy)
• Neurologic disorders such as spinal cord injury, stroke, dementia
Diarrhea may be a symptom of
• Diarrheal illness
• Hypermotility
• Medication side effects
• Alteration in digestive processes
• Intolerance of hyperosmolar or lactose-based enteral feedings
• Fecal impaction
• Neurologic disorders
• Endocrine disorders (e.g., hyperthyroidism, diabetic autonomic neuropathy)
Distinguish whether diarrhea stool elimination is under voluntary control or is eliminated involuntarily (fecal incontinence) | In fecal impaction, mucus and fluid are produced when hard stool irritates the rectum; this liquid seeps around the impaction, causing fecal incontinence; fecal incontinence may also be seen in patients with dementia, brain stroke, and rectal sphincter damage |

Table continued on following page

TABLE 7-1 Gastrointestinal Assessment Techniques, Tips, Geriatric Considerations *Continued*

Technique	Performance Tips	Description/Rationale	Geriatric Considerations
	Stool color	Stool color is influenced by substances in the fecal material; color changes may be due to • Blood: frank or occult • Excess fat, bilirubin • Drugs such as iron • Mucus, pus (infection) • Foods • Infestations	
2. Perianal inspection	*Look at* • Perianal area • Anal sphincter • Rectal lumen *ASSESSMENT TIPS* 1. If possible, position the patient on the left side with upper knee flexed	Examination of the perianal area may reveal hemorrhoids, a possible source of blood in stool When inserting the gloved finger through the external anal sphincter, note its tone; a weakened sphincter may be associated with fecal incontinence The index or middle finger will reach about 6–10 cm into the rectal	Rectal examination is a vagal maneuver that may increase parasympathetic activity in the heart, slowing conduction through the AV node; thus it may cause bradycardia or asystole in susceptible patients and should be done cautiously in the elderly and others with cardiac dysfunction

2. Lubricate a gloved finger with water-soluble gel
3. Apply pressure to the anal sphincter with the pad of the index or third finger of the dominant hand to relax it
4. Insert finger and examine the lumen and all four quadrants of the rectal wall
5. Note the size, shape, location, and consistency of any palpable mass or stool
6. Evaluate the position and consistency of any stool
7. Attempt to dislodge and break up stool if impacted
8. Test stool for occult blood as appropriate

lumen; stool, polyps, or strictures beyond this point cannot be assessed with this examination

The prostate gland can be palpated behind the ventral wall of the rectum; it is usually not examined in a critical care setting unless male urinary flow problems are present (see Chapter 8); palpation of the gland may produce a desire to urinate in the awake male; in the presence of prostatitis this examination will cause the awake male discomfort; a rectal examination that stimulates the prostate gland should not be done within 24 hours prior to drawing of a PSA (prostate specific antigen)

Table continued on following page

TABLE 7-1 Gastrointestinal Assessment Techniques, Tips, Geriatric Considerations *Continued*

Technique	Performance Tips	Description/Rationale	Geriatric Considerations
	Optional prostate examination in the male		
	1. Palpate the ventral (anterior) wall of the rectum for a firm, smooth area the consistency of a pencil eraser		
	2. Palpate for two lobes and a median sulcus		
	3. The gland should not protrude more than 1 cm into the rectal lumen		

GASTROINTESTINAL DISORDERS

Disorders of the gastrointestinal tract most commonly seen in the critically ill adult include gastrointestinal hemorrhage, hepatic failure, and acute pancreatitis.

 Gastrointestinal Hemorrhage

Pathophysiology

Gastrointestinal (GI) hemorrhage may be classified as upper or lower in origin. Upper GI hemorrhage refers to the loss of blood from a site above the ligament of Treitz at the duodenojejunal junction. Lower GI hemorrhage refers to the loss of blood from a site below the ligament of Treitz.

Upper GI Hemorrhage

Upper GI hemorrhage is more frequently seen than lower GI hemorrhage in the critically ill adult. Sources of upper GI hemorrhage include bleeding from the esophagus, stomach, or small intestine. Esophageal varices (see Hepatic Failure) are normally the cause of massive bleeding from the esophagus, although retching and vomiting may cause tearing of the esophageal or gastric mucosa (Mallory-Weiss syndrome).

Peptic ulcers are the most common cause of bleeding from the stomach and duodenum (gastric and duodenal ulcers). Ulcers may be caused by substances that cause an excessive production of hydrochloric acid and irritate the GI tract, such as caffeine, substances that break down the protective mucosal barrier, such as aspirin and alcohol, or ischemia to the GI tract related to trauma or sepsis.

Lower GI Hemorrhage

Lower GI hemorrhage involves bleeding from the colon. Lower GI bleeds may be associated with cancer, diverticulitis, ulcerative colitis, and polyps.

Assessment

Clinical manifestations of GI hemorrhage vary with the speed and the amount of blood loss (see Clinical Findings 7–1). An acute blood loss (greater than 15–20% of the total blood volume) may lead to hypovolemic shock (see Clinical Findings 12–3).

POINTS TO REMEMBER

▶ Because the critically ill adult may present with an upper GI hemorrhage, and is also susceptible to the development of an upper GI bleed associated with stress-related mucosal damage (hypersecretion of acid or decreased gastric blood flow), anticoagulant therapy, or bleeding disorders such as disseminated intravascular coagulation (see Clinical Findings 10–1), a thorough nursing history (see Tables 1–1 and 7–1 and Clinical Findings 7–1) is crucial to assist in identifying the cause, source, and extent of the bleed as well as to detect patients at risk.

▶ In addition to the initial and baseline assessments (see Table 2–1) and a focused assessment of the underlying disorder, focused gastrointestinal, respiratory, and cardiovascular assessments (see Tables 2–1, 7–1, 4–1, and 5–1) should be completed as often as the patient's condition dictates to detect or anticipate and prevent complications such as cardiovascular decompensation and hypovolemic shock (see Clinical Findings 12–3).

▶ Ongoing assessment incorporates the evaluation of responses to diagnostic procedures and therapeutic interventions aimed at detecting the source and extent of the bleed and the restoration of circulating blood volume; it includes collaboration with other members of the health team to control the hemorrhage and prevent further bleeding.

Clinical Findings 7–1 *Gastrointestinal Hemorrhage*

I. HISTORY

A. Predisposing factors

1. Previous history of ulcer or liver disease
2. Alcohol
3. Caffeine
4. Aspirin
5. Nonsteroidal anti-inflammatory drugs
6. Anticoagulants
7. Multiple trauma
8. Burns
9. Head injury
10. Spinal cord injury

11. Sepsis
12. Adult respiratory distress syndrome (ARDS)
13. Renal failure

B. Subjective findings
1. Thirst related to fluid loss
2. Nausea or vomiting related to gastrointestinal irritation
3. Dizziness related to deceased circulating blood volume and decreased cerebral perfusion
4. Fatigue related to decreased circulating blood volume and decreased perfusion of skeletal muscles
5. Epigastric pain related to inflammation or mucosal lesions

II. LABORATORY AND BEDSIDE MONITORING FINDINGS

A. Endoscopy: May be used to reveal the site of upper GI bleeding, the degree of ulceration, and the amount of tissue injury, or to control bleeding (sigmoidoscopy or colonoscopy may reveal the site of lower GI bleeding)

B. Laboratory studies
1. Decreasing hemoglobin (Hgb) and hematocrit (Hct) may reflect blood loss (the initial values may not reflect blood loss; see Table 13–8 for related information on Hgb and Hct)
2. Electrolyte imbalances may include hypokalemia and hyponatremia related to nasogastric suction, vomiting, or diarrhea (see Table 13–5 for related information on electrolyte imbalances)
3. WBC count may be elevated (return to normal 24 to 48 hours after bleed stops; see Table 13–9 for related information on WBC count)
4. Blood urea nitrogen (BUN) may be elevated, related to the absorption of blood from the GI tract or dehydration (see Table 13–6 for related information on BUN)
5. Prolonged clotting times may be related to hepatic impairment or anticoagulants (see Table 13–8 for related information on coagulation studies)

C. ECG (see Table 14–3 for related information on dysrhythmias): Tachycardia or dysrhythmias may be present, related to hypovolemia, myocardial ischemia, electrolyte imbalances, or drug therapy such as vasopressin

D. Hemodynamic parameters (see Chapter 14, Table 14–2, and Fig. 14–2 for related information on hemodynamic parameters)
1. Hypotension related to decreased circulating blood volume
2. Decreased right ventricular and left ventricular filling pressures related to hypovolemia (increased pressures may indicate fluid overload)
3. Decreased cardiac output related to hypovolemia

III. **Physical Assessment Findings**

A. General observations (inspection)

1. *Mental status:* Lethargy, drowsiness, confusion, irritability, or restlessness may be present, related to hypovolemia and decreased cerebral blood flow (blood loss in excess of 1000 ml or 20% of blood volume)

2. *Respiratory pattern:* Tachypnea may be present, related to the need to move more oxygen (the loss of blood and red blood cells decreases the oxygen-carrying capacity)

3. *Skin*
   - Conjunctivae, mucous membranes, skin, or nail beds may be pale, related to the loss of blood
   - Sclerae and skin may be yellow (jaundice) if the bleed is related to esophageal varices
   - Petechiae, ecchymosis, or purpuric lesions may be present if bleed is related to blood dyscrasias
   - Palmar erythema, spider angiomas, and ecchymosis may be present if bleed is related to esophageal varices

4. *Abdomen:* Abdominal distention (ascites) may be present if the bleed is related to esophageal varices

5. *Emesis:* Hematemesis or gross vomiting of blood (blood may be bright red or coffee ground in color) may be present with an upper GI bleed

6. *Stool*
   - Hematochezia, or passage of bright red blood via the rectum, may be present with a massive upper GI bleed, as the blood may not have time to be acted upon by the digestive enzymes (associated signs of hypovolemia will be present)
   - Melena, or black, tarry stools with a foul odor, are usually related to an upper GI bleed (with a lower GI bleed, stools are bloody but nonfetid)

7. *Urine:* Urine output may be less than 30 ml per hour, related to hypovolemia and decreased blood flow to the kidneys

8. *Temperature:* Fever may be present, related to dehydration

B. Auscultation

1. *Abnormal breath sounds:* Diminished breath sounds may be present, related to decreased respiratory excursion associated with ascites or areas of atelectasis

2. *Adventitious sounds:* Crackles or wheezes may be present, related to retained secretions associated with ineffective breathing patterns (splinting or reduced diaphragmatic excursion related to abdominal tenderness or ascites) or to aspiration of stomach contents (pneumonia, ARDS)

3. *Bowel sounds*

- Hyperactive bowel sounds may be present with an upper GI bleed
- Hypoactive bowel sounds may be present with a lower GI bleed
(see Table 7–1 for related information on evaluation of bowel sounds)

C. Palpation
1. *Skin:* May be cool and clammy related to hypovolemia and decreased peripheral blood flow (blood loss in excess of 1000 ml or 20% of blood volume)
2. *Peripheral pulses*
   - Pulse may be rapid and thready with blood loss in excess of 1000 ml or 20% of blood volume
   - Postural signs may be present (a decrease in the systolic blood pressure of greater than 20 mm Hg, a decrease in the diastolic pressure of greater than 10 mm Hg, or an increase in the pulse rate greater than 20 beats per minute with a change from the lying to the sitting position) with a blood loss greater than 20% of blood volume
3. *Abdomen:* The epigastric area may be tender to light palpation if the bleed is related to an ulcer

Hepatic Failure

Pathophysiology

Hepatic failure occurs when the liver becomes dysfunctional. The effects of hepatic failure on liver function include the following:

Normal Liver Function	Effect of Hepatic Failure
A. Vascular function	
1. Blood storage: The liver sinusoids store up to 400 ml of blood, which can be released into the systemic circulation as needed to maintain blood volume	The loss of this compensatory mechanism may be crucial in critical situations such as hypovolemic or hemorrhagic shock
2. Blood filtration: Kupffer's cells remove bacteria as the blood is filtered through the liver	• Kupffer's cells may be unable to remove bacteria • The patient may be prone to infection or bacteremia
B. Secretory function: Hepatocytes produce bile; the major components of bile are bile salts, bilirubin, and cholesterol	

Normal Liver Function	Effect of Hepatic Failure
1. Bile salts aid in the absorption of fats	• A decreased amount of bile salts may reach the intestine, resulting in the decreased emulsification of fats
	• The decreased emulsification of fats may lead to excessive loss of fat in the stools (steatorrhea), contributing to a malnourished state, and the decreased absorption of the fat-soluble vitamins A, D, E, and K
	• An increased amount of bile salts in the plasma may contribute to pruritus (the liver is unable to extract bile salts that are produced from the portal venous system)
2. Bilirubin is a breakdown product of hemoglobin: • Bilirubin is transported to the liver to be conjugated (made water-soluble) for excretion by the kidneys and the intestine • In the intestines, bacteria convert the yellow pigment to brown, and bilirubin is excreted with the feces • In the kidneys, bilirubin is filtered from the blood and is excreted with the urine, giving the urine a yellow color • Excess bilirubin is deposited in the body tissues, producing jaundice	• Jaundice and an elevated indirect bilirubin may reflect the liver's inability to conjugate bilirubin • Jaundice and an elevated direct bilirubin may reflect fibrotic obstruction to bile flow, resulting in reabsorption of conjugated bilirubin into the blood

Normal Liver Function	Effect of Hepatic Failure

C. Metabolic function

1. Carbohydrate metabolism: The liver
   - Metabolizes simple sugars to produce energy (glycogenesis)
   - Stores excess simple sugars as glycogen
   - Converts stored glycogen to glucose for additional energy (glycogenolysis)
   - Converts amino acids from proteins and glycerol and fatty acids from fats to glucose when necessary to maintain a normal blood glucose level (gluconeogenesis)

- Altered blood glucose levels may result from decreased metabolism
- Breakdown of muscle protein for conversion to glucose may contribute to weight loss and cachectic appearance
- The stress response may be decreased related to the lack of available glucose

2. Fat metabolism
   - The liver breaks down and synthesizes fats to fatty acids and glycerol to provide an energy source for the body cells
   - The liver is responsible for the formation of lipoproteins, cholesterol, and phospho-lipids
   - The liver converts carbohydrates to triglycerides and stores them in the adipose tissue

- Decreased fat metabolism may lead to fatigue and decreased activity tolerance
- Accumulation of fat in the liver may lead to fatty liver
- Serum lipid levels (especially cholesterol) may rise due to decreased excretion in the bile and failure of negative feedback control
- Xanthomas (deposits of fatty substances on the eyelids and skin) may be present

3. Protein metabolism: The liver is responsible for
   - The synthesis of serum proteins (albumin, α- and β-globulins, and fibrinogen)

- Albumin synthesis may decrease, contributing to fluid shifts from the vascular to the interstitial spaces (lack of protein decreases the colloid osmotic pressure in the

Normal Liver Function	Effect of Hepatic Failure
• The synthesis of clotting factors and the removal of activated clotting factors • The deamination of amino acids, producing ammonia, and for the conversion of ammonia to urea	blood vessels), resulting in edema and ascites • The decreased metabolism of fibrinogen and the decreased synthesis of clotting factors may lead to bruising, spontaneous bleeding, or hemorrhage • The inability of the liver to remove clotting factors may lead to the formation of microemboli, consumption of platelets, and disseminated intravascular coagulation (DIC; see Clinical Findings 10–1)

4. Detoxification of hormones and drugs: The liver is responsible for
  • Detoxifying harmful substances such as drugs into harmless substances to be excreted by the kidneys
  • The inactivation of many hormones, including the sex hormones (estrogen and testosterone), mineralocorticoids (aldosterone), and glucocorticoids (cortisol)
	• The liver's inability to metabolize drugs may prohibit the use of hepatotoxic medications (these medications may cause hepatic failure in the patient with compromised liver function)
	• Impotence, decreased libido, testicular atrophy, gynecomastia, and amenorrhea can result from the ineffectively metabolized hormones
	• Spider angiomas (nevi) and palmar erythema may be present, related to an excessive amount of estrogen
	• The continued circulation of aldosterone and antidiuretic hormone (ADH) may result in fluid and electrolyte imbalances and sodium and water retention (increased capillary hydrostatic pressure), contributing to complications of hepatic disease, including portal hypertension and ascites

Normal Liver Function	Effect of Hepatic Failure
D. Storage function: The liver is responsible for storing vitamins A, B_{12}, D, E, K, and minerals (copper, iron, and magnesium)	• The decreased absorption of vitamin D may cause hypocalcemia • Hypocalcemia stimulates the parathyroids, and increased amounts of calcium may be reabsorbed from the bone, contributing to osteomalacia, kyphosis, and fractures • Diminished amounts of vitamin K may contribute to bleeding tendencies • Diminished amounts of vitamin B may contribute to anemia and neurological problems

Hepatic failure can occur suddenly (acute fulminating hepatic failure), or it can have a more insidious onset. Disorders that may result in hepatic failure include hepatitis and cirrhosis (see Clinical Findings 7–2 for other predisposing factors).

Hepatitis

Hepatitis is the widespread inflammation and necrosis of liver cells. The most common cause of hepatitis is viral infection. (Other sources include drugs, chemicals, and transfusion reactions.) In nonfatal hepatitis, regeneration of liver cells begins almost with the onset of the disease. In overwhelming (fulminating) hepatitis, the virus may progress rapidly, causing liver shrinkage and necrosis.

Hepatitis A. Hepatitis A (infectious hepatitis) is the most common form of hepatitis. The virus is usually spread through the ingestion of food, water, and shellfish that have been contaminated with fecal contaminates. The course of the disease is usually mild (flu-like symptoms) with full recovery.

Hepatitis B. Hepatitis B (serum hepatitis) is a more severe form of hepatitis. The virus is spread by blood, blood products, saliva, and semen. The course of the disease is variable, and recovery may take several weeks or months. Hepatitis B may result in chronic hepatitis, cirrhosis, or liver cancer.

Hepatitis C. Hepatitis C (non-A, non-B hepatitis) is similar to hepatitis B but usually has a more insidious course (incubation period may vary from weeks to months). The virus is transmitted by blood, blood products, and sexual contact. This form of the virus may also lead to chronic hepatitis and cirrhosis.

Hepatitis D. Hepatitis D (delta hepatitis) is transmitted parenterally in the presence of hepatitis B. Hepatitis D may accelerate the progression of liver disease, including the damage to the compromised organ.

Hepatitis E. Hepatitis E is enterically transmitted (fecal or oral). The clinical presentation may be extremely virulent and progress to fulminating hepatitis. The incidence and prevalence are highest in underdeveloped countries.

Cirrhosis

Cirrhosis is a term applied to chronic liver disease that is characterized by diffuse inflammation and fibrosis of the liver, resulting in structural changes that may affect normal function. Laënnec's (alcoholic) cirrhosis is the most common form, although hepatitis, acute infection or inflammation (postnecrotic cirrhosis), cardiac failure (cardiac cirrhosis), metabolic disorders, and obstruction of the extrahepatic biliary tract (biliary cirrhosis) may also cause cirrhosis.

Physiological Changes Associated with Hepatic Failure

In addition to a loss of ability to perform normal functions, hepatic failure may lead to portal hypertension, encephalopathy, and hepatorenal syndrome.

Portal Hypertension

Obstruction of blood flow through the liver elevates portal pressure:

- Blood flow through the spleen may be delayed, which results in splenomegaly.
- Collateral channels may be formed to direct venous blood into areas of lower resistance, including the lower esophagus and upper stomach, rectum, and abdominal wall.
- Enlargement of the vessels in these areas results in the development of esophageal varices, hemorrhoids, and caput medusae (dilated abdominal veins).

- Blood flow to the liver is depleted, and detoxification and metabolic functions may be further compromised.
- Varices, especially esophageal, are fragile, and rupture may lead to gastrointestinal hemorrhage (see Clinical Findings 7–1).

The increased portal pressure may increase the capillary hydrostatic pressure and promote the shift of fluid into the peritoneal cavity, which may contribute to the formation of **ascites.** The decreased production of albumin may result in a decrease in the colloid osmotic pressure, which may promote more fluid loss into the peritoneal cavity. Increased hepatic lymph formation may exceed the removal capacity of the hepatic lymph ducts, which may promote additional fluid loss into the peritoneal cavity.

The decreased volume of circulating blood stimulates the kidneys, and the renin-angiotensin cascade may be activated (see Chapter 5 and Chapter 8 for related information on the renin-angiotensin cascade). Increased amounts of aldosterone and ADH may contribute to sodium and water retention and to fluid and electrolyte imbalances. The sodium and water retention may increase the circulating blood volume, which in turn may increase the portal venous pressure and the capillary hydrostatic pressure, so that even more fluid may be lost into the peritoneal cavity. The decreased intravascular volume may again stimulate the kidneys, the renin-angiotensin cascade may again be activated, and the cycle perpetuates itself.

Encephalopathy

The inability of the liver to convert ammonia to urea causes an increase in serum ammonia levels. The increased level of ammonia is thought to be a significant cause of alteration in cerebral metabolism in patients with advanced liver disease. Other predisposing factors may include hypoxia, hypercarbia, alkalosis, hypovolemia (GI bleeds), electrolyte abnormalities (hypokalemia, hyponatremia), alterations in renal function, infection, constipation, and drugs such as alcohol, sedatives, and anesthetics.

Neuromuscular manifestations may vary from personality and behavior changes (stage I), to confusion and disorientation to person, place, and time (stage II), drowsiness with noisy or violent periods when awake (stage III), and unresponsiveness to painful stimuli (stage IV). Speech may be slow and slurred in the early stages, and "liver flap," or asterixis (flapping tremor of the hands), may be apparent.

Clinical manifestations in the later stages may include posturing, Babinski's sign, seizures, and dilated pupils. The neuromuscular status should be continuously assessed, because the patient's clinical condition may fluctuate between the four stages.

Hepatorenal Syndrome

Renal failure may develop in association with liver disease in a person with previously healthy kidneys (see Chapter 8 for related information on renal failure). Decreases in the circulating blood volume (renal hypoperfusion), vasoconstrictive mechanisms such as the renin-angiotensin-cascade, circulating endotoxins such as thromboxanes and prostaglandins, and diversion of blood in the kidney (the development of shunts in the kidney diverts blood from the renal cortex to the medulla, decreasing the glomerular filtration rate) are causative factors implicated. Patients usually have end-stage liver disease with increased albumin and portal hypertension.

Assessment

Clinical manifestations of hepatic failure vary with the severity of liver destruction and the associated physiological changes (see Clinical Findings 7–2).

POINTS TO REMEMBER

▶ Because the critically ill adult may present with acute fulminating hepatic failure (no previous history of liver disease) or with a complication such as gastrointestinal hemorrhage related to chronic hepatic failure and because the critically ill adult may develop hepatic failure as a complication of another disorder such as sepsis or shock (see Chapter 12), a thorough nursing history (see Tables 1–1 and 7–1 and Clinical Findings 7–2 and 12–3) is crucial to assist in identifying the cause and extent of hepatic failure and in detecting patients at risk for the development of hepatic failure.

▶ Because of the many functions of the liver, hepatic failure may affect all body systems.

▶ In addition to the initial and baseline assessments (see Table 2–1) and a focused gastrointestinal assessment (see Tables 2–1 and 7–1), focused assessments of the respiratory, cardiovascular, neuromuscular, genitourinary, and integumentary systems (see Tables 4–1, 5–1, 6–1, 8–1, and 11–1) should be completed as often as the patient's condition dictates to detect or anticipate and prevent complications such as infection, gastrointestinal hemorrhage (see Clinical Findings 7–1) and renal failure (see Clinical Findings 8–1).

▶ Ongoing assessment incorporates the evaluation of responses to diagnostic procedures and therapeutic interventions aimed at supporting liver function and minimizing portal hypertension, ascites, and encephalopathy; it includes collaboration with other members of the health team to maintain vital functions such as fluid and electrolyte balance, acid-base balance, and nutrition.

Clinical Findings 7–2 *Hepatic Failure*

I. History

A. Predisposing factors

1. Alcohol abuse
2. Viral hepatitis
3. Biliary disease
4. Heart failure
5. Gallbladder disease
6. Hepatotoxic drugs, including acetaminophen, anesthetics, and antibiotics
7. Poisonous mushrooms
8. Tumors
9. Metastatic cancer
10. Chemicals such as industrial toxins, pesticides, and herbicides
11. Sepsis
12. Shock
13. Budd-Chiari syndrome
14. Wilson's disease
15. Reye's syndrome
16. Fatty liver of pregnancy
17. Portal vein thrombosis

B. Subjective findings

1. Weakness and fatigue related to alterations in metabolism or to anemia
2. Weight loss related to loss of appetite and muscle breakdown
3. Nausea and vomiting related to abdominal distention and electrolyte imbalances
4. Abdominal discomfort related to an enlarged liver or spleen or to ascites

   5. Pruritus related to metabolic dysfunction and increased amount of circulating bile salts
   6. Sexual dysfunction related to endocrine imbalances

II. LABORATORY AND BEDSIDE MONITORING FINDINGS

A. **Arterial blood gas studies** (see Chapter 13 for related information on arterial blood gas studies, acid-base disorders, and serum lactate levels)
   1. Hypoxemia may be present, related to decreased lung expansion secondary to ascites, hypoventilation secondary to hypokalemia, or anemia associated with a decreased number of red blood cells
   2. Metabolic alkalosis may be present, related to hypokalemia
   3. Metabolic acidosis may be present, related to increased lactic acid production secondary to decreased tissue perfusion, the inability of the liver to metabolize lactic acid, or to hyperkalemia associated with hepatorenal failure
   4. Respiratory acidosis may be present, related to hypoventilation associated with ascites, hypokalemia, or altered levels of consciousness
   5. Respiratory alkalosis may be present, related to hyperventilation associated with fever or tachypnea

B. **Liver function studies** (see Table 13–4 for related information on liver function studies)
   1. An elevated aspartate aminotransaminase (AST; formerly serum glutamic-oxaloacetic transaminase [SGOT]) and an elevated alanine aminotransferase (ALT; formerly serum glutamate pyruvate transaminase [SGPT]) may be present, related to the destruction of liver cells
   2. An elevated alkaline phosphatase may be present, related to reduced excretion in the bile associated with liver disease or biliary obstruction
   3. Elevated direct and total bilirubin may be related to hepatic cell destruction or obstruction of the biliary tract (the urine bilirubin and urobilinogen may also be increased)
   4. Increased cholesterol levels may be present, related to the decreased excretion of cholesterol in the bile
   5. Elevated ammonia levels may be present, related to the inability of the liver to convert ammonia to urea
   6. Elevated total globulins may be present, related to the inflammatory response of the liver
   7. Decreased plasma proteins (albumin and fibrinogen) may be present, related to decreased synthesis by the liver
   8. Prolongation of prothrombin time may be present, related to decreased synthesis of prothrombin by the liver

C. Electrolyte imbalances (see Table 13–5 for related information on electrolyte imbalances)

1. Dilutional hyponatremia may be present, related to increased ADH circulation and water retention
2. Hypernatremia may be present, related to increased aldosterone circulation or decreased intravascular volume
3. Hypocalcemia may be present, related to decreased absorption of vitamin D
4. Hypomagnesemia may be present, related to the decreased ability of the liver to store magnesium
5. Hypokalemia may be present, related to increased aldosterone circulation, diarrhea, or diuresis
6. Hyperkalemia may be present, related to hepatorenal failure

D. Other laboratory studies

1. Hypoglycemia may be present, related to the inability of the liver to perform glycogenolysis and glucogenolysis
2. Elevated BUN may be present, related to bleeding
3. Elevated creatinine may be present, related to decreased renal perfusion (see Table 13–6 for related information on BUN and creatinine)
4. An increased number of WBCs may be present, related to infection (increased susceptibility to infection related to the inability of the Kupffer's cells to filter bacteria)
5. Leukopenia may be present, related to hypersplenism (see Table 13–9 for related information on WBCs)
6. A decreased number of RBCs may be present, related to bleeding from the GI tract or destruction of RBCs secondary to hypersplenism (see Table 13–8 for related information on RBCs)

E. ECG

1. Tachycardia may be present, related to a hyperdynamic circulation (cardiac output is increased to compensate for collateral vessel development, anemia, and generalized vasodilation)
2. Dysrhythmias may be present, related to acid-base or electrolyte imbalances

F. Hemodynamic parameters: Hypotension may be present, related to decreased systemic vascular resistance (generalized vasodilation) or hypovolemia

III. Physical Assessment Findings

A. General observations (inspection): In general, there is a malnourished, cachectic appearance related to alterations in metabolism or anorexia; fetor hepaticus may be present, related to liver disease (see Table 7–1 for related information on evaluation of breath odors)

1. *Mental status:* Slurred speech, confusion, disorientation, drowsiness, behavior changes, and lack of response to verbal or painful stimuli may be present, related to encephalopathy
2. *Motor and sensory function*
   - Asterixis may be present, related to encephalopathy
   - Sensory and peripheral nerve alterations may be present, related to decreased synthesis of vitamin B
3. *Respiratory pattern*
   - Bradypnea or hypoventilation may be present, related to metabolic alkalosis or pressure on the diaphragm associated with ascites
   - Tachypnea or hyperventilation may be present, related to hypoxemia, metabolic acidosis, or fever
4. *Skin*
   - Skin may be flushed, related to hyperdynamic circulation
   - Jaundice may be present, related to increased bilirubin
   - Spider angiomas or palmar erythema may be present, related to endocrine imbalances
   - Gynecomastia, decreased body hair, or testicular atrophy may be present related to endocrine imbalancés
   - Bruising; spontaneous bleeding from the nose, skin, or gums; emesis, bloody stools, or frank hemorrhage may be present, related to decreased synthesis of clotting factors, prolonged prothrombin times, or varices
5. *Abdomen*
   - Distended abdominal veins may be present, related to shunting of blood secondary to increased portal pressure (caput medusae)
   - Abdominal distention may be present, related to ascites
6. *Edema:* Dependent edema may be present, related to decreased colloid osmotic pressure or increased capillary hydrostatic pressure
7. *Neck veins:* Jugular venous distention (JVD) may be present, related to hyperdynamic circulation or increased right ventricular filling pressures associated with pressure exerted on the heart from an elevated diaphragm related to ascites
8. *Urine:* Urine output may be decreased, related to decreased renal perfusion or hepatorenal failure
9. *Fever:* Temperature may be increased, related to liver inflammation or infections of ascitic or pleural effusion fluid (or other systemic infections)

B. Auscultation
   1. *Abnormal breath sounds:* Breath sounds may be diminished or absent with decreased lung expansion secondary to ascites, hypokalemia, or pleural

effusion (see Clinical Findings 4–5 for related information on pleural effusion)

2. *Adventitious breath sounds:* Crackles may be present, related to hyperdynamic circulation or retained secretions associated with ineffective breathing patterns or airway clearance

3. *Heart sounds*
   - Loud precordial impulse related to hyperdynamic circulation
   - Rapid or irregular heart sounds related to hyperdynamic circulation or dysrhythmias

4. *Bowel sounds:* May be hyperactive related to diarrhea or GI bleed

C. Percussion

1. In the supine position the dependent portion of the abdomen may be dull to percussion related to ascites

2. In the side-lying position, dullness (fluid) will shift to the dependent side (see Fig. 7–5 for related information)

D. Palpation

1. *Chest wall and thorax:* Chest expansion may be decreased or asymmetrical, related to ascites, hypokalemia, or a pleural effusion

2. *Peripheral pulses:* Pulses may be bounding, related to hyperdynamic circulation

3. *Abdomen*
   - Abdomen may be distended, related to ascites
   - Abdomen may be tender, related to splenomegaly or hepatomegaly

Acute Pancreatitis

Pathophysiology

Activation of pancreatic enzymes within the pancreas results in inflammation and autodigestion of the pancreas. (Normally, pancreatic enzymes are released from the pancreas in an inactive state and are activated in the duodenum.) Toxic agents such as drugs and alcohol, reflux of pancreatic enzymes from the duodenum, and obstruction of biliary ducts are mechanisms that have been implicated for the precipitation of the disease.

Local Effects

The activated enzymes (trypsin, elastase, and phospholipase A) break down tissue and cell membranes, causing edema (edematous pancreatitis) and escape of pancreatic enzymes into the surrounding tissue and peritoneal cavity. Peritonitis may result from spillage of pancreatic enzymes into the peritoneal cavity.

Progression to hemorrhage and necrosis of the pancreas and surrounding tissue often follows. Large amounts of plasma may be lost in the pancreas, peritoneal cavity, and retroperitoneal tissue.

Inflammation and necrosis of fat around the pancreas may lead to the formation of free fatty acids, which may result in hyperlipidemia and the binding of calcium. This may result in hypocalcemia (calcium is excreted with fat in the stool). Thrombosis, formation of a pseudocyst (pancreatic juice may become enclosed by a wall of fibrous or granulation tissue), and abscess (collection of pus within the abdomen) may also occur.

Systemic Effects

These toxic enzymes are also released into the vascular system and may stimulate other enzymes and kinins (vasoactive substances), resulting in increased vascular permeability and vasodilation. Increased vascular permeability may lead to the loss of plasma volume (albumin) and contribute to the collection of fluid within the peritoneal cavity, pleural effusion (see Clinical Findings 4–5), and ARDS (see Clinical Findings 4–1). Loss of plasma volume and vasodilation may also lead to hypovolemia, hypotension, and shock (see Clinical Findings 12–3). Acute renal failure may develop from decreased blood flow to the kidneys (see Clinical Findings 8–1).

Assessment

Clinical manifestations vary with the severity of the involvement of the pancreas and surrounding structures, and with the systemic effects perpetuated by the disorder (see Clinical Findings 7–3).

POINTS TO REMEMBER

▶ A thorough nursing history (see Tables 1–1 and 7–1 and Clinical Findings 7–3) is crucial to identify the cause of pancreatitis and the extent of damage.

▶ In addition to the initial and baseline assessments (see Table 2–1) and a focused gastrointestinal assessment (see Tables 2–1 and 7–1), focused respiratory, cardiovascular, neuromuscular, genitourinary, and integumentary assessments (see Tables 4–1, 5–1, 6–1, 8–1, and 11–1) should be completed as often as the patient's con dition dictates to detect or anticipate and prevent systemic complications.

▶ Diaphoresis, tachypnea, and tachycardia may be early warning signs of shock (see Clinical Findings 12–3).

▶ Ongoing assessment incorporates the evaluation of responses to diagnostic procedures and therapeutic interventions aimed at identifying the cause of pancreatitis and minimizing pancreatic destruction; it includes collaboration with other members of the health team to maintain fluid volume and cardiac output, and prevent respiratory and renal complications that may contribute to mortality.

Clinical Findings 7–3   *Acute Pancreatitis*

I. HISTORY

A. Predisposing factors

1. Alcohol ingestion
2. Gallstones
3. Idiopathic
4. Peptic ulcer
5. Drugs, including steroids, thiazides, furosemide, estrogen, methyldopa, sulfonamides, tetracycline, mercaptopurine, excessive vitamin D, and procainamide
6. Pregnancy
7. Cancer
8. Hyperlipidemia
9. Hypercalcemia
10. Ingestion of a high-fat meal
11. Blunt trauma to the abdomen
12. Infections (viral or bacterial)
13. Sepsis
14. Shock

B. Subjective findings

1. Severe abdominal pain (usually midepigastric; may radiate to the back) related to edema of the pancreas, inflammation of the peritoneum, and irritation or obstruction of the biliary tract
2. Nausea and vomiting related to bowel hypomotility or paralytic ileus secondary to peritonitis
3. Dyspnea related to irritation of the diaphragm

II. LABORATORY AND BEDSIDE MONITORING FINDINGS

A. CT scan or MRI: May reveal inflammation, swelling, biliary tract obstruction, pancreatic pseudocyst or abscess

B. Arterial blood gas studies: Hypoxemia may be present, related to hypoventilation secondary to abdominal distention or to respiratory complications such as ARDS (see Clinical Findings 4–1)

C. Other laboratory studies
   1. Elevated serum and urine amylase may be present, related to damaged pancreatic cells
   2. Elevated serum and urine lipase may be present, related to damaged pancreatic cells (see Table 13–4 for related information on amylase and lipase)
   3. Increased WBCs may be present, related to inflammation of the pancreas or peritonitis (see Table 13–9 for related information on WBCs)
   4. Hyperglycemia may be present, related to dysfunction of the beta cells of the pancreas, which make insulin, to dysfunction of the alpha cells, which secrete glucagon, or to the stress response
   5. Hypocalcemia may be present, related to fat necrosis or hypoalbuminemia
   6. Hypomagnesemia may be present, related to vomiting, nasogastric suction, or malnutrition
   7. Hypokalemia may be present, related to vomiting or nasogastric suction (see Table 13–5 for related information on electrolyte imbalances)
   8. Hyperlipidemia may be present, related to an increase in free fatty acids from fat necrosis (hyperlipidemia may also be a cause of pancreatitis)

D. ECG
   1. Tachycardia may be present, related to decreased circulating blood volume, hypoxemia, or fever
   2. Dysrhythmias may be present, related to hypoxemia, acid-base, or electrolyte imbalances

E. Hemodynamic parameters: Hypotension may be present, related to hypovolemia or vasodilation

III. PHYSICAL ASSESSMENT FINDINGS

A. General observations (inspection)
   1. *Mental status*
      - If able, the patient may sit and lean forward or maintain a knee-chest position (fetal) to relieve pain
      - Confusion or disorientation may be present, related to hypoxemia or hypovolemia and decreased cerebral blood flow
   2. *Respiratory pattern:* Tachypnea may be present, related to hypoxemia or hypovolemia

3. *Skin:* Jaundice may be present, related to biliary obstruction
4. *Abdomen*
   - Ecchymosis (grayish discoloration) may be present in the flanks (Grey Turner's sign) or around the umbilicus (Cullen's sign), related to hemorrhage and accumulation of blood in these areas (see Table 7–1 for related information on evaluation of these signs)
   - Abdominal distention may be present, related to bowel hypomotility, increased fluid in the peritoneal cavity, or paralytic ileus
5. *Motor and sensory function*
   - Chvostek's sign (twitching of the facial muscle when the cheek is tapped) and Trousseau's sign (inflation of the blood pressure cuff for longer than 3 minutes produces spasm of the hand) may be present, related to hypocalcemia
   - Muscular twitching, jerking, or irritability may be present, related to hypocalcemia
6. *Fever:* Elevated temperature and chills may be present, related to the inflammatory process
7. *Stool:* Steatorrhea (foul-smelling, gray stools) may be present, related to fat excretion

B. Auscultation
1. *Abnormal breath sounds:* Diminished breath sounds may be present, related to decreased lung expansion secondary to abdominal distention
2. *Adventitious breath sounds:* Crackles or wheezes may be present, related to retained secretions secondary to ineffective airway clearance or to pulmonary complications such as atelectasis, pneumonia, or ARDS
3. *Heart sounds:* May be rapid or irregular related to hypoxemia, hypovolemia, or dysrhythmias
4. *Bowel sounds:* May be decreased or absent, related to decreased bowel motility or paralytic ileus

C. Palpation
1. *Skin:* May be cool and clammy related to diaphoresis and peripheral vasoconstriction (sympathetic nervous system response)
2. *Chest wall and thorax:* Chest expansion may be decreased or asymmetrical, related to abdominal distention, ARDS (see Clinical Findings 4–1), or atelectasis (see Clinical Findings 4–3)
3. *Abdomen:* May be rigid, related to paralytic ileus

8

Renal Assessment

FUNCTION OF THE RENAL SYSTEM

The primary purposes of the renal system are maintenance of the fluid, electrolyte, and acid-base balance of extracellular fluid, and excretion of waste products of metabolism from the blood plasma. This is accomplished in approximately 2 million **nephrons**—the basic functional units of the kidneys. In the nephron blood plasma from the renal artery, a branch of the abdominal aorta, carried by afferent arterioles, is filtered through a compact complex of capillaries in the renal cortex known as a **glomerulus.** Large protein molecules and blood cells are usually not filtered. Smaller molecules, including nutrient and drug metabolites, toxins, and water enter the **Bowman's capsule** and the convoluted **renal tubule** associated with each glomerulus (see Fig. 8–1). Reabsorption and secretion of water and solutes takes place along the **proximal tubule, loop of Henle,** and **distal renal tubule** of each nephron by active and passive transport mechanisms (see Fig. 8–2). The final osmolality and composition of urine in the collecting ducts of the kidney is also controlled by **antidiuretic hormone** (ADH) secreted by the pituitary gland. Retained substances are returned to the general circulation through efferent arterioles to the renal veins and then to the inferior vena cava.

Blood flow through the kidneys is about 20% to 25% of cardiac output, or about 1200 ml/min. Assuming a normal hematocrit, this represents about 660 ml of plasma. Normal glomerular filtration rate (GFR) is approximately 100–125 ml of plasma per minute. This remains constant within a wide range of blood pressures because of

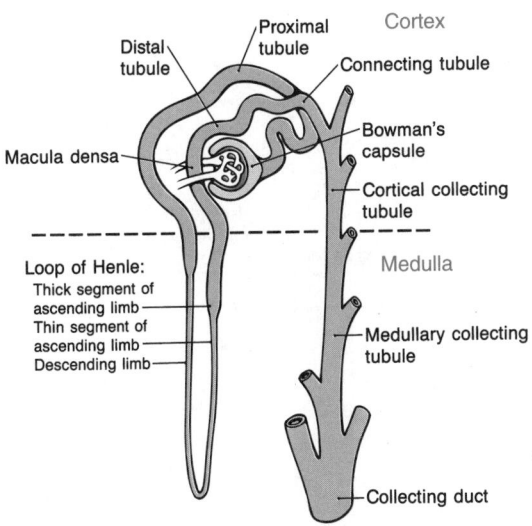

FIGURE 8–1

Basic tubular segments of the nephron. (From Guyton, A. C., & Hall, J. E. [1997]. *Human physiology and mechanisms of disease* [6th ed., p. 214]. Philadelphia: W. B. Saunders.)

autoregulation of renal arteriolar pressure. In severe compromise, however, blood will be shunted to heart, brain, or skeletal muscles at the expense of the kidneys. This may potentiate renal failure.

Renal function is routinely measured by the ability of kidneys to freely filter certain end-products of protein metabolism from the blood stream. **Creatinine** is a nonprotein product of anaerobic metabolism in skeletal muscle. It is produced and excreted continuously. Its clearance can be measured in urine and in blood as a reflection of GFR. **Urea nitrogen** is formed by the breakdown of protein in the liver. Its blood (plasma) concentration also approximates GFR.

The juxtaglomerular cells of the kidneys also have endocrine functions and play a significant role in other regulatory processes, including the following:

- **Blood pressure control,** through the synthesis of renin, which regulates angiotensin and aldosterone production and sodium retention

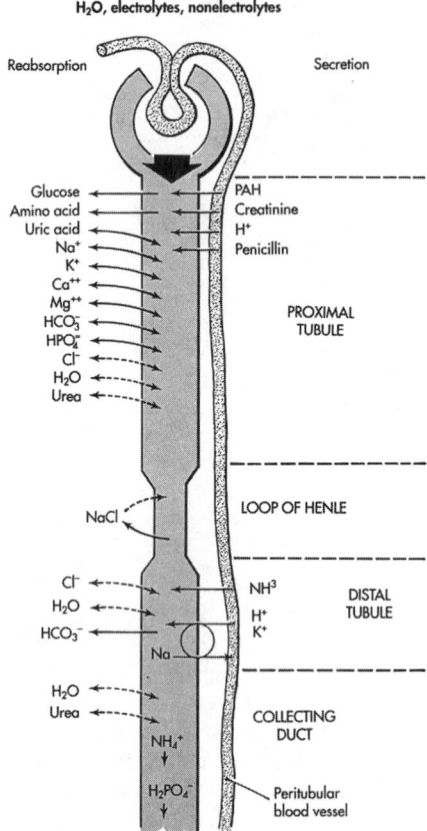

H₂O, electrolytes, nonelectrolytes

Reabsorption   Secretion

Glucose	PAH
Amino acid	Creatinine
Uric acid	H⁺
Na⁺	Penicillin

FIGURE 8–2

Tubular reabsorption and secretion along the glomerular nephron. *Solid arrows* indicate active transport, and *broken arrows* indicate passive transport. (From Price, S. A., & Wilson, L. M. [1992]. *Pathophysiology: Clinical concepts of disease processes* [4th ed., p. 620]. New York: McGraw-Hill.)

- **Red blood cell manufacture,** through the production of erythropoietin to stimulate bone marrow in the presence of hypoxia
- **Calcium absorption in the GI tract** (and, indirectly, extracellular phosphate balance) through the production of biologically active vitamin D
- **Insulin degradation**
- **Vasodilation** through the production of prostaglandins A and E-2

The kidneys are located behind the peritoneum at each side of the vertebral column in the lower thoracic–upper lumbar area. They are partially protected by the lower ribcage, fat pads, and the lower back muscles.

Excess water and solutes, including uric acid and creatinine from protein metabolism, flow through each renal pelvis and ureter for storage in the **bladder.** The bladder sits within the pelvic cavity behind the symphysis pubis and, unless severely distended, is inaccessible to examination through the abdominal wall. Approximately 500 ml of urine in the bladder stimulates impulses from the central (pons) and peripheral (spinal and autonomic) nervous systems to produce sphincter relaxation and bladder contraction. Urine is eliminated through the **urethra.** The length of the urethra in the female is about 1.5 inches, while in the male it is about 8 inches. In the male the proximal urethral wall below the neck of the bladder is formed by the **prostate gland,** which surrounds it.

Renal failure can occur due to intrinsic renal disease (renal stenosis, hemolysis, tumor, local infection), nephrotoxic substances, or neurologic or endocrine compromise. It can also be caused by prerenal conditions that cause poor renal perfusion (cardiac failure, shock, surgery, trauma, dehydration, multisystem failure) or by postrenal uropathies or obstructions to urine outflow.

Changes with Aging

Renal blood flow decreases at about 10% per decade beginning at about age 30. Glomerular filtration rate also progressively diminishes, which probably is due to the following factors:

- Decrease in size and weight of kidneys by 20%–30%
- Shrinking of nephron structures
- Loss of nephrons (30%–50%)
- Changes in the thickness of glomerular and tubular membranes affecting the filtering surface area

- Arteriosclerosis and atherosclerosis of blood vessels
- Diminished renal blood flow by shunting from afferent to efferent arterioles, thus bypassing glomeruli

Trace proteinuria may occur due to altered permeability of glomeruli. **Creatinine clearance declines** with aging (see Chapter 3 for formula). Blood urea nitrogen (BUN) and creatinine values, however, remain normal, probably due to lower muscle mass with aging, or to lower protein intake. Tubular changes may also increase the threshold for glycosuria. Decreased drug clearance in the kidneys increases susceptibility to toxicity from certain drugs at usual adult dosages.

Altered tubular permeability is the likely cause of **a diminished ability to concentrate and dilute urine** in the presence of dehydration or fluid overload despite normal or elevated levels of ADH. Decreased thirst sensation with aging further contributes to water imbalance. With aging there is also a **decreased active renin** concentration to stimulate angiotensin II and the production of aldosterone. This affects the ability of the kidneys to conserve sodium (and water) and excrete potassium. These changes make the older person **less tolerant of fluid and electrolyte deprivation** or overload. Recovery from metabolic acidosis may also take longer than in younger adults.

Changes in the kidney in the absence of disease are usually not symptomatic and are tolerated well at normal functional levels. Older persons who are exposed to environmental stressors, illnesses that alter mobility, diet, fluid intake, circulatory or mental status, or who take or are given multiple drugs may have insufficient functional reserve capacity within the renal system to maintain homeostasis. Changes with age and disease may also cause the elderly person in acute renal failure to present without the characteristic oliguria.

Bladder compliance and capacity decrease to approximately 250 ml with aging. This may cause relative urinary frequency and urgency. Weakened bladder muscles and pelvic support structures may contribute to loss of urine with increased intra-abdominal pressure (stress incontinence), especially in females. In addition, formation of bladder diverticula may cause hesitancy, diminished force of stream, or urine retention. Urinary incontinence is *not* a predictable change with aging. Bladder incontinence, however, is a common reason for institutionalization of the elderly person. **Common reversible and irreversible causes of urinary incontinence in the elderly** follow:

D Dementia, delirium, depression
    Drugs
R Retention (drugs, obstruction)
    Restricted mobility
I Infection, inflammation
    Intra-abdominal pressure
    Impaction
P Polyuria
    Prostatic enlargement (male)
S Stroke or other neurologic disorder

Additionally, **asymptomatic bacteriuria** is present in about 10%–20% of older persons, especially postmenopausal females.

Benign prostatic hyperplasia is present in about one third of elderly males. Gland growth usually occurs medially and laterally and may obstruct urine flow.

While the most reliable indicators of fluid and electrolyte balance, pH, and drug toxicity are laboratory tests, the critical care nurse should anticipate potential changes and look for signs and symptoms of alterations during the initial, baseline, focused, and ongoing assessment of the patient (Table 8–1). Lethargy or confusion in an elderly person may be an early sign of altered fluid or electrolyte balance or of urinary tract infection. This must be carefully distinguished from signs of sensory deprivation or overload, depression, or dementia.

TABLE 8-1 Renal Assessment Techniques, Tips, and Geriatric Considerations

Technique	Performance Tips	Description/Rationale	Geriatric Considerations
Pertinent History **1. Related medical history**	Review the patient's known medical history for **actual or potential disease states** that may affect renal function Do not disregard simple explanations for urine flow problems: • Urinary tract infection (UTI) • Changes in voiding volume with aging • History of chronic renal failure Look for prerenal, renal, and postrenal causes of acute renal failure (see Clinical Findings 8–1)	It is important to rule out common causes of urine flow problems that may be overlooked in critical care settings; identification of such problems can save the patient and health care providers unnecessary diagnostic procedures, treatments, and expense The nurse caring for the critically ill must also be alert to the need to assess all patients for renal compromise; any critically ill patient has the potential for acute renal failure, since most present with, or develop, conditions that can predispose them to it in the course of a critical illness	Common causes of reversible and irreversible urinary incontinence are presented on page 485, identifying possible sources of incontinence will facilitate appropriate treatment Renal failure or the potential for it should be suspected in all older patients; changes in renal function with age predispose the patient to acute renal failure secondary to most critical illnesses A common cause of renal failure in the elderly is diabetic nephropathy

2. Related drug history

Review the patient's recent past and current **drug therapy** for medications that may

- Increase renal signs and symptoms
- Mask renal signs and symptoms

Many drugs given in acute and critical care settings and in advanced cardiac life-support situations are renal-toxic in large doses; such drug administration should alert the nurse to the possibility of renal failure (see Clinical Findings 8–1)

The elderly patient is especially prone to renal toxicity associated with drug administration because of reduced renal clearance of drugs with age (see Chapter 3)

The elderly are also more likely to routinely take drugs that have the potential to be renal toxic

Conversely, drug toxicity due to acute renal failure may be missed because of the absence of oliguria in the acute phase

Table continued on following page

487

TABLE 8-1 Renal Assessment Techniques, Tips, and Geriatric Considerations *Continued*

Technique	Performance Tips	Description/Rationale	Geriatric Considerations
3. Common complaints and observations that indicate the need for a focused assessment of the renal system	*ASSESSMENT TIPS* 1. Interview the alert patient about the exact nature of any discomfort 2. Use appropriate portions of the following mnemonic to assure that all major aspects and characteristics of the symptoms have been evaluated **P** Precipitating factors, prodrome **Q** Quality, quantity **R** Region, radiation **S** Associated symptoms, setting **T** Timing, treatment effects	The most common symptoms of renal dysfunction include • Flank, lower back, suprapubic, or perineal discomfort or pain • Dysuria • Polyuria, oliguria, anuria • Frequency • Urgency • Hesitancy • Difficulty initiating the urine stream • Change in the caliber of the stream • Incontinence • Urine odor • Color changes	

If a urinary catheter is in place, the history will not be able to elicit information on current symptoms that are common in urinary tract problems; assessment of symptoms preceding hospitalization may be helpful		

Physical Examination
1. Evaluation of urine

• Amount of urine, flow rate	Look for correlation of intake and output: • Oral intake • Parenteral intake • Urinary output • Gastrointestinal system losses • Insensible losses – Respiration – Diaphoresis	Volume is high in hyperosmolar states (e.g., hyperglycemia, hypercalcemia, hypermagnesemia), adrenal crisis, diuretic therapy, diabetes insipidus, and in the diuretic phase of acute renal failure Volume is low in urinary tract obstruction, dehydration, hypovolemia, vasopressin (ADH) administration, and in the oliguric phase of renal failure	In the elderly, volume may be high during the oliguric phase of acute renal failure because of the loss of concentrating ability in the kidney

Table continued on following page

TABLE 8-1 Renal Assessment Techniques, Tips, and Geriatric Considerations *Continued*

Technique	Performance Tips	Description/Rationale	Geriatric Considerations
• Obstruction to urine flow	*ASSESSMENT TIPS* 1. If a urinary catheter is in place, check it for patency 2. If insertion of a catheter is not possible in a male patient, check for a history of prostate enlargement	May be caused by a • Stricture of urinary organs related to anatomy, injury, scarring • Obstruction related to infection, tumor, calculus • Obstructed urinary catheter • Neurogenic bladder (in the uncatheterized; e.g., diabetic neuropathy) • Psychogenic causes (rare)	Urinary tract obstruction is a postrenal cause of acute renal failure in the older patient; in males this is often due to prostatic hypertrophy or malignancy; in females, obstruction may be due to gynecologic problems or malignancy
— Color		*Examples of Substances and Conditions That May Affect Color:*	
		Pale — Dilute urine, overhydration, diuresis, diabetes insipidus	
		Amber, yellow, orange — Concentrated urine, dehydration, bilirubin, urobilinogen, pyridium, laxatives with anthraquinones, phenothiazines, rifampicin, phenacetin, tetracycline, sulfasalazine	
		Pink, red — Hemoglobin, myoglobin, blood, drugs, foods such as beetroot, prophyrins, phenolphthaleins	

490

	Brown, black	Standing melanin, standing myoglobin, methemoglobin, l-dopa, phenols, metronidazole, nitrofurantoin porphyrinuria, carmine dye, cascara, fecaluria, Addison's disease
	Green	Bacterial infection, some vitamins
	Blue-green	Methylene blue, *Pseudomonas* UTI, amitriptyline, nitrofurans
	Cloudy	Cells, bacteria, leukocytes, fat, urate crystals, casts, insoluble phosphates, catheter sediment
	Foamy	Proteinuria
— Specific gravity		Specific gravity is a measure of urine solute and an approximation of extracellular osmolality; distilled water has a specific gravity of 1.000; the normal specific gravity of urine is approximately 1.010 to 1.030
— Consistency and composition		Urine is thick in the presence of large numbers of bacteria, leukocytes, or casts and large amounts of sediment or mucus
◦ pH		Normal pH should be somewhat acidic; many pathogens survive in alkaline urine and may cause urinary tract or vaginal infection
◦ Glucose		Glucose in urine indicates a blood glucose above the normal threshold for elimination
		This threshold, however, varies among individuals and is not reliable
		Without hyperglycemia, glycosuria may indicate renal tubular disease
		Severe hyperglycemia may exist without glycosuria because of an increased threshold for glycosuria with aging

Table continued on following page

TABLE 8–1 Renal Assessment Techniques, Tips, and Geriatric Considerations *Continued*

Technique	Performance Tips	Description/Rationale	Geriatric Considerations

○ Blood: hematuria	Blood or its components in urine may be the result of
	• Trauma to organs of the renal system
	• Bladder or kidney tumor or stones
	• Prostatic disease
	• Irritated urethra
	  – Trauma, infection
	  – Urinary catheter
	  – Diagnostic procedures
	• Vaginal or rectal conditions in the uncatheterized patient
	• Systemic disorders
	  – Coagulopathies
	  – Sickle cell disease
	• Trauma
	• Drugs		

○ Protein: proteinuria	May indicate • Renal disease • Nephrotic syndrome • Diabetes • Drugs, toxins	• Infectious diseases • Malignancy • Multisystem disease • Fever • Idiopathic (non-pathologic) states	Trace proteinuria may be a usual finding in the geriatric patient because of altered permeability of renal blood vessels, allowing filtration of large molecules

○ Ketones	May indicate uncontrolled diabetes mellitus, starvation, or ethanol intoxication
○ Bilirubin, urobilinogen	A product of hemoglobin breakdown, conjugated bilirubin or urobilinogen may enter the bloodstream in hepatic or obstructive jaundice or hemolysis and be eliminated in urine
○ Nitrites	Some pathogens convert dietary nitrates in protein to nitrites; the presence of nitrite is indicative of urinary tract infection; absence of nitrite does not, however, preclude a UTI
○ Cells	More than a few cells suggest disease: • RBCs: inflammation, infection, tumor, stones • WBCs: inflammation, infection
○ Casts	A cast is a mold of an area of the nephron named for substances that comprise it: • RBC: glomerulonephritis • WBC: renal inflammatory processes such as pyelonephritis • Hyaline: present in normal urine, ARF • Waxy: advanced renal disease
○ Bacteria	Bacterial infection is suggested by the presence of 4–5 bacteria per high-powered field or cultures containing 10^5 colony-forming units (CFU)/ml; urinary tract catheterization is a common cause of infection in patients

Table continued on following page

TABLE 8-1 Renal Assessment Techniques, Tips, and Geriatric Considerations *Continued*

Technique	Performance Tips	Description/Rationale	Geriatric Considerations
2. Genitourinary discomfort	Perform palpation to evaluate for flank, costovertebral angle (CVA), suprapubic, or perineal discomfort	Kidney pain may be present with renal disease or injury Suprapubic or perineal aching may be present with a distended bladder, UTI, prostatitis Inflammatory or infectious diseases are usually accompanied by fever	Signs and symptoms of inflammation may be absent in the older patient
3. General condition • Mental status	*Look for* • Lethargy • Confusion • Agitation	Renal causes of altered mental status may be fluid and sodium imbalances: • Hyponatremia may cause cerebral edema • Hypernatremia may cause cerebral dehydration	A common presenting symptom or sign of urine flow problems is alteration in mental status In the elderly patient it is important to establish information on prehospital mental status to better assess changes that might be attributed to acute renal failure, fluid and electrolyte imbalances, or urinary tract infection

	Look for	
		Change in mental status may be the first or only presenting symptom of UTI or renal failure in the elderly
		The elderly are prone to dehydration related to decreased thirst sensation and decreased mobility

• Skin and mucous membranes	*Look for*
	• Hydration
	  – Moisture
	  – Turgor
	(See Table 5–1 for assessment tips for the evaluation of moisture and turgor)
	• Uremic crystals on the skin
	  – Itching
	  – Scratch marks
		Dry skin and mucous membranes and poor skin turgor (see Table 5–1) indicate dehydration due to hypovolemia or hypoperfusion; this may predispose the patient to renal failure
		
		Severe azotemia (excessive nitrogenous waste in blood plasma) may cause deposits of urate crystals on the skin; this may be accompanied by or preceded by itching and scratching

• Perfusion	*Look for* • Color of skin and mucous membranes • Skin temperature • Capillary refill	Signs of decreased perfusion may indicate hypovolemia or hypoperfusion, which are prenatal causes of acute renal failure (see Clinical Findings 8–1) The diminished response to volume depletion due to changes in renin secretion and ADH response may further predispose patients to azotemia due to nausea, vomiting, diarrhea, nasogastric suctioning, hyperglycemia, or congestive heart failure (CHF)

Table continued on following page

495

TABLE 8–1 Renal Assessment Techniques, Tips, and Geriatric Considerations *Continued*

Technique	Performance Tips	Description/Rationale	Geriatric Considerations
	• Blood pressure • Edema: periorbital, peripheral • Dyspnea, tachypnea • Lung sounds: crackles • Abnormal heart sounds (S_3, S_4) • Neck veins (see Tables 4–1 and 5–1 for assessment tips)	Tachypnea may be a sign of anemia or acidosis Neck vein distention occurs with hypervolemia or heart failure Flat neck veins with recumbency occur with hypovolemia	

• GI and abdominal examination	*Look for*
	• Bladder distention above the symphysis pubis
	• Signs of obstruction in abdominal organs
	  – Nausea, vomiting
	  – Abdominal pain
	  – Absent bowel sounds, borborygmi
	  – Constipation
		Gastrointestinal problems may predispose the patient to hypovolemia
		Lower abdominal obstructions or tumors may obstruct urine flow
		Increased capillary hydrostatic pressure in renal failure may result in ascites because of the increased pressure within the hepatic circulation, which forces fluid and plasma proteins into the interstitium and abdominal cavity	

- Ascites

    Auscultate renal arteries for bruits (see Table 7–1 for assessment tips)

    See Section III, Chapter 13 and Table 13–5, for a discussion of physical findings associated with electrolyte imbalances

4. Electrolyte changes

Renal artery stenosis may cause hypertension and diminished blood flow to kidneys

Renal impairment causes fluid and electrolyte imbalances that can be life-threatening

Because of changes in renal function and the frequent use of drugs that affect fluid and electrolyte balance, the elderly patient must be aggressively evaluated for imbalances

RENAL DISORDERS

Among the disorders of the renal system most commonly seen in the critically ill adult is acute renal failure. Acute renal failure may affect all body systems.

Acute Renal Failure

Pathophysiology

Acute renal failure (ARF) is a sudden reduction in renal function. The decreased ability of the kidney to form and excrete urine may lead to metabolic acidosis, electrolyte imbalances, and the accumulation of nitrogenous waste products such as BUN, creatinine, uric acid, and amino acids (azotemia). ARF may be classified as prerenal, renal, and postrenal.

Prerenal Failure

Prerenal failure results from decreased renal blood flow. External losses of circulating blood volume, redistribution of circulating blood volume, and decreased cardiac output are the most common causes of prerenal failure in the critically ill adult (see Clinical Findings 8–1).

The kidney reacts to the decrease in blood flow by decreasing the glomerular filtration rate (GFR). As well, sodium and water are reabsorbed as a compensatory mechanism to increase the circulating blood volume. Consequently, the urine output declines.

Nephron function usually remains intact. The oliguria may be reversed if renal perfusion is restored *before* ischemic changes take place in the kidney.

Renal Failure

Renal failure results from tissue damage that may occur to the glomeruli, tubules, or vessels. Prolonged periods of hypoperfusion, nephrotoxic substances, contrast media, and endogenous toxins are causes of renal failure in the critically ill adult (see Clinical Findings 8–1).

Acute tubular necrosis (ATN) is the most common form of ARF in the critically ill adult. The most common cause of ATN is renal ischemia. It is thought that renal ischemia causes damage to the nephron (necrotic patchy areas) and sloughing of the nephron cells. The cellular debris collects in the renal tubules and leads to intratubular obstruction and a damaged tubular epithelium, which allows back-leak of glomerular filtrate and oliguria. As well, renal ischemia may activate the compensatory mechanisms (renin-angiotensin cascade) and cause intrarenal vasoconstriction, which contributes to an increased pressure within the nephron, a decrease in the GFR, and oliguria.

Postrenal Failure

Postrenal failure results from obstruction of the urinary collecting system. Diseases, trauma, or obstructions that block the outflow of urine from the body are common causes of postrenal failure in the critically ill adult (see Clinical Findings 8–1).

The obstruction increases the intratubular pressure and causes the Bowman's capsule pressure to become elevated. The increased Bowman's capsule pressure decreases the GFR. The increased intratubular pressure also damages the tubular cells and may lead to permanent nephron dysfunction if the cause is not corrected.

Assessment

ARF may be oliguric (<400 ml/24 h) or nonoliguric (>400 ml/24 h). Nonoliguric failure has a better prognosis than oliguric failure, because there is less damage to the tubules.

Oliguric failure is more common than nonoliguric failure. Oliguric failure passes through four phases: onset, oliguric, diuretic, and recovery. Nonoliguric failure passes through three phases: onset, nonoliguric, and recovery.

The clinical manifestations of ARF vary with the underlying nature of the disorder (prerenal, renal, or postrenal failure) and with the presence of oliguric or nonoliguric failure (see Clinical Findings 8–1).

POINTS TO REMEMBER

▶ Because the critically ill adult may present with ARF and is also susceptible to the development of ARF as a devastating sequela of critical illness and trauma (mortality rates may be as high as 40%–50%), a thorough nursing history (see Tables 1–1 and 8–1 and Clinical Findings 8–1) is crucial to assist in identifying the cause and extent of ARF and to detect patients at risk for the development of ARF. (The critically ill adult may have a history of renal insufficiency or chronic renal failure unrelated to a presenting disorder. Clinical manifestations may be similar to those of ARF but more pronounced.)

▶ Because ARF can be prevented or reversed if the clinical manifestations are recognized early, and because uremic symptoms may be manifested in every body system, in addition to the initial and baseline assessments (see Table 2–1) and a focused genitourinary assessment (see Tables 2–1 and 8–1), focused respiratory, cardiovascular, neuromuscular, gastrointestinal, and integumentary assessments (see Tables 4–1, 5–1, 6–1, 7–1, and 11–1) should be completed as often as the patient's condition dictates to detect or anticipate and prevent complications such as pulmonary edema (see Clinical Findings 4–2), heart failure (see Clinical Findings 5–1 and 5–2), pericarditis (see Chapter 5), seizures (see Clinical Findings 6–2), peptic ulcer (see Clinical Findings 7–1), skin breakdown, and infection.

▶ Ongoing assessment incorporates the evaluation of responses to diagnostic procedures and therapeutic interventions aimed at identifying the cause of ARF and the prevention of nephron damage; it includes collaboration with other members of the health team to maintain fluid, electrolyte, and acid-base balance, and to prevent or minimize uremic toxicity.

Clinical Findings 8–1 *Acute Renal Failure*

I. HISTORY

A. Predisposing factors

1. *Prerenal factors* (hypovolemia or hypoperfusion)
   - External losses
     - Hemorrhage (GI, postsurgical, traumatic)
     - Vomiting
     - Diarrhea
     - GI drainage tubes
     - Diuresis
     - Diabetes insipidus (DI)
     - Diabetic ketoacidosis (DKA)
     - Hyperosmolar, hyperglycemic, nonketotic coma (HHNKC)
     - Burns
   - Redistribution of blood flow
     - Sepsis
     - Anaphylactic shock
     - Vasodilator drugs

- Acute pancreatitis
- Bowel obstruction
- Soft-tissue injury
- Decreased cardiac output
  - Cardiogenic shock
  - Heart failure
  - Cardiomyopathy
  - Pulmonary embolism
  - Cardiac tamponade

2. *Renal factors*
   - Prolonged periods of hypoperfusion (see prerenal predisposing factors)
   - Vasoconstrictive drugs such as dopamine
   - Renal artery thrombosis
   - Nephrotoxic drugs such as aminoglycosides, cephalosporins, amphotericin, penicillin, and tetracycline
   - Chemicals such as radiographic contrast media, carbon tetrachloride, methyl alcohol, ethylene alcohol, phenols, heavy metals (gold, lead, mercury, arsenic), pesticides, and fungicides
   - Endogenous toxins such as myoglobinuria (related to rhabdomyolysis), hemoglobinuria (related to hemolytic transfusion reactions), and septic endotoxins

3. *Postrenal factors*
   - Urethral stenosis
   - Ureteral obstruction (calculi, clots, or tumors)
   - Prostatic hypertrophy
   - Bladder infection or cancer
   - Cervical cancer
   - Spinal cord injury (neurogenic bladder)
   - Trauma (bladder or ureter tear)

B. Subjective findings

1. Flank pain may be present, related to obstruction of the urinary outflow tract
2. Abdominal pain may be present, related to obstruction of the urinary outflow tract or development of a peptic ulcer due to uremia
3. Fatigue related to uremia or anemia
4. Thirst related to hypovolemia
5. Itching related to uremia
6. Weight loss may be present, related to dehydration or a catabolic state
7. Weight gain may be present, related to an increased fluid load
8. Dyspnea may be present, related to fluid overload or complications such as pulmonary edema and heart failure

II. LABORATORY AND BEDSIDE MONITORING FINDINGS

A. Oliguric and nonoliguric failure

1. The urine output may be <400 ml/24 h and the GFR may be <1 ml/min related to oliguric failure
2. The urine output may be >400 ml/24 h and the GFR may be 2–10 ml/min related to nonoliguric failure
3. The urine output may be <100 ml/24 h with anuria

B. Prerenal, renal, and postrenal failure

1. *Prerenal failure*
   - Urine (because of the decreased GFR, the filtrate moves more slowly through the tubules, allowing more water and Na to be absorbed and resulting in highly concentrated urine with a minimal amount of Na)
     - Urine volume: <400 ml/24 h
     - Specific gravity (SG): >1.020
     - Sodium: <20 mEq/L
     - Urine osmolality: >500 mOsm/L
     - Little proteinuria or sediment
   - Blood: BUN : creatinine >20 : 1 (BUN elevation is greater than the rise in creatinine, reflecting the decreased GFR and the increased reabsorption of sodium, water, and urea)
2. *Renal failure*
   - Urine (because of tubular damage, the kidney loses the ability to concentrate urine and reabsorb Na, resulting in urine that is high in Na and has a similar concentration to plasma)
     - Urine volume
       <400 ml/24 h (oliguric)
       >400 ml/24 h (nonoliguric)
     - SG: Fixed 1.008 to 1.012
     - Na: >40 mEq/L
     - Urine osmolality: <350 mOsm/L
     - Increased protein, casts, tubular epithelial cells
   - Blood: BUN : creatinine 10 – 15 : 1 (BUN and creatinine rise proportionately, reflecting the damage to the nephrons and the inability to process glomerular filtrate)
3. *Postrenal failure*
   - Urine (with persistent obstruction, the concentration of the urine may decrease, and the excretion of Na may increase)
     - Urine volume: variable, depending on the cause of the obstruction
     - SG: fixed 1.008–1.012
     - Na: >40 mEq/L

- Urine osmolality: <350 mOsm/L
- Minimal protein and sediment
- Blood: BUN:creatinine 10–15:1 (BUN and creatinine rise proportionately, reflecting cessation in glomerular filtration from back pressure in the tubules)

C. Oliguric, diuretic, and recovery phases (see Table 13–2 for related information on acid-base disorders and Table 13–5 for related information on electrolyte imbalances)

1. *Oliguric phase* (may last 1 to 3 weeks)
   - Metabolic acidosis (pH <7.35 and HCO_3 <15–20 mEq/L) related to the inability of the kidney to excrete hydrogen ions
   - Hyponatremia related to
     - An increase in water associated with the inability of the kidney to excrete water (dilutional)
     - The release of water as cells are destroyed in catabolic patients (dilutional)
     - Failure of the Na-K pump and the movement of intracellular K out of the cell while Na and water move inward (transport)
   - Hyperkalemia related to
     - Increased K released into the extracellular fluid (ECF) with cell injury
     - Metabolic acidosis, which aggravates the problem as hydrogen moves into the cell and drives K out
     - Hyperglycemia, which aggravates the problem by decreasing glycolysis in the cell and causing the Na-K pump to fail from lack of energy
     - Hemolysis, catabolism, and tissue breakdown, which increase the K load that the kidney is unable to excrete
   - Hyperphosphatemia related to
     - The inability of the kidney to excrete phosphate
     - Catabolic and injured tissue, which release phosphate and aggravate the problem
     - Acidosis, which interferes with cellular glycolysis and causes phosphate to be released into the ECF
   - Hypocalcemia related to
     - Extra phosphate ions that bind with Ca and form Ca-P salts, which are deposited in the tissue
     - The inability of the kidney to synthesize vitamin D, which contributes to decreased mobilization of Ca from the bone and decreased absorption of Ca from the intestine (hypocalcemia stimulates the parathyroid hormone [PTH], causing hyperparathyroidism and leading to demineralization of the bone)

- Anemia (decreased hemoglobin and hematocrit) related to
  - Underlying blood loss (trauma, surgery, or GI bleed)
  - Azotemia, which causes hemolysis of RBCs
  - The diminished secretion of erythropoietin by the kidney
- Thrombocytopenia, platelet dysfunction, and abnormal prothrombin consumption related to azotemia (these abnormalities may contribute to bleeding tendencies in the critically ill adult)
- Leukopenia related to azotemia, which causes a reduction in leukocytes, cell-mediated immunity, and diminished phagocytosis (infection may lead to septicemia and death in the uremic critically ill adult)

2. *Diuretic phase* (may last 1 to 3 weeks)
   - Large volumes of urine may be excreted (may be cloudy or muddy brown related to the washout of cellular debris)
   - BUN and serum creatinine levels gradually begin to fall
   - Hypokalemia may occur, related to the loss of K in the urine
   - Hypophosphatemia may occur, related to loss of phosphate in the urine
   - Hypercalcemia may occur (reciprocal to phosphate)

3. *Recovery phase* (may last 3 to 12 months)
   - Serum BUN and creatinine return to normal
   - Defects in filtration and concentration may persist for an undetermined period

D. Other laboratory findings

1. *Arterial blood gas studies*
   - Hypoxemia may be present, related to anemia, an underlying disorder, or a complication such as pulmonary edema or heart failure
   - Metabolic acidosis may be present, related to kidney failure

2. *BUN and creatinine* (see Table 13–6 for related information on BUN and creatinine)
   - Creatinine >2 mg/dl related to the inability of the kidney to excrete creatinine; the creatinine may increase 1–2 mg/dl/d in noncatabolic states
   - BUN >30 mg/dl related to the increased absorption of urea and the catabolic state of the patient:
     - BUN may increase 10–20 mg/dl/d in mildly catabolic patients and 40–50 mg/dl/d in severely catabolic patients
     - In the critically ill adult, conditions such as the severity of illness, traumatic injury, fever, and infection may stimulate the stress response and increase the amount of circulating catecholamines, cortisol, and glucagon, which leads to an increase in the breakdown of

      protein and decreased protein synthesis, and contributes to the rise
in BUN

E. ECG (see Table 14–3 for related information on dysrhythmias): A
variety of dysrhythmias may be present, related to acid-base or electrolyte
imbalances

F. Hemodynamic parameters (see Table 14–2 and Fig. 14–2 for related information on hemodynamic parameters)

1. *Oliguric phase:* May be increased central venous pressure (CVP), pulmonary capillary wedge pressure (PCWP), cardiac output (CO), and hypertension, related to overhydration or hyperdynamic circulation associated with anemia

2. *Diuretic phase:* May be decreased CVP, PCWP, CO, and hypotension, related to rapid fluid loss

III. PHYSICAL ASSESSMENT FINDINGS

A. General observations (inspection)

1. *Mental status:* Lethargy, drowsiness, irritability, disorientation, or coma may be present, related to uremia, electrolyte imbalances, or the underlying disorder

2. *Motor and sensory function:* Muscle twitching or seizures may be present, related to uremia, electrolyte imbalances, or the underlying disorder

3. *Respiratory pattern:* Tachypnea may be present, related to anemia, the underlying disorder, or complications such as pulmonary edema, heart failure, or pericarditis

4. *Skin*
   - Pale skin and mucous membranes may be present, related to anemia
   - Dry mucous membranes may be present, related to dehydration

5. *Nails:* Capillary refill may be >2 seconds, related to decreased peripheral blood flow secondary to decreased cardiac output

6. *Abdomen:* Abdominal distention may be present, related to a distended bladder secondary to obstruction

7. *Edema*
   - Generalized subcutaneous edema may be present, related to overhydration or decreased osmotic pressure secondary to the loss of protein in the urine
   - Dependent edema may be present, related to heart failure

8. *Neck veins*
   - Flat neck veins in the horizontal position may be present, related to dehydration

- Distended neck veins may be present, related to overhydration or heart failure
9. *Fever:* Temperature may be increased, related to infection
10. *Nausea and vomiting:* May be present, related to uremic toxins or electrolyte imbalances
11. *Stool:* Occult blood or frank blood may be present in the stool, related to a peptic ulcer secondary to uremia

B. Palpation
1. *Skin:* May be hot and dry related to fever
2. *Chest wall and thorax:* Decreased chest expansion may be present, related to pericarditis
3. *Peripheral pulses*
   - A rapid pulse may be present, related to dehydration, anemia, or hypoxia
   - Full and bounding pulses may be present, related to overhydration

C. Percussion: The abdomen may be dull to percussion, related to a full bladder secondary to obstruction of urine outflow

D. Auscultation
1. *Adventitious breath sounds:* Crackles may be present, related to fluid volume overload, pulmonary edema, or heart failure
2. *Heart sounds*
   - Irregular heart sounds may be present, related to dysrhythmias
   - A pericardial friction rub may be present, related to pericarditis (see Chapter 5 and Table 5–1 for related information on pericarditis and pericardial friction rub)

9

Endocrine Assessment

FUNCTION OF THE ENDOCRINE SYSTEM

The endocrine system is a complex biochemical network that regulates metabolism and sexual function, and assists in the maintenance of homeostasis. This is accomplished by cells that secrete hormones into the bloodstream to control the functions of target (receptor) cells, tissues, and organs. Hormone secretion is autoregulated by feedback loops that involve stimulating and inhibiting hormones or a direct response to the composition and concentrations of extracellular fluid (see Fig. 9–1).

The **pituitary gland, or hypophysis,** plays a major role in hormone secretion. It is located in the sella turcica, a bony cavity, about 1 cm below the optic chiasm at the base of the brain. Physiologically it is divided into two parts: the anterior pituitary, or adenohypophysis, and the posterior pituitary, or neurohypophysis.

Specific **releasing hormones** are secreted by neurons of the **hypothalamus** into a portal circulatory system connected to the anterior pituitary gland (hypothalamic-pituitary axis). In response, cells of the **anterior pituitary** secrete **specific stimulating hormones** into the general circulation; these in turn cause hormone production by distant target cells. The stimulating hormones include

- **Adrenocorticotropin (ACTH)** to stimulate the adrenal cortex to secrete the adrenocortical hormone cortisol and some melanocyte-stimulating hormone
- **Thyroid-stimulating hormone (TSH)** to stimulate the thyroid gland to secrete thyroxine (T_4) and triiodothyronine (T_3)

- **Gonad-stimulating hormones: follicle-stimulating hormone (FSH), and luteinizing hormone (LH)** to stimulate ovulation, sperm formation, and secretion of reproductive hormones by ovaries or testes

The hypothalamic-pituitary axis also secretes hormones that directly affect cells and organs, including

- **Growth hormone (GH, or somatotropin)** to stimulate the growth of body cells
- **Prolactin** to stimulate breast development and lactation

When many of the hormones reach a specific blood level, **inhibiting hormones** complete the feedback loop by stopping the production of the hormone. For example, somatostatin secreted by the hypothalamus inhibits the release of growth hormone and TSH from the anterior pituitary. It is also released from pancreatic islet cells and certain gastrointestinal cells to inhibit the release of insulin and glucagon.

The **posterior pituitary gland** stores and releases at least two hormones produced by specialized nuclei in the hypothalamus:

- **Antidiuretic hormone (ADH),** or vasopressin, to preserve extracellular fluid volume
- **Oxytocin** to stimulate uterine contraction and milk expression perinatally

Other hormones significant to the integrity of the body do not involve the pituitary gland directly. These include

- **Epinephrine and norepinephrine (catecholamines)** produced by the adrenal medulla in response to sympathetic nervous system stimulation to facilitate vasoconstriction and stress response
- **Insulin** secreted by the beta cells of the islets of Langerhans in the pancreas to promote glucose uptake, storage, and cellular metabolism
- **Glucagon** secreted by the alpha cells of the islets of Langerhans in the pancreas to promote glycogenolysis and gluconeogenesis in the liver in response to hypoglycemia
- **Parathormone** secreted by the parathyroid glands to increase calcium ion concentration in the blood by controlling gut absorption, stimulating bone resorption, and promoting kidney conservation of calcium, while promoting excretion of phosphate

- **Calcitonin** secreted by the thyroid gland to rapidly decrease calcium ion concentration in the blood by inhibiting bone resorption and osteoclast formation

Insulin is secreted in response to a rise in blood glucose, usually postprandially. Insulin secretion can also be stimulated by the sympathetic (β-2-adrenergic) and parasympathetic (muscarinic) receptors of the nervous system and by hormones in the gastrointestinal system. It is required to transport glucose across cell membranes except those of the brain, kidney parenchyma, liver, intestinal mucosa, and blood cells. In the liver insulin facilitates the storage of glucose as glycogen (glycogenesis), which can be converted to glucose (gluconeogenesis) during fasting or in situations requiring additional energy, such as exercise or stress. During situations of increased stress such as infection, trauma, burns, or other critical illness, increased amounts of cortisol are secreted, which stimulate the secretion of glucagon to further increase the blood sugar level.

In addition to metabolic and environmental stimuli, hormone secretion is also influenced by circadian rhythms and biological clocks. Functioning of the endocrine system can be affected by diseases of endocrine cells, tissues, or organs; by injury or disease of the nervous system; or by autoimmune disease.

Changes with Aging

There are changes in hormone production involving the hypothalamic-pituitary–receptor organ axes with aging. **Decreased growth hormone** and **somatostatin** secretion contribute to losses of bone and lean body mass. ACTH and glucocorticoid levels remain intact. Both T_4 production and metabolism fall, resulting in unchanged circulating blood levels. Despite reduction in the conversion of T_4 to T_3 the level of T_3 remains normal. The blood level of **TSH increases** with age but may not be symptomatic of thyroid disease. There is a greater increase in **ADH** levels in response to increased plasma osmolality, but reduced release with volume stimulation. Decreased renin and aldosterone levels with age as well as kidney disease may further diminish the ability to conserve sodium with plasma volume depletion (see Chapter 8).

Production of other hormones may also be affected by age. Plasma catecholamine levels rise due to an **increase in norepinephrine.** This may be related to a diminished response of target cells. **Calcitonin** levels remain within normal limits but response to hypercalcemia is slowed. **Parathormone** levels increase, probably due to decreased renal function.

There is a decreased ability to maintain glucose homeostasis with aging. Secretion of insulin by the beta cells of the pancreas remains normal, but may be slower in response to a glucose challenge (**impaired glucose tolerance**). There is a 1–2 mg/dl increase in fasting glucose level and a 5–10 mg/dl increase in 2-hour postprandial glucose per decade after age 40–50. There is also probably some increase in glycosylated hemoglobin (Hb-A$_{1c}$). In healthy elderly this is probably due to insulin resistance (**decreased insulin sensitivity**), causing a decreased ability to utilize glucose at the cellular level. Obesity (increased adipose tissue) and physical inactivity are common causes of impaired glucose tolerance and non-insulin-dependent diabetes mellitus in the elderly. Age-related changes in drug metabolism or ingestion of drugs with glycemic effects may also affect glucose metabolism (see Clinical Findings 9–1).

Hyperglycemia of aging (impaired glucose tolerance) as well as diabetes mellitus may have its first manifestations in the older patient with signs and symptoms of end organ disease affecting macrocirculation (atherosclerotic cardiovascular disease) or microcirculation (retinopathy, nephropathy, neuropathy). Hyperglycemic coma in the older, non-insulin-dependent diabetic is usually hyperosmolar and nonketotic because of concurrent dehydration and an increased threshold for renal excretion of glucose.

Hypoglycemia may occur in the elderly due to impaired counterregulatory mechanisms involving glucagon, growth hormone, and cortisol.

ENDOCRINE DISORDERS

Disorders of the endocrine system are related to either hyperfunction or hypofunction of the hormones released by the endocrine glands. Disruption in function of the hormone may be related to hypersecretion, hyposecretion, or lack of responsiveness by target cells (see Fig. 9–1).

Endocrine disorders may be classified as primary or secondary. Primary endocrine disorders are the result of malfunction of the endocrine gland itself. Secondary endocrine disorders occur when a condition outside the endocrine gland causes hypersecretion or hyposecretion of the hormone.

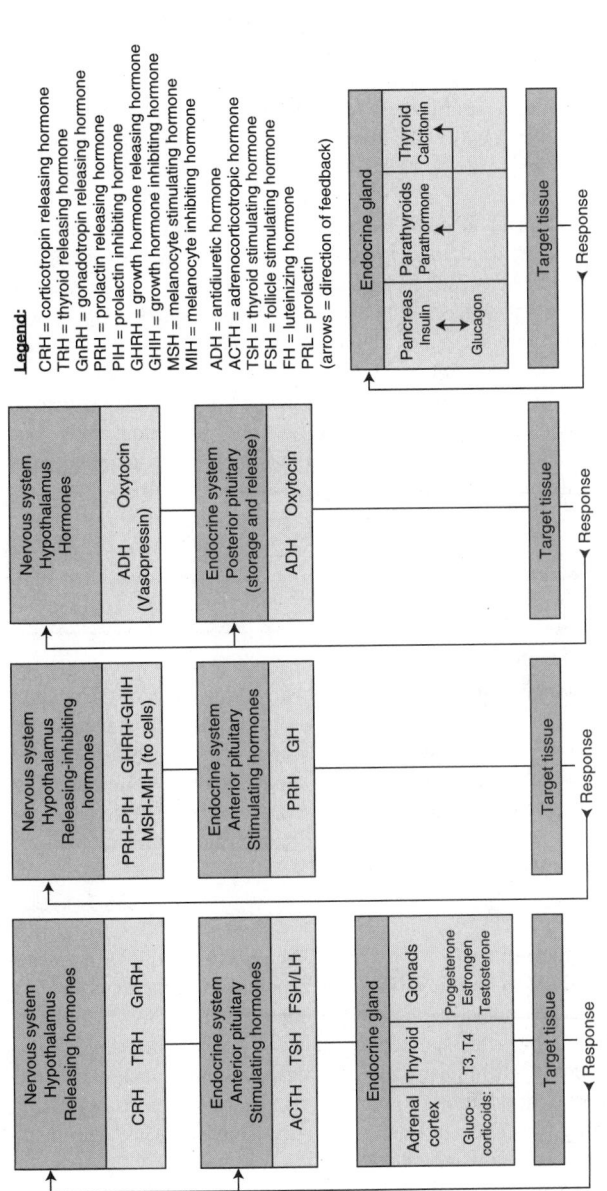

FIGURE 9-1

Mechanisms of endocrine system function and feedback loops.

Legend:

CRH = corticotropin releasing hormone
TRH = thyroid releasing hormone
GnRH = gonadotropin releasing hormone
PRH = prolactin releasing hormone
PIH = prolactin inhibiting hormone
GHRH = growth hormone releasing hormone
GHIH = growth hormone inhibiting hormone
MSH = melanocyte stimulating hormone
MIH = melanocyte inhibiting hormone

ADH = antidiuretic hormone
ACTH = adrenocorticotropic hormone
TSH = thyroid stimulating hormone
FSH = follicle stimulating hormone
FH = luteinizing hormone
PRL = prolactin
(arrows = direction of feedback)

511

Endocrine disorders may be further classified as functional disorders. Functional disorders are associated with the inability of the target organ to respond to the hormone. Lack of responsiveness may be related to defects at the receptor sites or lack of functional receptors on the target cells.

In the critically ill adult, endocrine disorders may be life-threatening crises, as acute decompensation of gland function may be precipitated by stressful events such as infections, trauma, head injuries, myocardial infarction, hypertension, heart failure, respiratory disorders, metastatic tumors, surgery, shock, alcohol withdrawal, adverse medication effects, and prolonged illness. Endocrine crises that may occur in the critically ill adult include adrenal crisis, pheochromocytoma, diabetic ketoacidosis, hyperosmolar hyperglycemic nonketotic syndrome, diabetes insipidus, syndrome of inappropriate antidiuretic secretion, thyroid storm, and myxedema coma.

Adrenal Crisis

Pathophysiology

The adrenal gland is composed of two hormonal units, the medulla and the cortex. The medulla is responsible for catecholamine secretion (epinephrine and norepinephrine) in response to sympathetic nervous system stimulation (see Pheochromocytoma for related information on epinephrine and norepinephrine). The cortex is responsible for secretion of the adrenocortical (steroid) hormones, including cortisol (glucocorticoid) and aldosterone (mineralocorticoid).

Cortisol

The release of cortisol is controlled almost entirely by the negative feedback system involving the hypothalamus, the anterior pituitary gland (adrenocorticotropin hormone), and the adrenal gland (see Fig. 9–1). Cortisol is secreted in response to stress. The primary function of cortisol is to raise the blood sugar and make glucose available for energy. In addition, cortisol exerts an anti-inflammatory effect, providing protection against potentially harmful toxins. The metabolic effects of cortisol include

- The stimulation of gluconeogenesis by the liver
- A decrease in the rate of glucose utilization by the cells

- An increase in blood glucose concentration
- Increased breakdown of proteins (decreased protein storage in all body cells except the liver)
- Increased plasma protein levels
- Increased mobilization of fatty acids to provide energy for cells in the absence of normal glucose
- A strong anti-inflammatory effect
  - Stabilizes lysosomal membranes of the inflammatory cells and prevents the release of inflammatory mediators
  - Decreases capillary permeability to prevent inflammatory edema
  - Depresses phagocytosis by the WBCs to reduce the release of inflammatory mediators
  - Suppresses the immune response (causes atrophy of lymphoid tissue, decreases eosinophils, decreases antibody formation, and decreases the development of cell-mediated immunity)
  - Reduces fever
  - Inhibits fibroblast activity
- Facilitates the response of catecholamines during trauma and extreme stress (must be present for catecholamines to produce arterial vasoconstriction)

Aldosterone

The release of aldosterone is primarily controlled by the renin-angiotensin cascade, an increased serum potassium level, decreased serum sodium levels, and adrenocorticotropin hormone (ACTH). The primary function of aldosterone is to maintain salt and water balance. Metabolic effects of aldosterone include

- The maintenance of extracellular fluid volume and electrolyte composition by the regulation of sodium and potassium concentrations
- The conservation of sodium and water to maintain blood pressure during the stress response

Adrenocortical Insufficiency

Adrenocortical insufficiency is the lack of sufficient glucocorticoids or mineralocorticoids to meet the demands of the cells. Adrenocortical insufficiency may be primary or secondary.

Primary Adrenocortical Insufficiency. Primary adrenocortical insufficiency results from disease of the adrenal gland itself (see Clinical

Findings 9–1 for predisposing factors). Destruction or hypofunction of the adrenal cortex leads to a decreased production of cortisol and aldosterone. Manifestations, including hypoglycemia, hyponatremia, hypovolemia, and hyperkalemia, reflect both cortisol and aldosterone deficiency.

Secondary Adrenocortical Insufficiency. Secondary adrenocortical insufficiency results from a pathological condition outside the adrenal glands that causes a deficiency of ACTH (see Clinical Findings 9–1 for predisposing factors). The major effect is on cortisol as the release of aldosterone continues to be stimulated by other methods, such as the renin-angiotensin cascade. Manifestations, including hypoglycemia and hypotension, are primarily related to cortisol deficiency.

Adrenal Crisis

Adrenal crisis may be precipitated in the patient with primary or secondary adrenocortical insufficiency during times of acute or prolonged stress:

- Cortisol and aldosterone are critical to the stress response.
- If the adrenal glands are unable to respond to the need for cortisol to maintain the blood glucose level and the blood pressure, and the need for aldosterone to maintain fluid and electrolyte balance, a potentially life-threatening situation such as profound hypotension and shock may occur.
- Adrenal crisis should be suspected in the critically ill adult for whom another cause for hypoglycemia and profound hypotension cannot be identified.

Assessment

The clinical manifestations of adrenal crisis may be related to the lack of cortisol and aldosterone (primary adrenocortical insufficiency), or the lack of cortisol (secondary adrenocortical insufficiency (see Clinical Findings 9–1). The effects of decreased aldosterone (fluid and electrolyte imbalances) may not be present in the critically ill adult with secondary adrenocortical insufficiency because of the continued presence of aldosterone.

POINTS TO REMEMBER

▶ The critically ill adult with chronic adrenocortical insufficiency (controlled with hormone replacement therapy) is at risk for adrenal crisis during times of increased physical or emotional stress (the diseased gland is unable to respond to increased demands for cortisol and aldosterone).

▶ The critically ill adult on long-term steroid therapy for a medical condition such as asthma or rheumatoid arthritis is at risk for adrenal crisis when maintenance steroids are not increased during times of stress, when exogenous steroids are withdrawn too rapidly or abruptly, or when there is atrophy of the adrenal glands related to prolonged suppression of the hypothalamic-pituitary axis by exogenous steroids.

▶ A thorough nursing history (see Table 1–1 and Clinical Findings 9–1) is crucial to identify patients at risk for the development of adrenal crisis or to identify the underlying cause of adrenal crisis.

▶ In addition to the initial and baseline assessments (see Table 2–1) and a focused assessment of the underlying disorder, focused cardiovascular and neuromuscular assessments (see Tables 2–1, 5–1, and 6–1) should be completed as often as the patient's condition dictates to detect or anticipate and prevent complications such as circulatory collapse or hypovolemic shock (see Clinical Findings 12–3).

▶ Ongoing assessment incorporates the evaluation of responses to diagnostic procedures and therapeutic interventions aimed at identifying adrenal crisis and restoring the circulating blood volume; it includes collaborating with other members of the health team to correct hormone and electrolyte imbalances, maintain blood pressure and peripheral blood flow, prevent infection, and provide patient education once the crisis has passed.

Clinical Findings 9–1 *Adrenal Crisis*

I. HISTORY

A. Predisposing factors

1. *Primary adrenocortical insufficiency*
   - Autoimmune disease (most common)
   - Infiltration of the adrenal glands by tuberculosis, histoplasmosis, blastomycosis, or sarcoidosis
   - Acquired immunodeficiency syndrome (cytomegalovirus)
   - Metastatic cancer

- Hemorrhage into the adrenal glands associated with anticoagulant therapy or infection (Waterhouse-Friderichsen syndrome)
- Bilateral adrenalectomy

2. *Secondary adrenocortical insufficiency*
- Exogenous steroid use
- Hypopituitarism (pituitary tumors, trauma, surgery, radiation, hemorrhage, and metastatic cancer involving the pituitary gland)
- Lesions in the hypothalamus (head trauma)

3. *Adrenal crisis*
- Infection
- Trauma
- Surgery
- Alcohol withdrawal
- Thyrotoxicosis
- Myxedema
- Abrupt withdrawal of steroids
- Inadequate replacement of steroids during stressful events such as surgery or infection

B. Subjective findings
- Profound weakness related to hypoglycemia
- Fatigue related to hypoglycemia
- Anorexia, nausea and vomiting, abdominal cramping, and diarrhea related to sodium and fluid loss, hyperkalemia, or hypoglycemia
- Headache or visual-field disturbances may be related to pituitary tumors

II. LABORATORY AND BEDSIDE MONITORING FINDINGS

A. Adrenal laboratory studies (see Table 13–7 for related information on adrenal laboratory studies)
1. A baseline cortisol level <20 μg/dl in the presence of stress is suggestive of the diminished or absent production of cortisol (with sufficient cortisol production, the baseline cortisol level should be >20 μg/dl in the presence of stress)
2. ACTH stimulation test may be used to screen for adrenocortical insufficiency and to distinguish between primary and secondary adrenocortical insufficiency

B. Other laboratory studies (see Table 13–5 for related information on electrolyte imbalances, Table 13–6 for related information on BUN, and Table 13–9 for related information on WBC count and differential)

1. Hypoglycemia (<75 mg/dl) may be present, related to the increased peripheral utilization of glucose, decreased hepatic gluconeogenesis, and decreased lipolysis (cortisol deficiency)
2. Hyponatremia (<135 mEq/L) may be present, related to aldosterone deficiency, which causes depletion of sodium and retention of potassium and hydrogen
3. Hyperkalemia (>5 mEq/L) may be present, related to aldosterone deficiency
4. Elevated BUN (>15 mg/dl) may be present, related to prerenal failure and azotemia secondary to hypovolemia
5. Eosinophilia may be present, related to cortisol deficiency and an increased immune response

C. Arterial blood gas studies (see Chapter 13 for related information on arterial blood gas studies and serum lactate levels)

1. HCO_3 <22 mEq/L and pH <7.35 may be present related to metabolic acidosis secondary to decreased peripheral blood flow
2. Serum lactate levels may be elevated, reflecting tissue oxygen deficits

D. ECG

1. Peaked T wave, widened QRS complex, prolongation of the PR interval, and decreased amplitude of the P wave may be present, related to decreased cortisol levels (may alter the normal excitability of the myocardium), hyperkalemia, and hyponatremia (may affect depolarization and repolarization of the myocardial cells)
2. Tachycardia may be present, related to vasodilation and hypotension (cortisol deficiency) and hypovolemia (aldosterone deficiency)
3. Dysrhythmias may be present, related to hyponatremia or hyperkalemia (aldosterone deficiency)

E. Hemodynamic parameters (see Chapter 14, Table 14–2, and Fig. 14–2 for related information on hemodynamic parameters)

1. Hypotension may be present, related to cortisol deficiency (vascular dilation) and aldosterone deficiency (hypovolemia)
2. CVP, PCWP, CO, and systemic vascular resistance (SVR) may be decreased, related to cortisol and aldosterone deficiency (vascular dilation and hypovolemia)

III. PHYSICAL ASSESSMENT FINDINGS

A. General observations (inspection)

1. *Mental status:* Emotional disturbances, depression, confusion, or coma may be present, related to hypoglycemia or dehydration

2. *Skin*
   - Hyperpigmentation of buccal mucosa, skin creases, scars, pressure sites, and areolae may be present, related to the excessive secretion of melanocyte-stimulating hormone (MSH), which is cosecreted by the pituitary with ACTH in response to low levels of cortisol
   - Vitiligo, areas of decreased pigmentation surrounded by areas of increased pigmentation, may be present, related to increased MSH secretion
3. *Fever:* Hyperthermia may be present, related to cortisol deficiency or the presence of infection (decreased anti-inflammatory response)
B. Palpation: Skin may be warm and dry, related to fever or dehydration
C. Auscultation: Heart sounds may be rapid and irregular, related to tachycardia and dysrhythmias

Pheochromocytoma

Pathophysiology

A pheochromocytoma is an encapsulated vascular tumor of chromaffin tissue. Pheochromocytomas occur primarily in the adrenal medulla.

Epinephrine

The adrenal medulla secretes catecholamines in response to sympathetic nervous system stimulation. Epinephrine accounts for 80% of the catecholamine secreted by the medulla. Epinephrine acts on alpha and beta receptors. Actions of epinephrine include

- Increased contractility and excitability of the heart muscle
- Facilitation of blood flow to the muscles, brain, and viscera
- Increased blood sugar (stimulates the conversion of glycogen to glucose in the liver)
- Decreased gastrointestinal function
- Bronchial dilation

Norepinephrine

Norepinephrine accounts for 20% of the catecholamine secreted by the medulla. Norepinephrine primarily acts on alpha receptors in the skeletal muscle vasculature, causing intense vasoconstriction. In addition, norepinephrine is the neurotransmitter produced by the postganglionic sympathetic fibers.

Like the adrenal medulla, the tumor cells of the pheochromocytoma produce and secrete epinephrine and norepinephrine. Secretion of the catecholamines may be triggered by sympathetic nervous system stimulation, or the release may be autonomous.

Assessment

Clinical manifestations of pheochromocytoma may vary with the predominance of epinephrine or norepinephrine and whether the hormones are secreted intermittently or on a continuous basis (see Table 13–7 for related information on catecholamines). Generally, pheochromocytomas secret a combination of epinephrine and norepinephrine, but norepinephrine is most often the hormone secreted in large amounts.

Epinephrine

Clinical manifestations associated with epinephrine secretion may reflect a hypermetabolic state and hyperglycemia; manifestations may include tachycardia, angina, cardiomegaly, diaphoresis, pallor or flushing, nervousness, increased blood glucose, polyuria, hypotension, dizziness, fainting, and syncopal episodes.

Norepinephrine

Clinical manifestations associated with norepinephrine secretion may include

- Persistent or paroxysmal hypertension, headache, visual disturbances, tremors, anxiety, and agitation.
- Classically, hypertension is the most common sign of pheochromocytoma.

General Findings

Weight loss, weakness, fatigue, anorexia, nausea, and vomiting may reflect a general response of the gastrointestinal tract to the increased sympathetic stimulation. The patient may also complain of abdominal pain.

POINTS TO REMEMBER

▶ The critically ill adult with pheochromocytoma may present with a severe hypertensive crisis. A thorough nursing history (see Table 1–1) is crucial to identify pheochromocytoma as the underlying cause of the hypertension.

▶ In addition to the initial and baseline assessments (see Table 2–1), focused cardiovascular and neuromuscular assessments (see Tables 2–1, 5–1, and 6–1) should be completed as often as the patient's condition dictates to detect or anticipate and prevent complications such as cardiovascular decompensation, myocardial ischemia or infarction (see Clinical Findings 5–3), heart failure (see Clinical Findings 5–1 and 5–2), seizures (see Clinical Findings 6–2), or a cerebrovascular accident (see Clinical Findings 6–5).

▶ Ongoing assessment incorporates the evaluation of responses to diagnostic procedures and therapeutic interventions aimed at stabilization of the blood pressure and fluid volume; it includes collaboration with other members of the health team to maintain a stress-free environment and prepare the patient for surgery (surgical removal of the tumor usually relieves the disorder).

Diabetic Ketoacidosis

Pathophysiology

Diabetic ketoacidosis (DKA) is a metabolic disorder associated with type I insulin-dependent diabetes mellitus (IDDM). DKA is usually abrupt in onset and is characterized by hyperglycemia, osmotic diuresis, and ketoacidosis.

Insulin

Insulin transports glucose into insulin-sensitive cells throughout the body to be used as an energy source. Insulin facilitates the storage of protein (amino acids) in the muscle, free fatty acids (triglycerides) in the adipose tissue, and glycogen in the liver.

Hyperglycemia and Osmotic Diuresis

In the absence of insulin, plasma glucose concentrations rise. When the absorptive capacity of the proximal tubules of the kidney is exceeded, glucose is excreted in the urine, resulting in an osmotic diuresis (polyuria). The thirst center in the brain is stimulated to increase fluid intake (polydipsia), and cellular starvation prompts polyphagia (increased intake of food).

Ketones

Continued insulin deficiency and cell starvation stimulates other hormonal influences. Increased levels of glucagon, catecholamines, growth hormone, and cortisol contribute to an accelerated production of glucose in the liver, and the breakdown of protein and fat (lipolysis). Free fatty acids are transported to the liver to be formed into ketones (keto acids).

Metabolic Acidosis

Under normal circumstances, keto acids are able to be neutralized by neural and muscle tissue in energy metabolism. However, when this normal pathway becomes saturated, the accumulation of ketones results in ketonemia, ketonuria, and metabolic acidosis.

Kussmaul's Respirations

The kidney attempts to buffer the acidosis with bicarbonate; however, the bicarbonate levels may be depleted as bicarbonate is also excreted with the osmotic diuresis. The respiratory system attempts to compensate for the acidosis by increasing the rate and depth of respiration (Kussmaul's respirations).

Electrolyte Imbalances

Electrolyte imbalances may be variable:

- Extracellular hydrogen ions are exchanged for intracellular potassium, ions which may result in a transient hyperkalemia.
- Large amount of fluid loss via vomiting or diuresis may result in hypokalemia.
- Polyuria, glycosuria, and ketonuria may lower the phosphate levels, since large amounts of phosphate may be lost in the urine.
- Severe hyperglycemia may pull water out of the cells into the extracellular fluid, resulting in a dilutional hyponatremia.
- Also, hypovolemia may stimulate the release of aldosterone, promoting the retention of sodium and leading to hypernatremia.

Assessment

The clinical manifestations of DKA are related to hyperglycemia, intracellular dehydration, hypovolemia, electrolyte imbalances, and ketoacidosis (see Clinical Findings 9–2 for clinical manifestations associated with the pathology of DKA, Table 13–7 for related information on blood glucose and serum and on urine osmolality, and Table 13–5 for related information on electrolyte imbalances).

Hyperglycemic Hyperosmolar Nonketotic Syndrome

Pathophysiology

Hyperglycemic hyperosmolar nonketotic syndrome (HHNK) is a metabolic disorder associated with type II non-insulin-dependent diabetes mellitus (NIDDM). HHNK is usually insidious in onset and is characterized by severe hyperglycemia with an absence of ketosis, severe dehydration, hyperosmolality, and alterations in the level of consciousness.

Hyperglycemia

Hyperglycemia is more pronounced in HHNK than DKA. It is thought that the severe hyperglycemia may be potentiated by the relative lack of insulin and stress-induced catecholamine and glucocorticoid secretion (catecholamines and glucocorticoids oppose the action of insulin and further decrease insulin secretion). The inability to produce enough insulin to transport glucose into the cells leads to an imbalance between the amount of glucose produced and the amount the body is able to utilize.

Osmotic Diuresis

Severe hyperglycemia leads to pronounced osmotic diuresis. Intracellular and extracellular dehydration may occur, resulting in a high serum osmolality. The high serum osmolality may lead to alterations in the level of consciousness. The fluid loss may lead to hypoperfusion of the kidneys and acute tubular necrosis. The kidneys may be unable to filter the urine, and the excretion of glucose is impaired, worsening the hyperglycemia.

Nonketosis

The lack of ketosis is most often attributed to the relative lack of insulin. It is thought that endogenous insulin is present in sufficient levels to prevent lipolysis and the formation of ketones. As well, it is postulated that there is an impaired hepatic synthesis of ketones from free fatty acids. In addition, serum levels of growth hormone and cortisol are lower in HHNK than DKA, which may also contribute to a possible cause of nonketosis in HHNK.

Assessment

The clinical manifestations associated with HHNK are related to severe hyperglycemia, pronounced osmotic diuresis (intracellular and extracellular dehydration), and hyperosmolality (see Clinical Findings 9–2 for clinical manifestations associated with HHNK; Table 13–7 for related information on blood glucose and serum, and on urine osmolality; and Table 13–5 for related information on electrolyte imbalances).

POINTS TO REMEMBER: DKA AND HHNK

▶ DKA and HHNK are complications of diabetes mellitus.

▶ The critically ill adult may present with DKA or HHNK as the presenting symptom of a new diagnosis of diabetes type I or type II.

▶ As well, the critically ill adult with known diabetes of type I or type II is susceptible to the development of DKA or HHNK.

▶ The critically ill or elderly adult unable to recognize or respond to thirst is particularly susceptible to the development of HHNK (see Chapter 3 for related information on changes with aging).

▶ A thorough nursing history (see Table 1–1 and Clinical Findings 9–2) is crucial to identify patients at risk for the development of DKA and HHNK, or to identify the underlying cause of DKA and HHNK.

▶ In addition to the initial and baseline assessments (see Table 2–1), focused cardiovascular and neuromuscular assessments (see Tables 2–1, 5–1, and 6–1) should be completed as often as the patient's condition dictates to detect or anticipate and prevent complications such as life-threatening dysrhythmias, thromboembolism related to hemoconcentration, hypovolemic shock (see Clinical Findings 12–3), or coma.

▶ Ongoing assessment incorporates the evaluation of responses to diagnostic procedures and therapeutic interventions aimed at identifying DKA or HHNK and the restoration of fluid volume; it includes collaboration with other members of the health team to correct blood glucose levels and electrolyte imbalances, maintain blood pressure and tissue perfusion, and provide patient education once the crisis has passed.

Clinical Findings 9–2 *DKA and HHNK*

DKA	HHNK

I. HISTORY

A. Predisposing factors
1. Infection (skin, respiratory and urinary tracts most common)
2. Surgery
3. Trauma
4. Emotional or physical stress
5. Inadequate doses of exogenous insulin or noncompliance to regimen

I. HISTORY

A. Predisposing factors
1. More common in older individuals (the elderly have a lower total body water content, which may compromise the ability to buffer changes in osmolality)
2. Associated with illnesses such as cardiovascular or renal disorders
3. Stress
4. Infections
5. Drugs that cause gluconeogenesis, insulin resistance, or inhibit insulin release, such as steroids, thiazide diuretics, epinephrine, calcium channel blockers, β-blockers, phenytoin, and immunosuppressive agents
6. Dialysis
7. Total parenteral nutrition
8. Surgery (anesthesia)
9. Inadequate fluids or lack of access to fluids (the elderly may have a decreased sense of thirst)

B. Subjective findings
1. Polydipsia related to osmotic diuresis and stimulation of the thirst mechanism
2. Polyphagia related to cellular starvation
3. Weight loss related to catabolism (breakdown of protein and fat for energy requirements)

B. Subjective findings
1. Same as DKA; however, polydipsia may not be present in the elderly critically ill adult or in the critically ill adult whose thirst center in the hypothalamus is impaired because of the high serum osmolality

DKA	HHNK

4. Fatigue, weakness, anorexia, nausea, and vomiting may be related to dehydration or electrolyte imbalances
5. Abdominal pain or cramps may be related to dehydration or electrolyte imbalances
6. Pleuritic chest pain may be present, related to dehydration

2. Fatigue or weakness related to dehydration or electrolyte imbalances

II. LABORATORY AND BEDSIDE MONITORING FINDINGS

A. Arterial blood gas studies
1. Metabolic acidosis (pH <7.30) related to ketoacidosis
2. HCO_3 <15 mEq/L related to compensation for ketoacidosis and osmotic diuresis
3. PCO_2 <35 mm Hg related to compensatory hyperventilation
4. PO_2 may be <80 mm Hg related to respiratory insufficiency

B. Other laboratory studies
1. Blood glucose >300 mg/dl (may average 300–800 mg/dl) related to the absolute lack of insulin, the inability of the cells to utilize glucose, and hormonal influences that increase the production of glucose

2. Serum osmolality 300–350 mOsm/kg related to hyperglycemia and excessive water loss

3. Sodium may be low (<135 mEq/L), related to an

II. LABORATORY AND BEDSIDE MONITORING FINDINGS

A. Arterial blood gas studies: No ketoacidosis; mild-to-moderate metabolic acidosis (pH <7.35 and HCO_3 <22 mEq/L) may be present, related to lactic acidosis associated with dehydration and decreased peripheral blood flow

B. Other laboratory studies
1. Blood glucose >800 mg/dl related to insulin deficiency, the inability of the cells to utilize glucose, hormonal influences that resist insulin and increase the production of glucose, and the inability of the kidney to excrete glucose

2. Serum osmolality >350 mOsm/kg related to the more severe hyperglycemia, water loss, and hypernatremia

3. Sodium same as DKA, but hypernatremia may be more pro-

DKA	HHNK
initial dilutional effect; normal; or high (>145 mEq/L), related to the increased secretion of aldosterone and sodium retention	nounced, related to the severe dehydration and increased secretion of aldosterone and sodium retention

DKA

4. Potassium may be high (>5 mEq/L) related to the movement of K into the extracellular fluid in exchange for hydrogen ions (transient change); normal; or low (<3.5 mEq/L), related to the loss of potassium with osmotic diuresis or vomiting

5. Phosphate may be <2.5 mg/dl related to osmotic diuresis

6. BUN >20 mg/dl related to dehydration or decreased renal perfusion associated with volume depletion

7. Creatinine may be >1.5 mg/dl, related to dehydration or decreased renal perfusion associated with volume depletion

8. Hemoglobin and hematocrit may be increased, related to dehydration

9. Leukocytosis may be related to increased catecholamine secretion or a preexisting infection

C. Urinalysis

1. Ketonuria (moderate to large amount) related to ketonemia and the excretion of ketones

2. Glucosuria related to hyperglycemia and the excretion of glucose

3. Specific gravity >1.025 related to loss of solutes

HHNK

4. Potassium same as DKA, but hypokalemia may be more pronounced, because potassium is excreted in the urine as aldosterone increases the absorption of sodium

5. Same as DKA

6. Same as DKA

7. Same as DKA

8. Same as DKA; however severe hemoconcentration may lead to coagulopathies

9. Same as DKA

C. Urinalysis

1. No ketones

2. Same as DKA

3. Same as DKA

DKA	HHNK

D. ECG

1. Peaked T waves, widened QRS complex, prolonged PR interval, and flattened P waves may be related to hyperkalemia
2. Flat or inverted T waves and depressed ST segments may be related to hypokalemia
3. Tachycardia related to dehydration
4. Dysrhythmias related to electrolyte imbalances or acidosis (see Table 14–3 for related information on dysrhythmias)

E. Hemodynamic parameters

1. Hypotension related to fluid loss
2. CVP, PCWP, and CO may be decreased, related to hypovolemia (see Chapter 14 and Table 14–2 for related information on hemodynamic parameters)

III. PHYSICAL ASSESSMENT FINDINGS

A. General observations (inspection): Fruity or sweet breath odor related to the acetones formed during the ketogenic process

1. *Mental status:* Altered levels of consciousness related to brain-cell dehydration (may vary from alert to lethargy, drowsiness, and unresponsiveness to painful stimuli)

D. ECG

1. Same as DKA
2. Same as DKA
3. Same as DKA
4. Same as DKA

E. Hemodynamic parameters

1. Same as DKA
2. Same as DKA, but values may be more pronounced, related to severe fluid loss

III. PHYSICAL ASSESSMENT FINDINGS

A. General observations (inspection): Absence of ketone odor to breath

1. *Mental status:* Same as DKA, but impaired levels of consciousness may be more pronounced, related to high serum osmolality and severe intracellular dehydration of the brain (seizures, positive Babinski's sign, and motor and sensory deficits such as hemiparesis may be present)

DKA	HHNK

2. *Respiratory pattern:* Kussmaul's respirations (deep and labored respirations) related to respiratory compensation for metabolic acidosis

2. *Respiratory pattern:* Tachypnea related to hypovolemia

3. *Skin:* Flushed, dry skin, dry mucous membranes, and sunken eyes related to dehydration

3. *Skin:* Dry mucous membranes, sunken eyes related to severe dehydration

4. *Fever:* Usually afebrile (increased temperature may be present related to the presence of an underlying infection)

4. *Fever:* Increased temperature may be present (the elderly may be afebrile in the presence of infection)

5. *Urine:* Polyuria related to osmotic diuresis

5. *Urine:* Same as DKA, but more pronounced

B. Palpation

1. *Skin:* Loss of skin turgor related to dehydration

B. Palpation

1. *Skin*
   - Same as DKA
   - Skin may be cool related to decreased perfusion

2. *Peripheral pulses:* May be rapid and thready related to dehydration

2. *Peripheral pulses:* Same as DKA

C. Auscultation

1. *Adventitious breath sounds*
   - Pleural friction rub may be present, related to dehydration
   - Crackles may be absent in the presence of an underlying pneumonia related to dehydration (may appear with rehydration)

C. Auscultation

1. *Adventitious breath sounds:* Crackles may be absent in the presence of an underlying pneumonia related to dehydration (may appear with rehydration)

2. *Heart sounds:* May be rapid or irregular, related to tachycardia and dysrhythmias

2. *Heart sounds:* Same as DKA

Diabetes Insipidus

Pathophysiology

Diabetes insipidus (DI) is a clinical syndrome that may result from a defect in the synthesis or secretion of antidiuretic hormone (neurogenic or central DI), or from an altered renal response to antidiuretic hormone (nephrogenic DI). DI is characterized by excessive urine output.

Antidiuretic Hormone (ADH)

Antidiuretic hormone (arginine vasopressin) assists in the regulation of plasma osmolality, blood volume, and blood pressure. The secretion of ADH is primarily regulated by osmotic receptors in the hypothalamus that mediate the suppression and release of ADH in response to the concentration of blood plasma. When the plasma becomes too concentrated, ADH is released from the posterior pituitary gland. In contrast, when the plasma is hypotonic, ADH secretion is suppressed (see Fig. 9–1).

Changes in extracellular fluid (ECF) volume also affect the release of ADH. Stretch receptors in the atria and pulmonary circulation feed back to the hypothalamus to mediate the suppression and release of ADH in response to decreases and increases in the ECF volume. When fluid volume is decreased, ADH secretion is increased to prevent hypovolemia. When fluid volume is increased, ADH secretion is suppressed to prevent volume overload.

ADH acts on receptors in the vascular smooth muscle (constricts arteriolar smooth muscle) and the distal renal tubules. Stimulation of the receptors in the distal renal tubules leads to the reabsorption of water in the kidneys and subsequent concentration of urine.

Water Loss

In the absence of ADH (neurogenic DI), or the inability of the kidney to respond to ADH (nephrogenic DI), the kidney is unable to conserve water. Large amounts of hypotonic fluid may be excreted. If the thirst mechanism is intact, fluid balance may be preserved. Dehydration, hypotension, hypernatremia, and neurological dysfunction may develop if increased water loss from the kidney is not replaced.

Assessment

The clinical manifestations of DI are related to water loss and hypernatremia (see Clinical Findings 9–3 for clinical manifestations associated with DI, Table 13–7 for related information on ADH and serum osmolality, and Table 13–5 for related information on hypernatremia).

POINTS TO REMEMBER

▶ The critically ill adult is susceptible to the development of neurogenic (most common) or nephrogenic DI. The critically ill adult unable to perceive or respond to thirst, or the critically ill adult receiving tube feeds or total parenteral nutrition, may be particularly vulnerable to water deficits.

▶ A thorough nursing history (see Table 1–1 and Clinical Findings 9–3) is crucial to identify patients at risk or to identify the underlying cause of DI.

▶ In addition to the initial and baseline assessments (see Table 2–1) and a focused assessment of the underlying disorder, focused cardiovascular and neuromuscular assessments (see Tables 2–1, 5–1, and 6–1) should be completed as often as the patient's condition dictates to detect or anticipate and prevent complications such as hypovolemic shock, thromboembolism related to hemoconcentration, and decreased cerebral perfusion pressure with subsequent deterioration in the level of consciousness in the head-injured patient (see Clinical Findings 6–3 for related information on head trauma).

▶ Ongoing assessment incorporates the evaluation of responses to diagnostic procedures and therapeutic interventions aimed at identifying the cause of DI and the restoration of hormone and fluid balance; it includes collaboration with other members of the health team to maintain cardiac output and cerebral and peripheral tissue perfusion, and to provide patient education once the crisis has passed.

Syndrome of Inappropriate Antidiuretic Hormone

Pathophysiology

The clinical syndrome of inappropriate antidiuretic hormone (SIADH) may result from the aberrant or sustained release of

ADH. SIADH is characterized by plasma hypotonicity and hyponatremia.

Water Gain

Ectopic production of ADH or failure in the negative feedback system regulating the release and suppression of the hormone leads to excessive amounts of circulating ADH (see Fig. 9–1). Despite low plasma osmolality and volume overload, the renal tubules continue to absorb water and excrete sodium. Lack of intervention may lead to water intoxication and dilutional hyponatremia.

Assessment

The clinical manifestations of SIADH are related to water intoxication and hyponatremia. (See Clinical Findings 9–3 for clinical manifestations associated with the syndrome of inappropriate ADH secretion, Table 13–7 for related information on ADH and serum osmolality, and Table 13–5 for related information on hyponatremia.)

POINTS TO REMEMBER

▶ Multiple conditions increase the susceptibility of the critically ill adult to the development of SIADH.

▶ A thorough nursing history (see Table 1–1 and Clinical Findings 9–3) is crucial to identify patients at risk or to identify the underlying cause of SIADH.

▶ In addition to the initial and baseline assessments (see Table 2–1) and a focused assessment of the underlying disorder, focused cardiovascular and neuromuscular assessments (see Tables 2–1, 5–1, and 6–1) should be completed as often as the patient's condition dictates to detect or anticipate and prevent complications such as hypervolemia, cerebral swelling, seizures (see Clinical Findings 6–2), and coma.

▶ Ongoing assessment incorporates the evaluation of responses to diagnostic procedures and therapeutic interventions aimed at identifying the cause of SIADH and the restoration of hormone and fluid balance; it includes collaborating with other members of the health team to prevent further injury related to impaired levels of consciousness and immobility, and to provide patient education once the crisis has passed.

Clinical Findings 9–3   *DI and SIADH*

DI	SIADH
I. HISTORY	**I. HISTORY**
A. Predisposing factors	**A. Predisposing factors**

DI

I. HISTORY

A. Predisposing factors
1. *Neurogenic DI*
   - Familial or idiopathic defect in the pituitary gland
   - Head injury (basilar skull fracture in particular)
   - Neurosurgical procedures
   - Hypothalamus or pituitary tumor or metastatic cancer (most commonly from the lung or breast)
   - Cerebrovascular accident (CVA)
   - Aneurysm
   - Cerebral bleed, such as subarachnoid hemorrhage
   - Cerebral infection such as meningitis and encephalitis
   - Drugs such as phenytoin, alcohol, and α-adrenergic agents, which suppress the release of ADH
2. *Nephrogenic DI*
   - Inherited
   - Renal disease
   - Renal transplant
   - Multisystem disease affecting the kidney, such as multiple myeloma, sickle cell disease, sarcoidosis
   - Electrolyte imbalances such as hypokalemia or hypocalcemia

SIADH

I. HISTORY

A. Predisposing factors
1. Tumors, including oat-cell carcinoma of the lung, thymomas, lymphomas (Hodgkin's and non-Hodgkin's), and cancer of the gastrointestinal tract, pancreas, and duodenum
2. Respiratory disorders such as viral pneumonia, tuberculosis, lung abscess, and chronic obstructive pulmonary disease (COPD)
3. Positive-pressure ventilation
4. Heart failure
5. Neuromuscular disorders such as Guillain-Barré syndrome, head trauma, brain tumors, cerebrovascular accidents, cerebral infections
6. Pituitary surgery
7. Drugs such as anesthetics, barbiturates, analgesics, antineoplastic drugs, tricyclic antidepressants, chlorpropamide, excessive exogenous vasopressin therapy, and nicotine
8. Excessive stress response related to conditions such as trauma, sepsis, and extensive surgery

DI	SIADH

- Drugs such as lithium and demeclocycline, which inhibit ADH action in the kidneys

B. Subjective findings
1. Thirst related to water loss
2. Fatigue, weakness, anorexia, and constipation related to dehydration
3. Weight loss related to profound water loss

B. Subjective findings
1. Headache, nausea and vomiting, abdominal cramps, fatigue, lethargy, or muscle cramps, related to hyponatremia and decreased osmolality
2. Weight gain related to increased water load (usually edema is absent, since the hypotonicity causes an osmotic shift of water into the cells)

II. LABORATORY AND BEDSIDE MONITORING FINDINGS

A. CT Scan: May reveal pituitary or hypothalamic tumor

B. Laboratory studies
1. Hypernatremia (sodium >145 mEq/L) related to water loss in excess of sodium
2. Elevated serum osmolality (>300 mOsm/kg) related to plasma concentration from fluid loss
3. BUN, creatinine, hemoglobin, and hematocrit may also be increased, related to water loss (dehydration)
4. Decreased urine osmolality (<200 mOsm/kg H_2O) and decreased specific gravity (SG) (<1.005) related to the in-

II. LABORATORY AND BEDSIDE MONITORING FINDINGS

A. X-ray, CT scan, and MRI: May reveal underlying cause such as tumor or head injury

B. Laboratory studies
1. Hyponatremia (sodium <130 mEq/L) related to reabsorption of water in excess of sodium
2. Decreased serum osmolality (<275 mOsm/kg) related to plasma dilution from an excess of water
3. BUN, creatinine, hemoglobin, and hematocrit may also be decreased, related to an excess of water (dilutional)
4. Increased urine osmolality (>150 mOsm/kg H_2O), or greater than the plasma osmolality), increased urine sodium

DI	SIADH

creased excretion of dilute urine

(>20 mmol/L), and increased SG (>1.030) related to the retention of water and excretion of sodium

C. ECG: Tachycardia related to hypovolemia

C. ECG: Tachycardia may be present, related to hypervolemia

D. Hemodynamic parameters (see Chapter 14, Table 14–1, and Fig. 14–2 for related information on hemodynamic parameters)
1. Hypotension related to decreased circulating volume

D. Hemodynamic parameters (see Chapter 14, Table 14–1, and Fig. 14–2 for related information on hemodynamic parameters)
1. Blood pressure may be normal, or hypertension may be present, related to increased circulating volume (the extracellular fluid volume may remain fairly normal)

2. Decreased CVP, PCWP, and CO related to hypovolemia

2. Increased CVP, PCWP, and CO may be present, related to hypervolemia (the extracellular fluid volume may remain fairly normal)

III. Physical Assessment Findings

A. General observations (inspection)
1. *Mental status*
   - Alterations in level of consciousness (LOC), including lethargy, confusion, and possibly coma related to cerebral dehydration

   - Seizures may be present, related to cerebral dehydration or neuromuscular excitability associated with hypernatremia

III. Physical Assessment Findings

A. General observations (inspection)
1. *Mental status*
   - Alterations in LOC progressing from confusion, disorientation, and personality changes, including hostility and irritability, to coma, related to the severity of hyponatremia and cerebral swelling
   - Muscle weakness or seizures may be present, related to the severity of hyponatremia (sodium is necessary for neuromuscular function)

DI	SIADH

2. *Skin:* Poor skin turgor, dry mucous membranes, decreased amounts of saliva and sweat, and sunken eyeballs may be present, related to dehydration
3. *Urine:* Polyuria related to lack of ADH or inability of the kidney to respond to ADH

B. Palpation
1. *Skin:* May be cool and clammy with severe hypovolemia
2. *Peripheral pulses:* May be rapid, weak, and thready with severe hypovolemia

C. Auscultation
1. *Heart sounds:* May be rapid and irregular, related to tachycardia and dysrhythmias
2. *Bowel sounds:* May be hypoactive, related to hypoperfusion

---

2. *Respiratory pattern:* Dyspnea on exertion or difficulty breathing may be present, related to weakness of respiratory muscles
3. *Urine:* Small amount of concentrated urine related to the reabsorption of water

B. Palpation
1. *Skin:* May be cool related to hypothermia
2. *Peripheral pulses:* May be full and bounding related to hypervolemia

C. Percussion: Sluggish or diminished deep tendon reflexes may be present, related to hyponatremia (sodium is necessary for neuromuscular function)

D. Auscultation
1. *Adventitious breath sounds:* Crackles may be present, related to fluid overload
2. *Bowel sounds:* May be hypoactive, related to decreased gastric motility associated with hyponatremia

Thyroid Storm

Pathophysiology

Thyroid storm is a rare, life-threatening thyrotoxicosis associated with excessive amounts of the thyroid hormones, thyroxine (T_4) and triiodothyronine (T_3). Thyroid storm is characterized by a critical increase in the metabolic rate.

The thyroid hormones are responsible for the metabolic regulation of body tissues including growth and maturation (necessary for the secretion of growth hormone), carbohydrate and lipid metabolism (increase the rate of absorption of carbohydrates from the GI tract and stimulate cholesterol synthesis), and development and maintenance of the nervous system. Thyroid hormones also promote the rate of insulin destruction and have a synergistic effect with the catecholamines.

Secretion of the thyroid hormones from the thyroid gland is regulated by the hypothalamic (thyroid-releasing hormone, TRH)-pituitary (thyroid-stimulating hormone, TSH)-thyroid feedback system (see Fig. 9–1). Any disruption in the feedback mechanism of thyroid hormone can cause an alteration in thyroid function.

Thyroid storm may be attributed to an abrupt release of thyroid hormones (an exacerbation of underlying hyperthyroidism), or an increased sensitivity of peripheral receptors to the circulating hormones. Thyroid storm may be spontaneous, but is usually associated with excessive physical or emotional stress.

Assessment

The clinical manifestations of thyroid storm are a reflection of hypermetabolism that may affect all body systems. Fluid and electrolyte imbalances, hyperthermia, cardiovascular collapse, and neuromuscular dysfunction may result (see Clinical Findings 9–4 for clinical findings associated with thyroid storm, Table 13–7 for related information on thyroid hormones, and Table 13–5 for related information on electrolyte imbalances).

POINTS TO REMEMBER

▶ The critically ill adult with known or unknown hyperthyroidism is susceptible to the development of thyroid storm.

▶ A thorough nursing history (see Table 1–1 and Clinical Findings 9–4) is crucial to identify patients at risk for thyroid storm or to identify the underlying cause of thyroid storm.

▶ In addition to the initial and baseline assessments (see Table 2–1) and a focused assessment of the underlying disorder, focused respiratory, cardiovascular, neuromuscular, gastrointestinal, genitourinary, and integumentary assessments (see Tables 2–1, 4–1, 5–1, 6–1, 7–1, 8–1, and 11–1) should be completed as often as the patient's condition dictates to detect or anticipate and prevent complications such as hyperthermia, dysrhythmias, high-output heart failure, increased oxygen consumption, central nervous system excitability, and hepatic dysfunction (chronic depletion of hepatic glycogen stores increases the susceptibility of the liver to injury).

▶ Ongoing assessment incorporates the evaluation of responses to diagnostic procedures and therapeutic interventions aimed at identifying the cause of thyroid storm and blocking the release, synthesis, and catecholamine-potentiated effects of the thyroid hormones; it includes collaborating with other members of the health team to maintain normal body temperature, cardiac output, tissue perfusion, and fluid and electrolyte balance, and to provide patient education once the crisis has passed.

Myxedema Coma

Pathophysiology

Myxedema coma is a rare, life-threatening thyroid deficiency resulting from decreased amounts of the thyroid hormones, T_3 and T_4. Myxedema coma is characterized by a critical decrease in the metabolic rate.

The slowed metabolism results in the accumulation of mucopolysaccharides in the tissue. The decreased cardiac output also leads to a decrease in the glomerular filtration rate and less body fluid is excreted. Increased capillary permeability and the osmotic pull of the mucopolysaccharides permits fluid to leak into the tissues, resulting in the cutaneous accumulation of water (nonpitting edema).

Any defect in the hypothalamic-pituitary-thyroid mechanism may cause myxedema coma. The primary cause of myxedema coma is the inability of the patient with hypothyroidism to adapt to physiological stress such as losses in blood volume or central nervous system dysfunction.

Assessment

The clinical manifestations of myxedema coma are related to hypometabolism that may affect all body systems. Fluid and electrolyte imbalances, hypothermia, cardiovascular collapse, and coma may result (see Clinical Findings 9–4 for clinical manifestations associated with myxedema coma, Table 13–7 for related information on thyroid hormones, and Table 13–5 for related information on electrolyte imbalances).

POINTS TO REMEMBER

▶ The critically ill adult with known hypothyroidism is susceptible to the development of myxedema coma, related to inadequate replacement of the hormones.

▶ The critically ill adult is susceptible to the development of hypothyroidism or myxedema coma related to trauma, infection, neoplasm, irradiation, or surgical procedures involving the hypothalamus, pituitary, or thyroid glands (as well, drugs such as dopamine may inhibit TSH release from the pituitary gland).

▶ A thorough nursing history (see Table 1–1 and Clinical Findings 9–4) is crucial to identify patients at risk or to identify the underlying cause of myxedema coma.

▶ In addition to the initial and baseline assessments (see Table 2–1) and a focused assessment of the underlying disorder, focused respiratory, cardiovascular, neuromuscular, gastrointestinal, genitourinary, and integumentary assessments (see Tables 2–1, 4–1, 5–1, 6–1, 7–1, 8–1, and 11–1) should be completed as often as the patient's condition dictates to detect or anticipate and prevent complications such as hypothermia, dysrhythmias, cardiovascular collapse, and coma.

▶ Ongoing assessment incorporates the evaluation of responses to diagnostic procedures and therapeutic interventions aimed at identifying the cause of myxedema coma and replacing thyroid hormone; it includes collaborating with other members of the health team to maintain normal body temperature, cardiac output, tissue perfusion, and fluid and electrolyte balance, and to provide patient education once the crisis has passed.

Clinical Findings 9–4 *Thyroid Storm and Myxedema Coma*

Thyroid Storm	Myxedema Coma
I. HISTORY	I. HISTORY
A. Predisposing factors	A. Predisposing factors
1. Hyperthyroidism (Grave's disease, an autoimmune thyroid disorder)	1. Hypothyroidism (Hashimoto's disease, or autoimmune thyroiditis)
2. Toxic multinodular goiter	2. Irradiation of the thyroid

Thyroid Storm	Myxedema Coma

3. Thyroid cancer
4. Increased thyroid-stimulating hormone (TSH-producing pituitary adenomas)

5. Ingestion of excessive thyroid hormone
6. Excessive stress such as that caused by pulmonary infections, trauma, surgery, myocardial infarction, pulmonary embolus, diabetic ketoacidosis, toxemia of pregnancy, or prolonged emotional trauma

B. Subjective findings
1. Palpitations related to tachycardia or tachydysrhythmias (hyperdynamic circulation)
2. Chest pain may be present related to myocardial ischemia secondary to tachycardia (decreased filling time for the coronary arteries)
3. Dyspnea related to intercostal muscle weakness

---

3. Removal of thyroid tissue
4. Decreased TSH or TRH related to infection, tumor, trauma, irradiation, or surgery associated with the hypothalamus or pituitary glands (dysfunction of the hypothalamic-pituitary axis)
5. Inadequate replacement of thyroid hormone
6. Excessive stress such as that caused by infection, trauma, prolonged critical illness, and exposure to cold

7. Drugs such as sedatives, narcotics, and anesthetics at dosages or frequencies the patient with hypothyroidism is unable to metabolize

B. Subjective findings
1. Headache related to hypometabolism and accumulation of water
2. Chest pain may be present, related to myocardial ischemia secondary to decreased contractility
3. Dyspnea related to a decreased ventilatory capacity associated with the interstitial accumulation of mucopolysaccharides and respiratory muscle weakness, and the decreased responsiveness of the central nervous system respiratory center to hypoxia and hypercarbia

Thyroid Storm	Myxedema Coma

4. Insomnia, inability to concentrate, nervousness, anxiety, emotional lability, or psychosis related to cerebral excitability (exaggerated adrenergic activity)
5. Heat intolerance related to hypermetabolism
6. Weight loss related to hypermetabolism (protein and fat catabolism to meet energy requirements)
7. Fatigue and weakness related to catabolism or increased energy requirements
8. Increased appetite related to hypermetabolism

4. Slowed cognitive ability, forgetfulness, dementia, or psychosis related to depressed metabolic processes
5. Cold intolerance related to hypometabolism
6. Weight gain related to hypometabolism
7. Fatigue and weakness related to hypoglycemia or hypometabolism
8. Anorexia related to hypometabolism

II. **LABORATORY AND BEDSIDE MONITORING FINDINGS**
A. **CT scan:** May reveal the presence of a thyroid or pituitary tumor
B. **Arterial blood gas studies**
   1. Hypoxemia ($PaO_2 < 80$ mm Hg) may be present, related to increased oxygen consumption
   2. Metabolic acidosis may be present, related to increased tissue demand for oxygen and decreased supply
C. **Other laboratory studies**
   1. Elevated serum T_4, T_3, and resin T_3 uptake (RT_3U) related to excessive amounts of the thyroid hormones in the circulation (see Table 13–7 for related information)

II. **LABORATORY AND BEDSIDE MONITORING FINDINGS**
A. **X-ray:** May reveal cardiomegaly
B. **Arterial blood gas studies**
   1. Hypoxemia ($PaO_2 < 80$ mm Hg) related to hypoventilation
   2. Hypercarbia ($PcO_2 > 45$ mm Hg) related to hypoventilation
   3. Respiratory and metabolic acidosis related to hypoventilation and decreased tissue perfusion
C. **Other laboratory studies**
   1. Decreased serum T_4, T_3, and RT_3U related to decreased amounts of thyroid hormone in the circulation

Thyroid Storm	Myxedema Coma
2. Decreased TSH and TRH related to increased amounts of circulating thyroid hormones (see Table 13–7 for related information)	2. Increased amount of TSH related to failure of the thyroid gland (an ACTH stimulation test [see Clinical Findings 9–1 and Table 13–7 for related information] should be completed to assure adrenal function; exogenous thyroid hormone in the presence of adrenal insufficiency may precipitate adrenal crisis)
3. Elevated radioiodine uptake related to Grave's disease (see Table 13–7 for related information)	
4. Decreased cholesterol and triglycerides related to increased excretion in the stool	3. Hypercholesterolemia related to decreased cholesterol synthesis
5. Liver function studies may be abnormal related to hepatic dysfunction (see Table 13–4 for related information)	
6. Hypercalcemia related to increased absorption of calcium from the bone secondary to thyroid overactivity and disruption of parathyroid hormone regulation (see Table 13–5 for related information)	4. Hyponatremia (dilutional) related to decreased glomerular filtration rate and subsequent decrease in excretion of water associated with hypometabolism (may develop a superimposed SIADH)
7. Hyperglycemia related to increased production of glucose to meet metabolic needs, and diminished sensitivity to insulin	5. Hypoglycemia related to decreased intake, decreased production of glucose, and decreased glucocorticoid effect secondary to decreased thyroid hormone
8. Elevated alkaline phosphatase related to hypermetabolism	

Thyroid Storm	Myxedema Coma

D. ECG

1. Tachycardia related to the increased demands on the myocardium to keep up with tissue oxygen consumption associated with the increased metabolic rate
2. Tachycardia and tachydysrhythmias such as atrial fibrillation and paroxysmal atrial tachycardia related to effect of thyroid hormones and increased catecholamine stimulation on the heart

E. Hemodynamic parameters (see Chapter 14, Table 14–2, and Fig. 14–2 for related information on hemodynamic parameters)

1. Hypertension related to the compensatory increase in cardiac output to meet metabolic demands, and increased catecholamine stimulation
2. Decreased peripheral vascular resistance related to vasodilation associated with the need to dissipate heat
3. Increased cardiac output related to increased metabolic demands (high-output failure may lead to cardiac decompensation and cardiovascular collapse; see Clinical Findings 5–1 and 5–2 for related information)
4. Diaphoresis, diarrhea, or vomiting may lead to hypovolemia

D. ECG

1. Bradycardia related to decreased myocardial contractility and decreased catecholamine effect
2. Low-voltage QRS complex, prolonged PR and QT intervals, and flattening of T waves related to decreased myocardial contractility

E. Hemodynamic parameters (see Chapter 14, Table 14–2, and Fig. 14–2 for related information on hemodynamic parameters)

1. Hypotension related to decreased myocardial contractility and decreased vascular tone secondary to decreased catecholamine effect
2. Decreased cardiac output related to decreased myocardial contractility (low-output failure may lead to cardiac decompensation and cardiovascular collapse; see Clinical Findings 5–1 and 5–2 for related information)

Thyroid Storm	**Myxedema Coma**

III. PHYSICAL ASSESSMENT FINDINGS
A. General observations (inspection)

1. *Mental status:* Restlessness, agitation, or tremors related to increased neuromuscular excitability

2. *Respiratory pattern*
   - Tachypnea related to the need to move more oxygen

   - Decreased respiratory excursion related to respiratory muscle weakness

3. *Skin, hair, and nails*
   - Pink skin related to vasodilation associated with hyperthermia
   - Jaundice may be present related to severe hepatic dysfunction (see Clinical Findings 7–2 for related information)
   - Visible muscle wasting may be present, related to catabolism
   - Soft, fine hair and friable nails related to protein catabolism

III. PHYSICAL ASSESSMENT FINDINGS
A. General observations (inspection)

1. *Mental status:*
   - Impaired level of consciousness, which may progress to coma related to neuromuscular depression
   - Seizures related to hyponatremia
   - Hoarse voice related to myxedematous swelling

2. *Respiratory pattern*
   - Hypoventilation related to decreased ventilatory capacity and respiratory muscle weakness, or impaired ventilatory response to hypoxia and hypercarbia
   - Decreased respiratory excursion related to hypoventilation and respiratory muscle weakness

3. *Skin, hair, and nails*
   - Pale or cyanotic skin related to vasoconstriction and decreased tissue perfusion with hypothermia
   - Facial puffiness and peripheral nonpitting edema related to the subcutaneous accumulation of water

   - Coarse hair and brittle nails related to hypometabolism

Thyroid Storm	**Myxedema Coma**
4. *Eyes:* Exophthalmos (bulging eyes), lid retraction, lid lag, or periorbital swelling may be present related to overactivity of Müller's muscle in the eye	4. *Eyes, ears, nose, and mouth:* • Puffy eyelids and periorbital tissue related to the subcutaneous accumulation of water (myxedematous swelling) • Diminished hearing related to myxedematous swelling of middle ear • Snoring related to myxedematous swelling of upper airway • Thick tongue related to myxedematous swelling
5. *Neck:* Goiter (enlarged thyroid) may be visible related to overactivity of the thyroid gland	5. *Neck:* Diffuse enlargement of the thyroid gland related to underactivity
6. *Temperature:* Hyperthermia (exceptionally elevated temperatures) related to the increased metabolic rate	6. *Temperature:* Hypothermia (exceptionally low temperatures) related to the decreased metabolic rate
7. *Emesis:* Nausea and vomiting related to autonomic hyperactivity	7. *Abdomen:* Abdominal distention related to paralytic ileus secondary to decreased autonomic activity or myxedematous swelling
8. *Urine:* Increased urine output related to compensatory increase in cardiac output and increased glomerular filtration rate	8. *Urine:* Decreased urine output related to decreased renal blood flow and decreased glomerular filtration rate
9. *Stool:* Diarrhea related to increased intestinal motility	9. *Stool:* Constipation related to decreased intestinal motility
B. Palpation 1. *Chest wall and thorax:* Decreased chest expansion related to respiratory muscle fatigue	**B. Palpation** 1. *Chest wall and thorax:* Decreased chest expansion related to hypoventilation and weakened respiratory muscles

Thyroid Storm	**Myxedema Coma**

2. *Skin and neck*
   - Hot and moist skin related to hyperthermia and diaphoresis

   - Enlarged thyroid gland related to overactivity of the thyroid gland

3. *Peripheral pulses*
   - May be full and bounding, related to increased cardiac output
   - May be irregular, related to dysrhythmias (pulse deficit may be present with atrial fibrillation)

C. Percussion: Hyperreflexia related to neuromuscular excitability

D. Auscultation
   1. *Abnormal breath sounds:* Diminished breath sounds may be present, related to decreased chest expansion
   2. *Adventitious breath sounds:* Crackles may be present, related to pulmonary edema (see Clinical Findings 4–2 for related information) or retained secretions associated with respiratory muscle fatigue and ineffective airway clearance
   3. *Heart sounds*
      - Rapid or irregular apex related to tachycardia and dysrhythmias
      - Loud heart sounds related to increased cardiac output

2. *Skin and neck*
   - Cool and dry skin related to hypothermia and the absence of sweating
   - Diffuse, enlarged thyroid gland or nonpalpable thyroid gland related to underactivity

3. *Peripheral pulses:* May be slow and weak, related to bradycardia and hypotension

C. Percussion: Hyporeflexia related to neuromuscular depression

D. Auscultation
   1. *Abnormal breath sounds:* Diminished breath sounds related to hypoventilation
   2. *Adventitious breath sounds:* Crackles may be present, related to hypoventilation or heart failure

   3. *Heart sounds*
      - Slow apical rate related to bradycardia
      - Distant heart sounds related to decreased myocardial contractility or pericardial or

Thyroid Storm	**Myxedema Coma**
(thyroid bruit may be present over the superior thyroid arteries related to hypermetabolism and increased cardiac output)	pleural effusion related to myxedematous fluid leakage
• S$_3$ may be present, related to heart failure (see Clinical Findings 5–1 and 5–2 for related information)	
4. *Bowel sounds:* May be hyperactive, related to increased intestinal motility	4. *Bowel sounds:* May be hypoactive, related to decreased intestinal motility or paralytic ileus

10

Hematologic Assessment

FUNCTION OF THE HEMATOLOGIC SYSTEM IN MAINTENANCE OF HEMOSTASIS

Hemostasis is a complex physiologic process that prevents or stops blood loss from the circulatory system. It is accomplished through the balancing of coagulation and anticoagulation sequences. The several steps in the process include

- **Vessel spasm:** Injury to blood vessel endothelium stimulates a myogenic, neurogenic, and humoral response that causes vasoconstriction at the site of injury, with resultant decrease in blood flow to the area.
- **Platelet plug formation:** Circulating blood platelets aggregate at the site of injury and attach to the subepithelial collagen. The process is aided by von Willebrand's factor, which is regularly produced by endothelial cells and attached to the circulating coagulation factor VIII, and by release of adenosine diphosphate, thrombin, thromboxane, and other substances from platelets. Platelets adhere to each other and to blood cells and trap plasma, loosely plugging the area of vessel disruption.
- **Clot formation:** The clotting process further traps red blood cells, platelets, and plasma to form a fibrin network. This is accomplished through chemical activation and inhibition of procoagulation factors in a cascade sequence. This may involve two pathways: the intrinsic pathway that responds to events within the blood vessel, and the extrinsic pathway that responds to tissue damage. Each pathway ends in a common pathway that

produces thrombin and fibrin to form an insoluble clot (see Fig. 10–1).

- **Clot retraction:** Through release of plasma from the fibrin structure and continued platelet aggregation and adherence, the edges of the clot are pulled together.

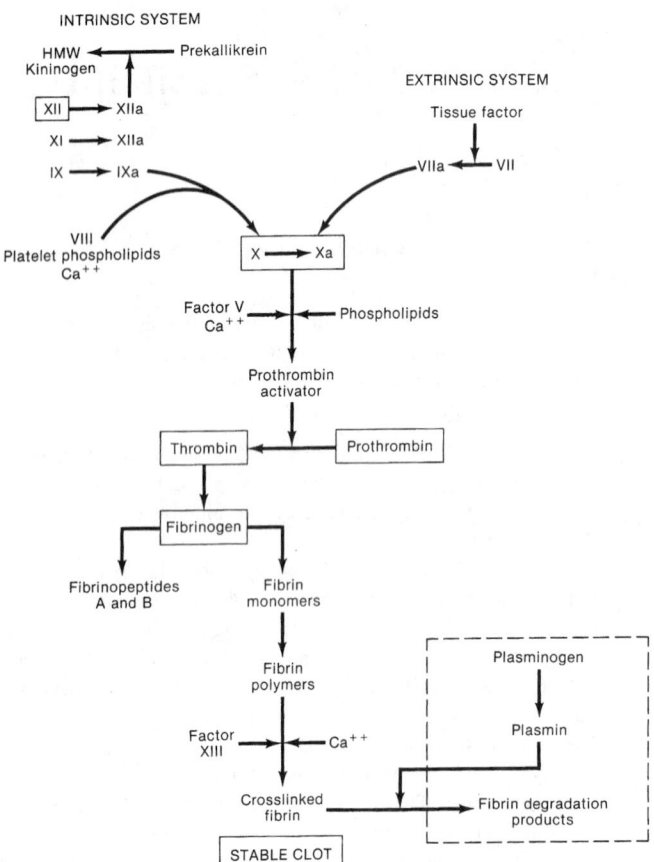

INTRINSIC SYSTEM

FIGURE 10–1

The coagulation process: HMW = high molecular weight. (From Clochesy, J. M., Breu, C., Cardin, S., Whittaker, A. A., & Rudy, E. B. [1996]. *Critical care nursing* [2nd ed., p. 1144]. Philadelphia: W. B. Saunders.)

- **Anticoagulation and fibrinolysis:** Following vessel-wall repair, a cascade of events occurs in which the plasma protein plasminogen (profibrinolysin) is converted to the proteolytic enzyme plasmin (fibrinolysin) by activators formed in vessel endothelium, liver, and kidneys. Plasmin interrupts the clotting mechanism by digesting clotting factors such as fibrinogen and factors V and VIII as well as the fibrin clot itself. This prevents vessel occlusion. Plasmin is deactivated by inhibitors synthesized by vascular endothelium and the liver.

Platelets are formed by megakaryocyte stem cells in bone marrow. They have an average circulating life of 10 days. All but three clotting factors (III, VIII, XIII) are synthesized in the liver. The clotting sequence requires both calcium and vitamin K and sufficient nutrients to supply plasma proteins essential to the clotting mechanisms. Bleeding disorders may be due to defective or diminished platelets (thrombocytopenia), deficiencies of clotting factors or their precursors or catalysts, or increased consumption of clotting factors. Bleeding problems may be associated with heredity, liver disease, impaired synthesis or storage of vitamin K (destruction of intestinal flora with antibiotic therapy, impaired fat absorption), drug effects and side effects (anticoagulants, aspirin, nonsteroidal anti-inflammatory drugs, chemotherapeutics, alcohol), or calcium deficiency.

Hypercoagulation states may be due to increased platelet activity (vessel-wall defects, trauma, atherosclerosis), slowed blood flow (immobility, shock), and increased clotting activity or decreased anticoagulant activity (drugs, pregnancy, malignancy, sepsis). Such states may lead to the formation of a stationery clot (thrombus) or a moving clot (embolus). Arterial thrombi are usually associated with platelet aggregation, while venous thrombi are more likely due to fibrin accumulation. These clots may occlude a blood vessel and disrupt blood flow to tissues or organs.

Changes with Aging

Hematopoiesis in healthy elders is similar to that in the younger person. With aging, however, there is a decrease in functional reserve capacity resulting in a diminished ability of bone marrow to compensate in the face of exposure to illness, toxins, nutritional abnormalities, certain drugs, or other stresses. There is an increased risk of atherosclerosis and blood vessel defects with age. Additionally there is some evidence for increased platelet aggregation with aging and for increased fibrinogen, factors VII, VIII, X, prekallikrein, and high molecular weight kininogen. Conversely there may be a decrease in antithrombin III and an increased plasminogen activator inhibitor, which may impair fibrinolysis. These may lead to increased risk of arterial and venous thrombotic and embolic diseases, especially in the presence of compromised circulation and decreased mobility.

NOTE: Integumentary assessment is integral to a focused assessment of the hematologic system (see Chapter 11 and Table 11–1).

HEMATOLOGIC DISORDERS

A coagulopathy is a disorder in which the primary cause of bleeding is a problem with the formation, stabilization, or lysis of the fibrin clot. Disorders of coagulation may be inherited or acquired.

Disseminated Intravascular Coagulation

Pathophysiology

Disseminated intravascular coagulation (DIC) is an acquired clotting disorder characterized by simultaneous thrombosis and hemorrhage. The pathophysiological processes that may be associated with the triggering of DIC include the release of procoagulant tissue factors into the circulation, damage to the vascular endothelium, and platelet aggregation.

Procoagulant Tissue Factors

Tissue damage that occurs in disorders such as burns, crush injuries, and major surgical procedures may cause tissue thromboplastin (factor III) to be released into the circulation. Tissue thromboplastin activates factor VII and the extrinsic clotting pathway (see Fig. 10–1).

Damage to the Vascular Endothelium and Platelet Aggregation

Endotoxins that are released from infectious agents in the septic process may injure the vascular endothelium and the red blood cells. The injury may stimulate excessive platelet aggregation as the platelets adhere to the exposed subendothelial collagen (contact activation).

Shock, acidosis, and hypoxemia associated with disorders such as adult respiratory distress syndrome (ARDS) may also damage the vascular endothelium. The damage may activate factors XII, XI, IX, and VIII and the intrinsic clotting pathway (see Fig. 10–1).

Coagulation

Regardless of the process, overwhelming stimulation of the clotting process (see Fig. 10–1) leads to the formation of multiple microclots that may embolize into the microcirculation and cause ischemia of organs and tissues. Coagulation factors such as prothrombin, platelets, factor V, and factor VIII are rapidly consumed.

Fibrinolysis and Anticoagulation

Simultaneously, the fibrinolytic system is activated to break down the clots. Plasminogen activators initiate fibrinolysis, and large amounts of fibrin degradation products (fibrin split products) are released. The fibrin split products exert an anticoagulant effect that leads to more bleeding.

Clotting factors are consumed faster than they are able to be replaced by the liver and bone marrow. The depletion of coagulation factors prevents the formation of a stable clot at a site of injury.

Effects

The cycle of coagulation, fibrinolysis, and anticoagulation may lead to vascular occlusion, hemorrhage, and shock. Hypoperfusion and stagnant blood flow may impair the ability of the reticuloendothelial system to clear fibrin, activated clotting factors, endotoxins, and fibrin split products from the circulation. The impaired clearance of these factors may potentiate excessive platelet aggregation, hypercoagulability and DIC. Multiple organ dysfunction may result.

Assessment

The clinical manifestations of DIC may vary with the underlying disorder, the extent of bleeding, and the amount of ischemic damage to tissues and organs (see Clinical Findings 10–1). In general, the patient with DIC usually presents with bleeding from multiple sites.

POINTS TO REMEMBER

▶ DIC always occurs secondary to another disorder.
▶ Numerous disorders place the critically ill adult at risk for DIC:

- The most common disorders include burns (see Clinical Findings 12–1), sepsis (see Chapter 12), and trauma (see Clinical Findings 12–2).
- ARDS (see Clinical Findings 4–1) and shock (Clinical Findings 12–3) may either precipitate or be a complication of DIC.

▶ A thorough nursing history (see Table 1–1 and Clinical Findings 10–1) is crucial to identify patients at risk for the development of DIC or to identify the cause of DIC.

▶ In addition to the initial and baseline assessments (see Table 2–1) and a focused assessment of the underlying disorder, focused assessments of all organ systems (see Tables 2–1, 4–1, 5–1, 6–1, 7–1, 8–1, and 11–1) should be completed as often as the patient's condition dictates to detect or anticipate and prevent complications such as hepatic failure (see Clinical Findings 7–2), renal failure (see Clinical Findings 8–1), shock (see Clinical Findings 12–3), and multiple organ dysfunction.

▶ Ongoing assessment incorporates the evaluation of responses to diagnostic procedures and therapeutic interventions aimed at identification and treatment of the underlying pathology; it includes collaboration with other members of the health team to maintain cardiac output and blood flow to the peripheral tissues and organs.

Clinical Findings 10–1 *Disseminated Intravascular Coagulation*

I. HISTORY

A. Predisposing factors

1. Sepsis and bacterial (gram-negative most common), viral, protozoal, mycotic, and rickettsial infectious agents
2. Burns
3. Trauma
4. Head injuries
5. Acidosis
6. Hypoxia
7. Shock
8. ARDS
9. Major surgical procedures

10. Extracorporeal circulation
11. Neoplasms
12. Fat embolism
13. Pulmonary embolism
14. Obstetric complications such as a dead fetus, abruptio placentae, septic abortion, and amniotic fluid embolism
15. Dissecting aneurysm
16. Hemolytic-uremic syndromes
17. Acute glomerulonephritis
18. Near drowning
19. Transfusion reaction
20. Organ transplant rejection
21. Sickle cell anemia
22. Snake bites

B. Subjective findings: In general, findings may include
1. Dyspnea related to respiratory insufficiency secondary to thrombi in the pulmonary microvasculature
2. Fatigue and weakness related to anemia secondary to blood loss
3. Abdominal pain related to thrombi or bleeding in the GI tract

II. Laboratory and Bedside Monitoring Findings

A. Chest x-ray: May reveal interstitial edema with diffuse deposition of microemboli in the lungs
B. Arterial blood gas studies (see Chapter 13 for related information on arterial blood gas studies and acid-base disorders)
1. Hypoxemia (PaO_2 <80 mm Hg) may be present, related to the underlying disorder, the presence of microemboli in the lungs, or hypovolemic shock
2. Respiratory or metabolic acidosis may be present, related to the underlying disorder, respiratory insufficiency, or decreased peripheral blood flow secondary to hypovolemic shock
3. Respiratory or metabolic alkalosis may be present, related to the underlying disorder
C. Coagulation studies (see Table 13–8 for related information on coagulation studies)
1. Elevated fibrin split products (may be >100 μg/ml)
2. Decreased platelet count (may be <50,000/μl)
3. Prolonged partial thromboplastin time (>60–90 seconds)
4. Prolonged prothrombin time (>15 seconds)
5. Prolonged thrombin time (>15–20 seconds)
6. Decreased fibrinogen level (<75–100 mg/dl)

7. Elevated D-dimer assay (>200 mg/ml)
8. Decreased factors V and VIII
9. Positive protamine sulfate test
D. Other laboratory studies: General findings may include:
1. Decreased hemoglobin and hematocrit related to significant blood loss (see Table 13–8 for related information on hemoglobin and hematocrit)
2. Elevated BUN and creatinine related to blood loss and hypovolemia or thrombi in the renal microvasculature (see Table 13–6 for related information on BUN and creatinine)
E. ECG
1. Heart rhythm and regularity will vary with the underlying disorder
2. Tachycardia may be present, related to hypoxemia or hypovolemic shock
3. Dysrhythmias may be present, related to hypoxemia, acidosis, or electrolyte imbalances (see Table 14–3 for related information on dysrhythmias)
F. Hemodynamic parameters (see Chapter 14, Table 14–2, and Fig. 14–2 for related information on hemodynamic parameters)
1. BP, CVP, PCWP, CO and SVR will vary with the underlying disorder
2. In general, a decreased CVP, PCWP, and CO, hypotension, and an elevated SVR may be present, related to hypovolemia

III. PHYSICAL ASSESSMENT FINDINGS

A. General observations (inspection): In general, findings may include the following
1. *Mental status*
   - Alterations in level of consciousness (LOC) related to blood loss and decreased cerebral blood flow or to cerebral hemorrhage or thrombosis
   - Seizures, paresis, or paralysis may be present, related to cerebral hemorrhage or thrombosis
2. *Respiratory pattern:* Tachypnea may be present, related to hypoxemia or hypovolemia
3. *Skin*
   - Petechiae, ecchymoses, or hematomas may be present, related to bleeding into the soft tissue
   - Cyanosis may be present, related to hypoxemia or peripheral vasoconstriction
   - Acrocyanosis (cold, mottled lips, nose, ears, fingers, and toes) may be present, related to obstruction of the microcirculation
   - Pallor may be present, related to significant blood loss
   - Jaundice may be present, related to microemboli in the hepatic circulation

- Overt bleeding may be present from all body orifices, intravenous and central line access sites, injection sites, incision lines, wounds, drainage tubing, and body exit sites related to decreased platelets and exhaustion of coagulation factors
4. *Epistaxis:* May be present, related to bleeding from nasopharynx
5. *Pulmonary secretions:* May be bloody, related to bleeding from upper airways and pulmonary interstitial bleeding
6. *Hematemesis:* May be present, related to gastrointestinal hemorrhage
7. *Urine*
   - Hematuria may be present, related to microthrombi in the renal vasculature
   - Decreased urine output may be present, related to hypovolemia and decreased glomerular filtration rate
   - Oliguria may be present, related to thrombosis of the kidneys
8. *Stool:* May show evidence of frank or occult bleeding related to GI hemorrhage or rupture of surface capillaries

B. Palpation: Pulses may be weak and thready related to bleeding

C. Auscultation
1. *Adventitious breath sounds:* Crackles may be present, related to thrombi in the pulmonary microcirculation
2. *Heart sounds:* May be rapid or irregular, related to tachycardia and dysrhythmias
3. *Bowel sounds*
   - Bowel sounds may be hyperactive, related to GI hemorrhage
   - Bowel sounds may be hypoactive, related to gastrointestinal shunting with hypovolemic shock

11

Immunologic Assessment

FUNCTION OF THE IMMUNE SYSTEM

The immune system is a complex network of specialized organs and cells that defends the body against exogenous and endogenous threats to its integrity and function. It includes the following:

- **Bone marrow,** which produces stem cells that differentiate into polymorphonuclear leukocytes (granulocytes), lymphocytes, and monocytes (macrophages) to identify and destroy invading organisms (see Fig. 11–1)
- **Lymphatic system,** including the thymus, spleen, lymph nodes, vessels, and other tissues, which mature lymphocytes and plasma cells to provide immunity against specific foreign substances called *antigens*
- **Complement proteins** that are integral to initiation of the inflammatory and immune responses and to cell-membrane lysis in preparation for phagocytosis
- **Cytokines,** or hormonal proteins (e.g., interleukin-2), produced by leukocytes to stimulate and regulate inflammatory and immune responses through activation of responder cells

The cells of the immune system must have self-tolerance, or the ability to distinguish self from nonself and destroy only foreign substances. This is accomplished because the cells of the immune system are capable of evaluating the surface proteins of cell membranes in their environment. These markers are unique to cells and tissue types and to each individual. They contain human leukocyte

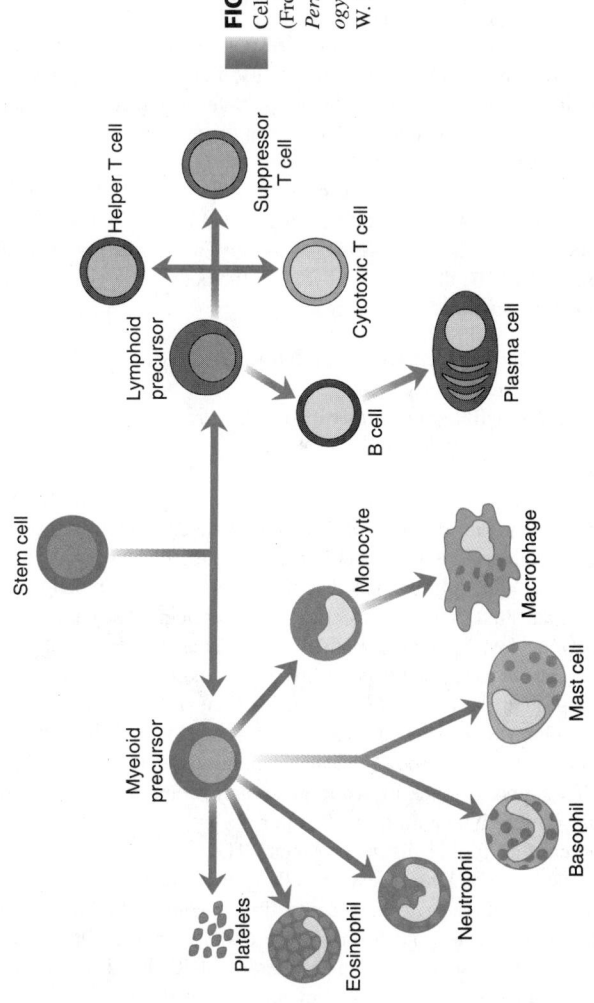

FIGURE 11-1

Cells of the immune system. (From Copstead, L. C. [1995]. *Perspectives on pathophysiology* [p. 174]. Philadelphia: W. B. Saunders.)

Stem cell

Lymphoid precursor

Myeloid precursor

Helper T cell

Suppressor T cell

Cytotoxic T cell

B cell

Plasma cell

Monocyte

Macrophage

Mast cell

Basophil

Neutrophil

Eosinophil

Platelets

557

antigens (HLAs), also known as human compatibility antigens, human transplantation antigens, or class I antigens. These antigens are inherited and produced on chromosome 6 by at least three gene pairs. This gene region is called the major histocompatibility complex (MHC). Major HLAs must be closely matched in organ transplantation.

Nonspecific immunity is a response to a threat that does not require recognition of a specific foreign substance. It comprises the chemical, cellular, and vascular responses of the inflammatory process, including the phagocytic actions of granular leukocytes (neutrophils, eosinophils, basophils) and mononuclear leukocytes (monocytes and tissue macrophages) that form the mononuclear phagocytic system (old reticuloendothelial system).

Specific (acquired) immunity is a response to a threat that requires recognition of a specific foreign protein or antigen by the lymphatic system. It occurs either naturally or through vaccination. Immunity can be developed actively by the body or be provided to it. Acquired immunity is of two types:

- **Humoral (antibody)-mediated immunity** involving activation of B lymphocytes.
- **Cell-mediated immunity** involving activation of T lymphocytes and natural killer cells.

B lymphocytes are formed in bone marrow and mature in lymphoid tissue. In the presence of complimentary antigens they transform into plasma cells that contain specific surface antibodies (immunoglobulin IgG, IgA, IgM, IgE, or IgD) that are secreted into the blood and extracellular fluid to destroy specific foreign proteins. They are most effective against bacteria and other infectious agents. Humoral immunity requires assistance from macrophages and helper T lymphocytes for optimum response. Compromise of the inflammatory process, T-lymphocyte damage, and protein or nutritional deficiencies can adversely effect antibody-mediated immunity.

T lymphocytes are formed in bone marrow and mature in the thymus or other lymphoid tissues. Mature cells contain surface antigen markers that further distinguish them. They respond to information provided by antigen-processing cells (APCs) such as macrophages. These cells share major histocompatibility complexes (MHCs) with the T lymphocytes and form antigen-MHC complexes that bind to T lymphocytes sharing the same class of MHC proteins, sensitizing them to the specific antigens. They are of three types:

- *Helper/inducer T cells* stimulate growth and activity of other leukocytes involved in inflammatory, humoral and cell-mediated immunity, through secretion of lymphokines. They are positive for surface antigen markers, including CD4+. Helper T lymphocytes are destroyed by the AIDS virus.
- *Killer (cytotoxic/cytolytic) T cells* bind to specific foreign cells, disrupt their cellular membranes, and secrete specific antibodies to disintegrate them. They are positive for CD8+ surface markers.
- *Suppressor T cells* act to inhibit the action of the other two by restricting antibody production. This prevents overreaction to specific antigens and probably controls autoimmune responses. A 2:1 ratio of helper to suppressor T cells maintains a balanced response to antigens. They are also positive for CD8+ markers.

T lymphocytes are effective against intracellular organisms, virus-infected cells, and fungi. They are also responsible for graft rejection. An additional cytotoxic cell, the *natural killer cell,* can destroy infected and mutated body cells without prior sensitization and specific MHC class compatibility.

B and T lymphocytes are cloned to include memory cells that sustain sensitivity to a specific antigen and attack any that recur. The inflammatory response and humoral and cell-mediated immunities are interdependent and unable to function efficiently if there are defects in the others. Immune responses may need to be suppressed in transplantation and allergic and autoimmune diseases. Immune responses may need to be enhanced medically and nutritionally to combat other diseases or the side effects of treatment (e.g., radiation, chemotherapy, corticosteroids).

Changes with Aging

While immunosenescence does occur as people age, the amount of immunocompromise is not predictable in any individual. Changes in inflammatory response with aging are discussed in the comparable section on focused respiratory assessment.

The major change occurs in cell-mediated immunity due to a decline in T-cell proliferation and response to antigen stimulation. This change is influenced by involution of the thymus gland and its hormone with aging, and by decreased production of the cytokine interleukin-2, a T-cell growth factor. This change is indicated by an increased incidence of anergy or a lack of a delayed hypersensitivity reaction with exposure to intradermally injected antigens.

Antibody-mediated immunity is also effected with aging. This includes decreased antibody production by B cells in response to antigenic exposure, and lower and less sustained serum antibodies following exposure or vaccination. There is a probable decrease in T-cell numbers and their ability to regulate B-cell function. This may also explain the increased numbers of autoantibodies found in aging individuals and may be implicated in the development of atherosclerosis as well as common autoimmune diseases in older persons.

Stress has also been implicated in decreased lymphocyte production and response in all age groups. Major life changes occur with increased frequency with aging, and the additional stress of critical illness may enhance immunocompromise. In all age groups decreased physical activity and the use of alcohol and nicotine have also been implicated in immunosuppression.

It is important that the nurse conduct a comprehensive initial, baseline, focused and ongoing assessment to look for indications of immunocompromise (Table 11–1). In the presence of immunocompromise the patient is increasingly susceptible to the development of infection and septicemia. It is not uncommon for the critically ill older adult to experience respiratory infection as part of a critical illness.

NOTE: Integumentary assessment is integral to a focused assessment of the immunologic system and will be reviewed here.

TABLE 11-1 Integumentary Assessment Techniques, Tips, Geriatric Considerations

Technique	Performance Tips	Description/Rationale	Geriatric Considerations
Pertinent History **1. Related medical history**	Review the patient's known medical history for **actual or potential disease states** that may affect the skin, skin glands, hair, or nails	It is important to rule out common skin disorders that may mask or mimic an acute problem of the integumentary system; some of these conditions may be chronic and present on admission, whereas others may be exacerbated by the stress of illness: • Psoriasis may affect skin and nails • Seborrheic dermatitis • Dermatitis, eczema • Tinea • Pemphigus • Herpes zoster • Erythema multiforme/Stevens-Johnson syndrome • Kaposi's sarcoma	Common disorders that may affect the skin and its appendages include • Seborrheic keratoses • Senile lentigines • Actinic keratoses • Xerosis (dry skin) • Seborrheic dermatitis • Stasis dermatitis/venous ulcers • Bullous pemphigoid • Pruritus • Delayed inflammatory response • Malignant neoplasms

Table continued on following page

TABLE 11-1 Integumentary Assessment Techniques, Tips, Geriatric Considerations Continued

Technique	Performance Tips	Description/Rationale	Geriatric Considerations
2. Related drug history	Review the patient's recent past and current **drug therapy** for medications that may • Increase skin signs and symptoms • Mask skin signs and symptoms *ASSESSMENT TIPS* 1. Attempt to correlate a new symptom with a recently administered drug or changed dose 2. Attempt to correlate improvement of a symptom with discontinuance of a	• Liver, gallbladder, hemolytic disease • Endocrine diseases Many drugs given in acute and critical care settings such as epinephrine, lidocaine, digoxin, or antibiotics may produce a cutaneous reaction Skin reactions may include • Generalized maculopapular eruptions • Urticaria (hives) • Erythema multiforme • Necrolysis • Sun-induced reactions to previously prescribed drugs that the patient may present with	The elderly patient is prone to skin eruptions associated with drug administration because of immunocompromise with age The elderly are also more likely to experience drug-related eruptions because they are routinely prescribed drugs that have the potential to cause eruptions and because of polypharmacy

	drug or with a changed dose	
3. Common complaints and observations that indicate the need for a focused assessment of the renal system	*ASSESSMENT TIPS* 1. Interview the alert patient about the exact nature of any discomfort 2. Use the following mnemonic to assure that all major aspects and characteristics of the symptoms have been evaluated: **P** Precipitating factors, prodrome **Q** Quality, quantity **R** Region, radiation **S** Associated symptoms, setting **T** Timing, treatment effects	The most common symptoms of skin disorders include • Skin lesions, rashes • Skin or hair color changes • Itching • Dryness • Scaling • Excess moisture

Table continued on following page

TABLE 11–1 Integumentary Assessment Techniques, Tips, Geriatric Considerations Continued

Technique	Performance Tips	Description/Rationale	Geriatric Considerations
Physical Examination: **Inspection and Palpation** **1. Color**	*ASSESSMENT TIPS* 1. Evaluate color in ambient (natural) light if possible; fluorescent light adds a blue cast; nonfluorescent, a yellow cast 2. Look for variations in color over different areas of the body and attempt to correlate with history or lifestyle	Skin color is influenced by skin pigment (melanin), surface vasculature, abnormal circulating pigments (bilirubin, carotene), local secretions (hemosiderin), altered tissue perfusion, and environmental exposures See Tables 4–1 and 5–1 for discussion of specific skin color changes related to respiratory and cardiovascular disease; Chapter 7 for liver, gallbladder, or hemolytic conditions that may produce jaundice; and Chapter 9 for endocrine diseases that may affect skin pigmentation (Addison's disease)	The skin, because of rapidly proliferating cells, shows the first visible effects of nutritional deficiencies in capillary fragility and poor wound healing Sun damage is common in aging skin that has been unprotected
2. Temperature	See Tables 4–1 and 5–1 for assessment of skin temperature and changes with aging		

3. Moisture

See Tables 4–1 and 5–1 for assessment of skin moisture and changes with aging

4. Texture

See Tables 4–1 and 5–1 for assessment of skin texture and changes with aging

5. Turgor and elasticity

See Tables 4–1 and 5–1 for assessment of skin turgor and elasticity and changes with aging

6. Skin lesions

ASSESSMENT TIPS

Lesions should be described according to the following characteristics and in the following order:

1. The number of lesions present if they are multiple and able to be counted easily

- Number

Table continued on following page

TABLE 11–1 Integumentary Assessment Techniques, Tips, Geriatric Considerations *Continued*

Technique	Performance Tips	Description/Rationale	Geriatric Considerations
• Color • Type	2. The color(s) of the lesions 3. See Table 11–2, page 568, for a description of the morphology of common primary and secondary lesions		
• Size	4. The size of a lesion or cluster of lesions is usually recorded in millimeters or centimeters of length, width, and diameter; a record of size allows for evaluation of increase or decrease in size with successive assessments		
• Configuration	5. Any discernible pattern of several lesions, e.g., annular, linear, clustered, dermatomal		

- Distribution
- Associated discharge

6. The distribution of lesions over the body surface, e.g., chest, groin, generalized

7. Vascular lesions

Look for
- Ecchymoses
- Erythema
- Petechiae, purpura
- Telangiectasia

Blunt trauma may rupture blood vessels, producing an ecchymosis; color progression from red-purple to brown to yellow-green can indicate the age of the lesion

Small violet-to-purple petechiae or larger purpurae are caused by rupture of superficial capillaries; this can be due to even mild trauma or certain medications

8. Nails and nail beds

See Tables 4–1 and 5–1 for assessment of nails and changes with aging

9. Hair

Look for
- General distribution over the body (vellus hair)
- Local distribution to scalp, eyebrows, nose, ears, face, axillae, groin, lower extremities
- Note any color change and its consistency with age
- Inspect for infestations

Hair cells reproduce rapidly and can be affected by heredity, disease, trauma, or medications

Graying, thinning, and loss of scalp and body hair occur with advancing age; increased growth of coarse hairs may occur in eyebrows, nares, and ears, especially in males; increased facial hair may occur in postmenopausal females

TABLE 11-2 The Morphology of Common Primary and Secondary Lesions

Lesions	Description
Primary Lesions	
Macule	Circumscribed, flat alteration in skin color ≤1 cm in diameter
Patch	Circumscribed alteration in skin color >1 cm in diameter
Papule	Raised, superficial, lesion ≤1 cm in diameter
Plaque	Coalesced papules >1 cm in diameter
Nodule	Raised lesion >1 cm in diameter, extending deeper into the dermis than a papule or plaque
Tumor	Raised lesion >2 cm in diameter, extending deeper into the dermis than a papule or plaque
Wheal	Raised, superficial, temporary, erythematous, edematous lesion
Urticaria	Coalesced wheals accompanied by pruritus
Vesicle	Raised, serum-filled lesion ≤1 cm in diameter
Bulla	Raised, fluid-filled lesion >1 cm in diameter
Cyst	Raised, fluid-filled, or semisolid sac extending deeper into the dermis than a vesicle or bulla
Pustule	Raised, pus-filled lesion
Secondary Lesions	
Crust	Dried exudate (blood, serum, pus)
Scale	Dried skin or keratin cells
Fissure	Linear crack in the skin, extending into the dermis
Excoriation	Superficial, usually self-induced scraping or abrasion of epidermis
Erosion	Moist, circumscribed loss of superficial epidermis
Ulcer	Bleeding, circumscribed or irregular loss of epidermis and dermis or more
Scar	Wound healing with connective tissue following normal tissue loss
Keloid	Hypertrophied scar
Lichenification	Thickened skin with prominent skin lines often following severe scratching

IMMUNOLOGIC DISORDERS

An immunodeficiency is a disorder in which the body is unable to defend itself against pathogens. Immunodeficiency disorders may be primary or secondary. Primary immunodeficiencies may be genetic, congenital, or acquired. Secondary immunodeficiencies may be attributable to a number of factors, including medications such as chemotherapy agents and steroids, excessive physical or emotional stress, and malnutrition.

Acquired Immunodeficiency Syndrome

Pathophysiology

Acquired immunodeficiency syndrome (AIDS) is an acquired, primary immunodeficiency disorder caused by the human immunodeficiency virus (HIV). The patient with AIDS has a T4 cell count less than $200/\mu L$.

Depletion of T4 Lymphocytes

HIV is a retrovirus that is attracted to cells with the CD4 surface receptor, primarily the helper T4 lymphocytes responsible for cell-mediated immunity. The virus integrates itself into the helper T4 lymphocyte, and viral RNA is transcribed into DNA, causing viral replication rather than normal cell reproduction. Consequently, the helper T4 lymphocytes become depleted. The progressive decline in T4 lymphocytes compromises the function of monocytes, macrophages, B cells, and cytotoxic and killer T cells, many of which depend on or interact with T4 lymphocytes to maintain effective immune function (see Fig. 11–1).

Opportunistic Infections

Disruption of cellular immunity predisposes the patient with HIV to numerous opportunistic infections. Opportunistic infections commonly associated with the diagnosis of AIDS include the following:

- Parasitic infections such as *Pneumocystis carinii* pneumonia (PCP), *Cryptosporidium* (intestinal infection), and *Toxoplasma gondii* (central nervous system infection)
- Bacterial infections such as *Mycobacterium tuberculosis*
- Fungal infections such as candidiasis (thrush, esophagitis) and cryptococcosis (cryptococcal meningitis)

- Viral infections such as herpes simplex, herpes zoster, and cytomegalovirus (cytomegalovirus retinitis, esophagitis, colitis, encephalitis)
- Malignancies such as Kaposi's sarcoma and non-Hodgkin's lymphoma

The HIV virus may be transmitted through blood, semen, vaginal and cervical secretions, amniotic fluid, and breast milk. The HIV virus may be present in saliva, tears, cerebrospinal fluid, urine, and feces but is not believed to be transmitted through these secretions.

Assessment

The clinical manifestations of AIDS may be directly related to the HIV virus (AIDS wasting syndrome and AIDS dementia complex), or associated with the opportunistic infections that may accompany the immune dysfunction (see Clinical Findings 11–1). In general, as AIDS is the end-stage of HIV infection, most body systems are affected.

POINTS TO REMEMBER

▶ The critically ill adult with AIDS may present with an acute episode of an opportunistic infection.
▶ The critically ill adult may present with a disorder unrelated to an underlying HIV infection.
▶ A thorough nursing history (see Table 1–1 and Clinical Findings 11–1) is crucial to detect past, current, or new onset opportunistic infections as well as to identify high-risk populations.
▶ Because opportunistic infections often compromise the patient's pulmonary, neuromuscular, or gastrointestinal systems, in addition to the initial and baseline assessments (see Table 2–1), focused assessments of all organ systems (see Tables 2–1, 4–1, 5–1, 6–1, 7–1, 8–1, and 11–1) should be completed as often as the patient's condition dictates to detect or anticipate and prevent complications such as ARDS (see Clinical Findings 4–1), fluid and electrolyte imbalances (see Table 13–5), AIDS wasting syndrome, AIDS dementia complex, or sepsis (see Chapter 12).
▶ Ongoing assessment incorporates the evaluation of responses to diagnostic procedures and therapeutic interventions aimed at identifying opportunistic infections or preventing additional opportunistic infections; it includes collaborating with other members of the health team to maintain fluid and electrolyte balance,

oxygenation, peripheral blood flow, nutrition, and integrity of the skin and mucous membranes, and to prevent transmission of the infection.

Clinical Findings 11–1   *AIDS*

I. HISTORY

A. Predisposing factors
1. High-risk groups, including homosexuals, bisexual males, and intravenous drug abusers
2. Unprotected sexual intercourse with an HIV-positive person, an individual in a high-risk group, or outside of a monogamous relationship
3. HIV mother to fetus or HIV mother to breast-feeding infant
4. HIV-contaminated blood or blood products

B. Subjective findings
1. Nausea, retrosternal pain with swallowing, or abdominal pain may be related to infectious agents such as cytomegalovirus (CMV), herpes simplex, *Candida*, or *Cryptosporidium*
2. Dyspnea or chest pain may be related to infectious agents such as *P. carinii* or cytomegalovirus
3. Night sweats may be related to HIV infection, tuberculosis, or non-Hodgkin's lymphoma
4. Lethargy, malaise, and weakness may be related to AIDS wasting syndrome
5. Headache and malaise may be related to infectious agents such as *Toxoplasma* and *Cryptococcus*
6. Forgetfulness, memory loss, impaired concentration, and apathy may be related to AIDS dementia complex
7. Blurred vision, floaters, or decreased visual acuity may be related to cytomegalovirus

II. LABORATORY AND BEDSIDE MONITORING FINDINGS

A. Chest x-ray
1. May reveal bilateral, diffuse, interstitial infiltrates related to PCP
2. May reveal presence of tuberculosis

B. Endoscopy: May reveal the presence of candidal esophagitis

C. Arterial blood gas studies: May reveal hypoxemia related to PCP

D. Other laboratory studies (see Tables 13–8 and 13–9 for related information)

1. Hemoglobin, WBCs, lymphocytes, and platelets may be decreased related to HIV infection
2. Helper/supressor T-cell ratio may be altered, related to HIV infection (helper T4 lymphocytes will be decreased, and supressor T8 lymphocytes will be increased)
3. Immunoglobulins (IgG and IgA) may be increased, but humoral antibody response (B cells) may be impaired related to HIV infection
4. Serum albumin may be decreased related to HIV infection and malnutrition (see Table 13–4 for related information on serum albumin)

E. ECG: Alterations in heart rate and rhythm may be present, related to hypoxemia due to PCP or fluid and electrolyte imbalances due to diarrhea and malnutrition (AIDS wasting)

F. Hemodynamic parameters: Hypotension may be present, related to fluid loss secondary to diarrhea

III. PHYSICAL ASSESSMENT FINDINGS

A. General observations (inspection)

1. *Mental status*
   - Confusion, disorientation, or coma may be present, related to AIDS dementia complex
   - Behavioral changes, including depression and mutism, may be present, related to AIDS dementia complex
   - Tremors, incontinence, hemiparesis, or paralysis may be present, related to AIDS dementia complex
   - Seizures or focal neurological deficits may be present, related to infectious agents such as *Toxoplasma*, non-Hodgkin's lymphoma, or AIDS dementia complex (see Clinical Findings 6–2 for related information on seizures)
   - Meningeal signs such as nuchal rigidity, Brudzinski's sign, and Kernig's sign may be present, related to cryptococcal meningitis (see Clinical Findings 6–6 for related information on meningitis)
   - Muscle wasting and weight loss may be present, related to numerous factors, including malnutrition or diarrhea (AIDS wasting)
2. *Respiratory pattern:* Tachypnea may be present, related to hypoxemia due to PCP (see Clinical Findings 4–4 for related information on pneumonia)
3. *Skin*
   - Pallor or cyanosis may be present, related to hypoxemia due to PCP
   - Seborrheic dermatitis or skin-colored papular eruptions may be present, related to allergies, infectious agents, or neoplasms (see Table 11–2, p 568)

- Painful red lesions may be present in the skin region of the affected dermatomes related to herpes zoster (shingles)
- Purplish lesions that may change to dark brown may be present on the face, scalp, mouth, extremities, penis, GI tract, or lungs, related to Kaposi's sarcoma

4. *Fever:* An increased temperature may be present, related to a number of opportunistic infections including *Cryptococcus* meningitis, PCP, *T. gondii,* and tuberculosis or non-Hodgkin's lymphoma

5. *Eyes:* Hemorrhages, exudates, and vasculitis may be present related to CMV retinitis

6. *Mouth*
   - White to gray lesions may be present on the tongue and buccal mucosa (oral hairy leukoplakia), related to the Epstein-Barr virus or human papillomavirus
   - Oral lesions may be present, related to herpes simplex
   - Creamy, curdlike patches may be present on the tongue and buccal mucosa (thrush) related to candidiasis

7. *Cough*
   - A dry cough may be present, related to PCP
   - A persistent cough may be present, related to tuberculosis

8. *Nausea and vomiting:* May be present related to a number of factors, including *Cryptococcus* infection (meningitis), gastritis, and drug therapy

9. *Stool:* Diarrhea may be present, related to a number of factors, including *Cryptosporidium* infection (watery diarrhea)

10. *Genitalia:* Lesions or discharge may be present, related to herpes simplex or candidiasis infection

B. Palpation

1. Skin may be warm related to the presence of fever
2. Lymphadenopathy of axillary, occipital, and cervical nodes may be present, related to HIV infection
3. Abdominal tenderness may be present, related to *Cryptosporidium* infection

C. Auscultation

1. *Adventitious breath sounds:* Crackles or wheezes may be present, related to PCP
2. *Bowel sounds:* Hyperactive bowel sounds may be present, related to *Cryptosporidium* infection and diarrhea

12

Multisystem Disorders

IMPLICATIONS OF MULTISYSTEM DISORDERS

When assessing multisystem disorders, one must take into consideration the basic anatomy and physiology of obviously involved systems as discussed throughout this book. Initial and baseline assessments will suggest the systems needing further evaluation. Focused and ongoing assessments will usually require continuing assessment of the cardiorespiratory, neuromuscular, and renal systems for life-threatening complications.

Changes with Aging

For the older person any illness has the potential to produce a cascade of events that will affect multiple body systems because of

- Normal changes with aging
- Decreased functional reserve when any organ or system is compromised
- Increased vulnerability of organs and systems to disease
- The likely presence of one or more chronic conditions in any older person

Most burn injuries in the elderly occur in the home. Increased sensitivity to cold, functional impairments (vision, hearing, pain sensation, balance, mobility), and mental impairment (drugs, depression, dementia, evolving infection, transient ischemic attack) can cause inattention to environmental hazards that may result in injury. Burn assessment in the elderly may be complicated by changes in the skin with aging, including

- Skin and capillary fragility
- Flattening of the epidermal-dermal junction with easier blistering
- Loss of dermal thickness, dermal microvasculature, and subcutaneous fat
- Stiffening of dermal elastin and collagen fibers, causing shearing injury
- Thinning, graying, and loss of scalp and fine vellus body hair
- Diminished inflammatory and stress responses
- Slowed healing processes

Smoke inhalation is complicated by diminished respiratory defense mechanisms (see Chapter 4). Fluid loss may be enhanced by presenting dehydration, and healing may be complicated by malnutrition.

Traumatic injury in the elderly may occur under less severe circumstances than in the younger person. The consequences of an impact injury on the musculoskeletal system may be more severe than expected due to the increased porosity (brittleness) of bones with age. Head injury may also be more severe than anticipated due to loss of brain bulk, causing more violent intracranial acceleration-deceleration events. Initial, baseline, focused, and ongoing assessment of the elderly multiple trauma victim must continually consider preexisting diseases and age-related changes in body systems discussed throughout this book. Currently there is no trauma scale that has been validated for the geriatric patient. Predicted outcomes are likely poorer for the elderly than for the younger victim on any scale in use.

In the older person the classic signs and symptoms of shock may be altered, blunted, or absent due to changes with age and disease in the cardiorespiratory system, thermoregulatory mechanisms, and inflammatory and stress responses. An altered level of consciousness may be the first or only clue to developing shock. Even this may be difficult to assess without input from significant others. A history of dementia will further complicate the evaluation. Hypovolemic shock may also progress more rapidly because of baseline malnutrition or dehydration. Hypotension will also be poorly tolerated by the geriatric patient and must be identified and corrected quickly.

MULTISYSTEM DISORDERS

Burns

Pathophysiology

A burn injury is damage to tissue resulting from contact with thermal, electrical, or chemical agents. Other causes include exposure to radiation or hot tar. Burns are commonly classified according to the depth of injury, extent of injury, and severity of injury.

Depth of Injury

Burn injury may be described as superficial (first-degree), superficial partial-thickness and deep partial-thickness (second-degree), or full-thickness (third-degree). Superficial injuries involve the outermost layer of the epidermis. Superficial partial-thickness injuries involve the epidermis and varying depths of the dermis. Deep partial-thickness injuries may involve the entire dermis, sparing the appendages such as hair follicles and sweat glands. Full-thickness injuries involve the entire epidermis and dermis and may extend into the subcutaneous tissue, muscle, or bone.

Extent of Burn Injury

The extent of burn injury may be determined by estimating the percentage of the total body surface area (TBSA) burned. The rule of nines (see Fig. 12–1*A*) or the Lund and Browder method (see Fig. 12–1*B*) may be used to calculate the amount of TBSA burned.

Severity of Burn Injury

The severity of burn injury is related to the depth and the extent of the burn. The severity of injury may be categorized as minor, moderate, and major (see Table 12–1).

First Phase of Burn Injury (Burn Shock)

Major burn injury may be divided into two phases. The first phase, burn shock, occurs within minutes following burn injury and may last up to 24 hours. Damage to the tissue in the area of the burn allows fluid to leak out of the body. Damage to the capillary membrane and the action of vasoactive substances such as histamine allow large amounts of

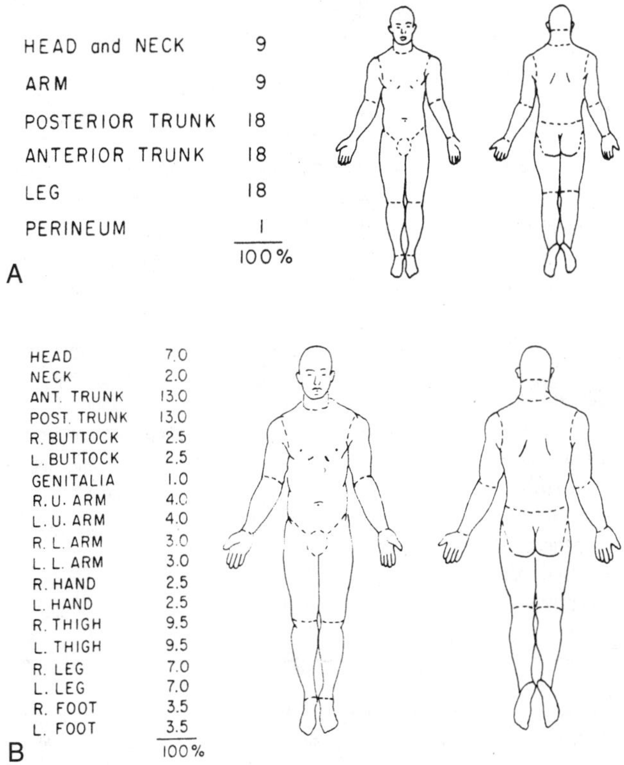

HEAD and NECK	9
ARM	9
POSTERIOR TRUNK	18
ANTERIOR TRUNK	18
LEG	18
PERINEUM	1
	100%

A

HEAD	7.0
NECK	2.0
ANT. TRUNK	13.0
POST. TRUNK	13.0
R. BUTTOCK	2.5
L. BUTTOCK	2.5
GENITALIA	1.0
R.U. ARM	4.0
L.U. ARM	4.0
R.L. ARM	3.0
L.L. ARM	3.0
R. HAND	2.5
L. HAND	2.5
R. THIGH	9.5
L. THIGH	9.5
R. LEG	7.0
L. LEG	7.0
R. FOOT	3.5
L. FOOT	3.5
	100%

B

FIGURE 12–1

A, The rule of nines is a commonly used assessment tool that permits timely and useful estimate of the percentage of the total body surface area burned. **B,** The Lund and Browder chart. The areas of the body are presented in section, which permits a more accurate estimation of burn size. (From Kravitz, M. [1988]. Thermal injuries. In V. D. Cardona, P. D. Hurn, P. J. Bastnagel Mason, A. M. Scanlon, & S. W. Veise-Berry [Eds.], *Trauma nursing: From resuscitation through rehabilitation* [p. 710]. Philadelphia: W. B. Saunders. **B** originally adapted from Lund, C. C., & Browder, N. C. [1944]. *Surg Gynecol Obstet, 79,* 352–358. By permission of *Surgery, Gynecology, and Obstetrics.*)

TABLE 12–1 American Burn Association: Criteria of Burn Injury Severity for Adults

Minor Burn Injury	Moderate (Uncomplicated) Burn Injury	Major Burn Injury
Second-degree injury: <15% TBSA*	Second-degree injury: 15%–25% TBSA	Second-degree injury: >25% TBSA
Third-degree injury: <2% TBSA not involving the eyes, ears, face, hands, feet, or perineum	Third-degree injury: <10% TBSA not involving the eyes, ears, face, hands, feet, or perineum	Third-degree injury • >10% TBSA • All burns involving the eyes, ears, face, hands, feet, or perineum
Excludes electrical injury, inhalation injury, complicated injuries such as fractures, and all poor-risk patients such as the elderly patient with concurrent illnesses	Excludes electrical injury, inhalation injury, complicated injuries such as fractures, and all poor-risk patients such as the elderly patient with concurrent illness	All inhalation, electrical, and complicated injuries, and all poor-risk patients

*TBSA, total body surface area.

From Kravitz, M. (1988). Thermal injuries. In V. D. Cardona, P. D. Hurn, P. J. Bastnagel Mason, A. M. Scanlon, & S. W. Veise-Berry (Eds.), *Trauma nursing: From resuscitation through rehabilitation* (p. 711). Philadelphia: W. B. Saunders.

plasma and proteins to shift from the intravascular to the interstitial space. The shift of protein decreases the osmotic pressure in the intravascular space. Consequently, as the capillary hydrostatic pressure continues to push fluid into the interstitial space, the decreased plasma colloid oncotic pressure is unable to pull fluid back into the vasculature. The lymphatic system becomes overwhelmed, and fluid retention leads to massive edema. The fluid loss may lead to decreased cardiac output and hypovolemic shock. In addition, the hematocrit may be greatly increased due to the increased number of red blood cells (too large to leak from the vasculature) relative to plasma. Compensatory vasoconstriction and increased viscosity may lead to increased peripheral vascular resistance.

Second Phase of Burn Injury (Burn Shock Subsides)

The second phase, fluid remobilization, occurs as capillary integrity begins to be restored, fluid loss ceases, and burn shock subsides (usually 24 to 36 hours after injury). The plasma colloid osmotic pressure becomes reestablished, and fluid is mobilized from the tissues back into the circulation. The lymphatic system is able to reabsorb fluid from the interstitium, and the edema decreases.

Assessment

Clinical manifestations vary with the depth, extent, severity, and phase of burn injury (see Clinical Findings 12–1). Primary considerations always begin with assessment of the airway, breathing, and circulation.

In the absence of alternative causes such as an associated head injury, a preexisting disorder, hypoxia, or drug or alcohol intoxication, the burn patient is usually awake, alert, and oriented immediately after burn injury:

- Therefore, even though the burn victim may not be able to see, hear, or speak (the eyes may be swollen shut with edema, hearing may be impaired because of edema in the auditory canals, and speech may be inhibited by swelling of the upper airway), airway obstruction is more likely to be related to edema than to the loss of consciousness.
- Generally, the internal edema will subside with the external edema.
- As the eyes become less swollen, the airway usually becomes less compromised.

POINTS TO REMEMBER

▶ Major burn injury causes numerous physiologic and hemodynamic changes that may affect every organ system.
▶ A massive physiologic stress response usually occurs at the time of burn injury and continues until wound closure:
  - The accompanying hyperdynamic and hypermetabolic state may lead to increased oxygen consumption and catabolism.
  - As well, the sustained stress response may potentiate adrenal insufficiency (see Clinical Findings 9–1).

► The release of histamine, serotonin, complement factors, prostaglandins, kinins, endotoxins, oxygen free radicals, catecholamines, and glucocorticoids may result in the impaired function of neutrophils, reduced humoral and cell-mediated immunity, activation and depletion of the complement system, and impaired helper T4 lymphocyte activity, decreasing the immune response and increasing the risk for sepsis.

► The elderly critically ill adult has decreased physiological reserve to respond to the overwhelming stress of burn injury and is therefore at greater risk for multiple organ dysfunction.

► Because numerous factors may affect the patient's treatment and recovery, a thorough nursing history (see Table 1–1 and Clinical Findings 12–1) should be completed as quickly as possible to obtain crucial information about the burn incident, associated factors, and preexisting disorders and allergies.

► In addition to the initial and baseline assessments (see Table 2–1), focused assessments of all organ systems (see Tables 2–1, 4–1, 5–1, 6–1, 7–1, 8–1, and 11–1) should be completed as often as the patient's condition dictates to detect or anticipate and prevent complications such as airway obstruction, hypovolemic shock (see Clinical Findings 12–3), sepsis (see Chapter 12), ARDS (see Clinical Findings 4–1), DIC (see Clinical Findings 10–1), gastrointestinal ulcer and hemorrhage (see Clinical Findings 7–1), and acute renal failure (see Clinical Findings 8–1).

► Ongoing assessment incorporates the evaluation of responses to diagnostic procedures and therapeutic interventions aimed at calculating the amount of fluid loss and the restoration of fluid volume; it includes collaboration with other members of the health team to maintain fluid and electrolyte balance, tissue perfusion, and oxygenation, and to prevent the development of infection.

Clinical Findings 12–1   *Major Burn Injury*

I. HISTORY

A. Predisposing factors

1. *Thermal injuries*
   - House fires (smoke inhalation)
   - Hot water scalds
   - Flammable liquids
   - Grease

- Vehicle fires
- Explosions
2. *Chemical injuries*
   - Oxidizing agents such as sodium hypochloride, chromic acid, and potassium permanganate
   - Reducing agents such as nitric acid and hydrochloric acid
   - Corrosive agents such as phenol, white phosphorus, sodium metals, and lyes
   - Protoplasmic poisons such as tannic acid, picric acid, formic acid, oxalic acid, and hydrofluoric acid
   - Desiccants such as sulfuric acid and muriatic acid
   - Vesicants such as cantharides, dimethylsulfoxide, and mustard gas
   - Gasoline burns
3. *Other injuries*
   - Electrical
   - Radiation
   - Tar

B. Subjective findings
1. Pain related to partial-thickness burns (tactile and pain sensors remain intact)
2. Pain may occur with full-thickness burns due to deep pain beyond the wound site, or partial-thickness burns adjoining full-thickness burns
3. Anxiety or panic may be present related to an altered body image or a fear of dying

II. Laboratory and Bedside Monitoring Findings
A. Chest x-ray: May be used 24 to 48 hours after injury to reveal areas of atelectasis, pulmonary edema, or diffuse bilateral infiltrates indicative of ARDS
B. Pulmonary function studies (see table 13–1 for related information on pulmonary function studies): Decreased vital capacity, tidal volume, and inspiratory force may be present with ARDS (see Clinical Findings 4–1 for related information on ARDS)
C. Arterial blood gas studies (see Chapter 13 for related information on arterial blood gas studies, acid-base disorders, the efficiency of gas exchange [intrapulmonary shunting], and serum lactate levels; see Chapter 14 for information on oxygen delivery and oxygen consumption parameters)
1. Hypoxemia may be present, related to decreased pulmonary blood flow, decreased pulmonary compliance, or increased oxygen consumption secondary to a hypermetabolic state

2. Respiratory alkalosis may be present, related to hyperventilation secondary to anxiety, pain or hypoxemia

3. Metabolic acidosis may be present, related to decreased peripheral blood flow or acute renal failure (electrical burn injuries may have profound metabolic acidosis related to tissue necrosis)

4. Base deficit may be < -2 mEq/L related to metabolic acidosis

5. Serum lactate level may be >2 mEq/L, reflecting tissue oxygen deficits

D. Other laboratory studies

1. Elevated carboxyhemoglobin levels (COHb $>10\%$) may be present, related to carbon monoxide inhalation (carbon monoxide has a greater affinity than oxygen for binding to hemoglobin and displaces the oxygen-carrying capacity of the hemoglobin)

2. Hyperkalemia may be present, related to the movement of sodium into the cells and potassium out of the cells (failure of the sodium-potassium pump may occur, related to hypovolemia and cellular ischemia) or exchange of extracellular hydrogen ions for potassium ions in the presence of metabolic acidosis

3. Hypokalemia may be present, related to the stress response and activation of aldosterone (potassium is excreted with the retention of sodium)

4. Hypernatremia may be present, related to hemoconcentration or activation of the stress response and the secretion of aldosterone (sodium and water retention)

5. Hyponatremia may be present, related to the loss of sodium through the site of burn injuries

6. Chloride may be elevated, related to hemoconcentration (see Table 13–5 for related information on electrolyte imbalances)

7. Hematocrit may be elevated, related to hemoconcentration

8. Hemoglobin may be decreased, related to bleeding from associated injuries or hemolysis of red blood cells (RBCs) (anemia may be masked by high levels of hematocrit associated with hemoconcentration, see Table 13–8 for related information on hemoglobin and hematocrit)

9. BUN may be elevated, related to hemoconcentration or acute renal failure

10. Creatinine kinase may be elevated, related to skeletal muscle damage, electrical burn injuries, or acute renal failure (see Table 13–6 for related information on BUN and creatinine)

11. Albumin may be decreased, related to the loss of protein through the site of the burn injuries and increased capillary permeability (see Table 13–4 for related information on albumin)

12. Leukocytosis may be present, related to stimulation of the sympathetic nervous system and activation of the stress response (WBC count may be as

high as 30,000/mm³ but usually resolves within 24 hours. Persistent elevation may be related to infection; see Table 13–9 for related information)

13. Hyperglycemia may be present, related to an increased stress response
    and an associated increased insulin resistance

14. Platelets may be decreased, related to fluid resuscitation, microvascular
    thrombosis, or disseminated intravascular coagulation (DIC, see Ta-
    ble 13–8 for related information on platelets and Clinical Findings 10–1
    for related information on DIC)

E. Urinalysis

1. Elevated specific gravity (SG) (>1.035) may be present, related to hypovolemia and dehydration

2. Increased protein may indicate that the patient is in a negative nitrogen
   balance (using protein stores for food)

3. Increased glucose may be related to the increased stress response, hypermetabolism, and decreased glucose utilization or to glucose intolerance
   related to sepsis

4. Rust- or burgundy-colored urine may be present, related to myoglobinuria
   associated with the breakdown of muscle tissue secondary to deep burn
   injury or electrical burn injury

5. Green urine may indicate the presence of *Pseudomonas* organisms

6. Urine tests positive for blood may be related to hemolysis from the initial
   injury or the presence of septic shock

F. ECG

1. Tachycardia may be present, related to hypoxemia or hypovolemia in the
   resuscitative phase or to hypermetabolism once burn shock has subsided
   (the elderly are less able to respond to stress with tachycardia and therefore may be inadequately perfused with a normal heart rate)

2. Dysrhythmias may be present related to hypoxemia or acid-base or electrolyte imbalances

3. Electrical burn injuries may cause ventricular fibrillation and cardiac arrest
   (the potential for cardiac arrest persists for 24 hours after electrical burn
   injury)

G. Hemodynamic parameters (see Chapter 14, Table 14–2, and Fig. 14–2 for
related information on hemodynamic parameters)

1. During burn shock, a decreased central venous pressure (CVP), pulmonary
   capillary wedge pressure (PCWP), cardiac output (CO), and hypotension
   may be present, related to hypovolemia

2. A decreased CO may persist, related to myocardial depressant factor, acidosis, right ventricular dysfunction (pulmonary vascular resistance [PVR]
   may be increased related to the release of vasoconstrictor mediators such

as serotonin and thromboxane which may lead to pulmonary hypertension and increased right ventricular workload), hypothermia, and increased systemic vascular resistance (SVR)

3. After burn shock, the CO may become supranormal related to the increased stress response, hypermetabolism, and hyperdynamic circulation

4. Because of the increased risk of sepsis associated with the use of invasive procedures, hemodynamic monitoring, including the use of mixed venous oxygen saturation ($S\bar{v}o_2$), may be reserved for the critically ill adult with severe burns, smoke inhalation, or underlying heart disease

III. PHYSICAL ASSESSMENT FINDINGS
A. General observations (inspection)

1. *Airway:* Hoarseness, stridor, and laryngeal edema may be present, related to smoke inhalation, burns to the head, face, and neck, and major body burns (The risk of airway obstruction increases during the first 24 hours with fluid shifts and resuscitation. Prophylactic endotracheal intubation may be required to prevent airway obstruction)

2. *Respiratory pattern*
   - Tachypnea may be present, related to anxiety, pain, or hypoxemia
   - Decreased chest excursion may be related to eschar formation in patients with circumferential, full-thickness injuries to the chest and neck (immediate escharotomy may be necessary to permit the chest wall to expand)

3. *Circulation*
   - Massive edema may be present, related to fluid shifts from the intravascular space to the interstitial space
   - Dark, amber urine (<30 ml/h) may indicate decreased peripheral and renal blood flow
   - Diuresis may occur once burn shock has subsided and fluid is remobilized into the intravascular space
   - Hypothermia may be present during burn shock related to vasoconstriction and loss of integumentary thermal regulation
   - An increased temperature following burn shock may be related to the hypermetabolic state maintained by hypothalamic regulation (the body resets the internal temperature upward to approximately 38.5° C)
   - An increased temperature (>38.9° C) may be related to infection (the cellular barrier that protects against bacterial invasion and wound sepsis is no longer intact)

4. *Mental status*
   - Confusion, disorientation, restlessness, or altered levels of consciousness may indicate decreased cerebral perfusion related to hypovolemia or hypoxemia
   - Memory loss, ataxia, or sensory deficits may be associated with electrical burn injuries and damage to neurons
5. *Eyes:* Corneal abrasions may be present associated with facial burns
6. *Nose and mouth:* Singed nasal hairs, carbon in the mouth and oropharynx, and carbonaceous sputum may be present, related to smoke inhalation
7. *Skin:* In general, findings may include
   - Erythema related to superficial burns
   - Fluid-filled blisters and red-to-pale ivory skin related to superficial partial-thickness burns
   - Flat, dry, tissue-paper blisters and waxy, white discoloration surrounded by pink or cherry red discoloration related to deep partial-thickness burns
   - Dry, leathery eschar (loss of dermal elasiticity) and thrombosed veins related to full-thickness burns
   - Copious amounts of plasmalike fluid may ooze through the wounds related to deep partial-thickness and full-thickness burns (the cellular barrier that protects the internal organs from the environment is no longer intact)
   - Gross tissue necrosis and heat-coagulated vessels related to electrical burn injuries (areas distal to the burn site will usually be without blood supply)
8. *Nails:* Capillary refill >2 seconds may indicate decreased peripheral blood flow (capillary refill <1 second may reflect improved tissue perfusion during resuscitation)
9. *Abdomen:* Abdominal distention may be present, related to slowed peristalsis and to ileus during burn shock (blood flow from the gut is redistributed to vital organs)
10. *Nausea and vomiting:* May be present, related to a slowed peristalsis and to ileus
11. *Gastric aspirate, emesis, and stool:* Blood may be present, related to duodenal or Curling's ulcer (sustained stress response may erode gastric and duodenal membranes)

B. Palpation

1. *Skin:* Partial-thickness burns may be painful to the touch throughout the burned areas

    2. *Peripheral pulses:* Decreased pulses may indicate decreased perfusion (strong pulses during the resuscitative phase may reflect improved perfusion)

C. Auscultation

    1. *Abnormal breath sounds:* Breath sounds may be decreased, related to decreased chest expansion

    2. *Adventitious breath sounds:* Crackles may be present, related to overzealous fluid administration, the inability to clear secretions, or decreased lung compliance

    3. *Bowel sounds:* May be absent during burn shock

Multiple Trauma

Pathophysiology

Trauma occurs when intentional or unintentional sources of energy come in contact with the body. The severity of trauma depends on the force of impact, the duration of contact, the mechanism of injury, and the portion or portions of the body injured. Trauma is commonly categorized as blunt or penetrating.

Blunt Trauma

Blunt trauma may damage tissue, organs, bones, and muscle structure through compression (crushing), shearing, rotary, acceleration, or deceleration forces. Common mechanisms of injury in blunt trauma include motor vehicle accidents, motorcycle and bicycle accidents, pedestrian-versus-vehicle accidents, falls, jumps, sports-related injuries, and assaults with blunt objects:

- In motor vehicle accidents,
  - Head-on collisions may result in chest, facial, abdominal, femur and hip injuries.
  - Rear-end collisons may result in hyperextension of the neck (whiplash injury).
  - Lateral collisions may result in left-sided fractures and splenic injury on the driver's side and right-sided injury and liver trauma on the passenger side.
  - Contralateral injuries may involve the head, neck, spine, pelvis, chest, and abdomen.

- Motorcycle and bicycle crashes may result in injuries to the head (particularly in the absence of helmets), neck, ribs, or extremities.
- Pedestrian-versus-vehicle collisions may result in femur fractures, chest injuries, and head injuries.
- Injuries from falls or jumps depend on the height, the landing, and the surface impacted. Spinal, head, and lower extremity traumas are common.

Penetrating Trauma

Penetrating trauma generally damages tissues, vessels, and organs along the path of penetration but may also cause blunt injuries to the affected structures. Common mechanisms of injuries in penetrating trauma include impaled objects (usually knives) and ballistic injuries (usually from guns). Wounds may be small and clean or involve gross tissue destruction and contamination as objects often pass through wood, glass, clothing, or other substances and introduce foreign particles into the body. High-velocity missles may change pathways and cause cavitation (destroy surrounding tissues and vessels).

Assessment

Clinical manifestations associated with the sequelae of multiple trauma vary with the severity of trauma, the body's response to injury and associated factors such as age, chronic illness, and alcohol and drug intoxication. In the prehospital and emergency phases, awareness of the patient's history and mechanism of injury assists in predicting, identifying, and stabilizing life-threatening injuries. In the critical care phase, awareness of the patient's history and the mechanism of injury assists in the continued stabilization of life-threatening injuries, the anticipation, prevention, or identification of additional, new, or recurrent injury, and secondary complications (see Clinical Findings 12–2).

Specific Injuries

Head trauma may include skull lacerations, fractures, and intracranial hemorrhage (see Clinical Findings 6–1, 6–3, and 6–4) or cervical spinal cord injury (see Clinical Findings 6–7). Chest trauma may include tracheobronchial injuries, diaphragmatic injuries, flail chest, pneumothorax (see Clinical Findings 4–6), tension pneumothorax (see

Clinical Findings 4–6), hemothorax (see Clinical Findings 4–5), pulmonary contusion, pericardial tamponade (see Chapter 5), aortic dissection (see Clinical Findings 5–4), blunt cardiac trauma (myocardial contusion) with or without dysrhythmia, or ruptured heart. Abdominal trauma may include splenic, liver, small bowel, pancreatic, renal, or bladder injuries. Musculoskeletal injuries may include thoracic or lumbar spinal cord injury (see Clinical Findings 6–7), pelvic and extremity fractures, amputation and soft tissue injury, and rectal, pelvic, perineal, and gluteal lacerations. Bleeding may be obvious (external hemorrhage) or occult.

Secondary Complications

Severe head trauma may lead to secondary complications such as ARDS (see Clinical Findings 4–1) and gastrointestinal ulceration (see Clinical Findings 7–1). Chest trauma such as pulmonary contusion may potentiate the development of ARDS. Blunt cardiac trauma (myocardial contusion) may cause cardiac tamponade (see Chapter 5). Abdominal and pelvic trauma increase the risk for infection and the development of sepsis (see pp. 597–611) and may cause abdominal compartment syndrome (impaired respiratory, cardiovascular, and renal function secondary to increased intra-abdominal pressure). Musculoskeletal injuries may also cause compartment syndrome (a nerve, tendon, or muscle may become trapped within a muscle sheath by external forces such as casts and surgical closures, or internal forces such as edema and bleeding, and compromise function to an already-injured extremity). Open wounds, fractures, and massive tissue injuries increase the risk for development of sepsis, fat embolism (see Clinical Findings 4–7), and DIC (see Clinical Findings 10–1).

Hypoperfusion increases the risk for development of shock (see Clinical Findings 12–3), ARDS (see Clinical Findings 4–1), and acute renal failure (see Clinical Findings 8–1). Hypovolemic shock, massive tissue destruction, gastric aspiration, and the systemic inflammatory response syndrome (SIRS) may potentiate the development of ARDS, and prolonged immobility may cause deep vein thrombosis (DVT) which may lead to pulmonary embolism (see Clinical Findings 4–7).

Stress Response

Following injury, an increased stress response induces a hypermetabolic state that may increase oxygen consumption and carbon dioxide production and trigger the breakdown of carbohydrates, proteins, and fat to meet the accelerated energy demands (the sympathetic nervous system response to injury varies with the individual). Without adequate nutritional replacement, metabolic deficiencies may lead to delayed wound healing, compromised immune function, and depletion of energy reserves and muscle mass.

POINTS TO REMEMBER

- ▶ Head trauma may be complicated by alcohol or drug intoxication.
- ▶ Hypoperfusion is a common initiator of hypovolemic shock and multiple organ dysfunction in the critically ill adult with multiple trauma.
- ▶ Disturbances in host defense mechanisms that may result from injury or therapy predispose the critically ill adult with multiple trauma to the development of sepsis and septic shock.
- ▶ A number of factors, including decreased physiologic reserve, decreased cardiac index, decreased pulmonary compliance, decreased glomerular filtration rate, preexisting diseases such as coronary artery disease and chronic obstructive lung disease, and an impaired release of growth hormone, insulin, and cortisol after injury may impact outcome and recovery in the elderly critically ill adult with multiple trauma.
- ▶ Because numerous factors may impact the patient's treatment and recovery, a nursing history (see Table 1–1 and Clinical Findings 12–2) should be completed as thoroughly and as quickly as possible to obtain crucial information about the mechanism of injury, associated factors, and preexisting disorders and allergies.
- ▶ In addition to the initial and baseline assessments (see Table 2–1), focused assessments of all organ systems (see Tables 2–1, 4–1, 5–1, 6–1, 7–1, 8–1, and 11–1) should be completed as often as the patient's condition dictates to detect or anticipate and prevent complications such as hypovolemic shock (see Clinical Findings 12–3), septic shock (see Clinical Findings 12–3), ARDS (see Clinical Findings 4–1), DIC (see Clinical Findings 10–1), pulmonary embolism (see Clinical Findings 4–7), fat embolism (see Clinical Findings 4–7), and acute renal failure (see Clinical Findings 8–1).

▶ Ongoing assessment incorporates the evaluation of responses to diagnostic procedures and therapeutic interventions aimed at the continued stabilization of injuries; it includes collaboration with other members of the health team to maintain oxygenation, peripheral blood flow, and nutritional support, and to prevent the development of infection.

Clinical Findings 12–2   *The Sequelae of Multiple Trauma*

I. HISTORY

A. Predisposing factors

1. *Unintentional injuries*
   - Motor vehicle accidents
   - Motorcycle accidents
   - Bicycle accidents
   - Pedestrian-versus-vehicle accidents
   - Sports-related accidents
   - Falls (especially in the elderly)
2. *Intentional injuries* (usually associated with violence, including homicide and suicide)
   - Assaults with blunt objects
   - Stabbings
   - Gunshot wounds
   - Jumps
3. *Associated risk factors*
   - Alcohol
   - Drugs
   - Age
   - Preexisting disorders

B. Subjective findings

1. Dyspnea may be present, related to respiratory impairment secondary to a variety of factors, including pneumothorax, tension pneumothorax, hemothorax, flail chest, tracheobronchial injury, pulmonary contusion, spinal cord injury, ARDS, pulmonary embolism, fat embolism, and abdominal compartment syndrome
2. Neck pain or tenderness may be present, related to cervical spine injury
3. Excruciating chest pain radiating to the jaw, shoulder, or left arm may be present, related to blunt cardiac trauma (myocardial contusion)
4. Severe chest or back pain may be present, related to aortic dissection

5. Chest pain with chest wall movement may be present related to rib fractures
6. Sudden onset of chest pain may be related to pulmonary embolism
7. Thoracic, lumbar, or sacral spine pain or tenderness may be present, related to spinal cord injury
8. Abdominal tenderness, rigidity, and involuntary guarding may be present related to injury, inflammation, or peritonitis
9. Left, upper quadrant pain and peritonitis may be present, related to splenic injury (suspect with left lower rib fractures)
10. Periumbilical pain radiating to the shoulders, testicular pain in males, and peritonitis may be present, related to small bowel injury
11. Flank pain or tenderness may be present, related to renal injuries
12. Lower abdominal pain may be present, related to bladder injury or rupture
13. Pain and tenderness in a lower extremity may be related to DVT
14. Pain out of proportion to a limb injury and not relieved by narcotics may be related to compartment syndrome
15. Anxiety may be present, related to the fear of dying
16. Hoarseness or dysphagia may be present, related to aortic dissection

II. Laboratory and Bedside Monitoring Findings

A. Cervical, thoracic, and lumbar spine x-ray and CT scan: If injury to the cervical, thoracic, or lumbar regions of the spine has not been cleared, spinal precautions are maintained as ordered

B. Chest x-ray
1. May reveal reexpansion of the lung following initiation of chest drainage for pneumothorax, tension pneumothorax, or hemothorax
2. May reveal new or recurrent pneumothorax, tension pneumothorax, or hemothorax
3. Widened mediastinum may be present, related to aortic dissection
4. Solid or air-filled viscus above the diaphragm may be present, related to diaphragmatic injury
5. Diffuse bilateral infiltrates may be present, related to ARDS
6. Pulmonary infiltrates may be present, related to fat embolism

C. Abdominal x-ray: May reveal free air in the abdomen related to bowel injuries

D. Serial CT scans: May be used to monitor blunt hepatic, splenic, and renal trauma in the hemodynamically stable patient

E. Arterial blood gas studies (see Chapter 13 for related information on arterial blood gas studies, the efficiency of gas exchange, and serum lactate levels; see Chapter 14 and Table 14-1 for related information on oxygen delivery and consumption parameters)

1. Hypoxemia may be present, related to a variety of factors including hemorrhage (decreased oxygen-carrying capacity); pulmonary contusion, ARDS, pulmonary embolism, and fat embolism (intrapulmonary shunting); and increased oxygen consumption secondary to hypermetabolism
2. Hypercapnia may be present, related to respiratory depression secondary to a variety of factors, including head injury, spinal cord injury, alcohol or drug intoxication
3. Hypocapnia may be present, related to tachypnea or hyperventilation secondary to a variety of factors, including hypoxemia, head injury, pneumothorax, tension pneumothorax, hemothorax, sepsis, ARDS, pulmonary embolism, fat embolism, pain, and anxiety
4. Respiratory acidosis may be present, related to hypercapnia
5. Respiratory alkalosis may be present, related to hypocapnia
6. Metabolic acidosis may be present, related to lactic acidosis secondary to hypovolemic shock, septic shock, cardiovascular dysfunction, or crush injuries
7. Base deficit may be < -2 mEq/L related to metabolic acidosis
8. Serum lactate level may be >2 mEq/L, reflecting tissue oxygen deficits

F. Other laboratory studies
1. Leukocytosis (WBC $>12,000/mm^3$), leukopenia (WBC $<4000/mm^3$), or the presence of $>10\%$ immature neutrophils (see Table 13–9) may be present, related to the systemic inflammatory response syndrome (SIRS)
2. Abnormal liver function studies (see Table 13–4) may be present, related to liver injuries, sepsis, or shock
3. Elevated serum and urine amylase (see Table 13–7) may be present, related to pancreatic injury
4. Progressively decreasing hemoglobin and hematocrit (see Table 13–8) may be present, related to obvious or occult bleeding
5. Abnormal coagulation studies (see Table 13–8) may be present, related to coagulopathies or DIC
6. Alterations in BUN and creatinine (see Table 13–6) may be present, related to acute renal failure
7. Electrolyte imbalances (see Table 13–5) may be present, related to factors such as hypovolemia, massive tissue injury (hyperkalemia), or acute renal failure
8. Cardiac enzymes (see Table 13–3) may be elevated, related to blunt cardiac trauma

G. ECG
1. Tachycardia may be present, related to numerous factors, including hypovolemia, hypoxemia, pain, anxiety, fever, anemia, fat embolism, and the hypermetabolic state induced by the sympathetic nervous system response

2. Bradycardia may be present, related to neurogenic shock
3. Dysrhythmias may be present, related to numerous factors, including blunt cardiac trauma, hypoxemia, acid-base imbalances, and fluid and electrolyte imbalances (see Table 14–3 for related information on dysrhythmias)

H. Hemodynamic parameters (see Chapter 14, Table 14–2, and Fig. 14–2 for related information on hemodynamics and formulas for calculation of parameters such as SVR, PVR, and left and right ventricular stroke work indexes)

1. A difference in blood pressure between the right and left extremities may be present, related to aortic dissection (suspect with first rib or sternal fracture, see Clinical Findings 5–4)
2. Pulsus paradoxus may be present, related to cardiac tamponade (see Chapter 5)
3. Hypotension may be present, related to a variety of factors, including hemorrhage, cardiac tamponade, pulmonary emboli, fat emboli, and shock (hypotension is a late stage of shock)
4. Decreased CVP, RA, PCWP, CO, and BP, and increased SVR may be present, related to hypovolemic shock (PA pressure may be low, related to decreased circulating blood volume)
5. Decreased CVP, RA, PA, PCWP, and BP, and normal or increased CO, and decreased SVR may be present, related to the early (warm) stage of septic shock (as septic shock continues, the CO falls and RA and PCWP may increase related to incomplete systolic emptying. As well, the PA pressure may increase, related to the transmission of elevated left ventricular pressures, hypoxic pulmonary artery vasoconstriction, and the effect of toxic inflammatory mediators)
6. Decreased CVP, RA, PA, PCWP, CO, BP, and SVR may be present, related to neurogenic shock (massive vasodilation)
7. Increased CVP, increased PCWP, decreased CO and BP, and increased or normal SVR may be present, related to decreased ventricular compliance associated with conditions such as myocardial ischemia and cardiac tamponade
8. Increased CO may be present related to overzealous fluid resuscitation or a hypermetabolic state

III. PHYSICAL ASSESSMENT FINDINGS

A. General observations (inspection)

1. *Mental status*
   - Lethargy, restlessness, agitation, disorientation, or confusion may be present, related to hypoxemia, hypoperfusion, head injury, alcohol intoxication, or drug intoxication

- Altered levels of consciousness, including lack of response to painful stimuli and posturing may be present related to head injury (see Table 6–6, GCS)
- An abrupt change in the level of consciousness may be related to pulmonary embolism or fat embolism
- Alterations in motor or sensory function may be present, related to head trauma (see Clinical Findings 6–1, 6–3, and 6–4), spinal cord injury (see Clinical Findings 6–7), or musculoskeletal injuries
- Seizures (see Clinical Findings 6–2) may be present, related to head trauma

2. *Scalp, skull, face, eyes, ears, nose, and mouth:* Scalp wounds, deformities, hematomas, facial edema, asymmetry of face, periorbital edema, racoon eyes, Battle's sign, bloody drainage, otorrhea, rhinorrhea, and cranial nerve dysfunction such as alterations in pupil size and reaction, visual acuity, and extraocular movements may be present, related to head or facial trauma

3. *Neck*
   - Jugular venous distention (JVD) may be present, related to conditions such as pericardial tamponade or tension pneumothorax (may not be present if the patient is hypovolemic)
   - Flat neck veins in the horizontal position may be related to hypovolemia
   - Tracheal deviation may be present, related to tension pneumothorax (toward the unaffected side), or hematoma and swelling (soft tissue injury)
   - Subcutaneous emphysema may be present, related to laryngotracheal disruption, esophageal tear, or tracheobronchial injuries

4. *Respiratory pattern* (many patients are intubated and receiving ventilatory assistance)
   - Tachypnea may be present, related to a variety of factors, including hemorrhage, hypoxemia (ARDS), pneumothorax, tension pneumothorax, hemothorax, sepsis, pulmonary embolism, and fat embolism
   - Bradypnea may be present related to head injury or alcohol or drug intoxication
   - A variety of respiratory patterns may be present with head injury (see Table 6–1 and Fig. 6–3)
   - Paradoxical respirations (uncoordinated movement of the chest wall with ventilation) may be present, related to flail chest

5. *Respiratory excursion:* Asymmetrical chest expansion may be present, related to factors such as pneumothorax, hemothorax, rib fractures, sternal fractures, and flail chest

6. *Chest*
   - Subcutaneous emphysema may be present, related to rib fractures, tracheobronchial injuries, and lung injury
   - Ecchymosis, lacerations, swelling, and seat belt marks may be present, related to soft tissue injury
7. *Abdomen and flanks*
   - Abdominal distention or suprapubic masses may be present related to abdominal and peritoneal injuries or peritonitis
   - Ecchymosis, lacerations, swelling, and seat belt marks may be present, related to soft tissue injury (may be underlying organ injury)
   - Ecchymosis in the flank area may reflect pancreatic injury (Grey Turner's sign) or renal injury
8. *Perineum*
   - Ecchymosis, lacerations, and swelling of external genitalia may be present, related to soft tissue injury
   - Blood at the urinary meatus may reflect renal or bladder injury
9. *Extremities*
   - Bony deformities, ecchymosis, lacerations, and swelling may be present in upper or lower extremities, related to open or closed fractures or soft tissue injury
   - Pallor in an extremity and paresthesia along the muscle compartment may indicate compartment syndrome
   - Redness, swelling, and discrepancy in the girth of right and left extremities may be indicative of DVT
10. *Skin*
    - Cyanosis (late sign) may be present, related to decreased tissue perfusion secondary to factors such as hypovolemia, cardiac tamponade, and pulmonary embolism
    - Peripheral cyanosis may be present, related to vasoconstriction
    - Petechiae and pallor may be present, related to fat embolism
    - Pallor may be present, related to blood loss
11. *Nails:* Capillary refill may be >2 seconds, related to decreased peripheral blood flow
12. *Temperature*
    - Fever may be present, related to factors such as fat embolism, SIRS (>38° C), and sepsis
    - Hypothermia may be present, related to factors such as hypoperfusion, vasoconstriction, and SIRS (<36° C)

13. *Urine*
- Hematuria may be present, related to renal or bladder injury
- A decrease in urine output may be related to acute renal failure (protein, myoglobin, and red or white blood cells may be present in the urine)
- Decreased urine output may be present, related to hypovolemic shock

B. Palpation

1. *Head, scalp, and face*
   - Soft tissue injury, bony deformities, pain, tenderness, or loss of sensation may be present, related to underlying injury
   - Crepitus may be palpable over areas of subcutaneous emphysema

2. *Chest wall and thorax*
   - Decreased chest expansion may be present, related to hypoventilation secondary to high-level thoracic spinal cord injury, rib fractures (splinting), altered levels of consciousness associated with head injury or alcohol or drug intoxication, abdominal distention, or tight dressings or binders
   - Point tenderness may be present, related to rib fracture (injuries to the first and second ribs may be associated with major vascular injury; injuries to right-sided lower ribs may involve liver injury; injuries to the left-sided lower ribs may involve splenic injury)
   - Crepitus may be palpable over areas of subcutaneous emphysema

3. *Abdomen:* Auscultation is performed before palpation and percussion. Palpation and percussion should not be performed if splenic, liver, or aortic injury is suspected or present
   - Pain and tenderness on palpation may be related to hematomas, peritonitis, or pelvic fracture
   - Rigidity may be present, related to peritonitis

4. *Extremities*
   - Weak and thready peripheral pulses may be present, related to hemorrhage or hypovolemia
   - A pulseless extremity may be related to compartment syndrome (late sign)
   - Tenderness, crepitance, and abnormal movements may be present at fracture sites
   - Pain, tenderness, and warmth over an area of redness and swelling may be related to DVT

C. Percussion

1. *Chest wall and thorax*
   - Hyperresonance may be present, related to pneumothorax
   - Dullness may be present, related to hemothorax

  2. *Abdomen*
     - Hyperresonance may be present, related to the presence of free air in the abdomen (bowel injury)
     - Dullness to percussion may be related to the presence of intrabdominal fluid (usually blood)

D. Auscultation

  1. *Abnormal breath sounds:* Diminished breath sounds may be present, related to pneumothorax, hemothorax, pulmonary contusion, or hypoventilation (see palpation)
  2. *Adventitious breath sounds:* Crackles and wheezes may be present, related to factors such as pulmonary contusion, ARDS, fat embolism, or overzealous fluid resuscitation
  3. *Heart sounds:* Distant or muffled heart sounds may be related to the presence of pericardial tamponade
  4. *Bowel sounds:* Decreased or absent bowel sounds may be related to gastrointestinal shunting (redistribution of blood flow to vital organs) and paralytic ileus

Shock

Pathophysiology

Shock is defined as a complex syndrome of hypoperfusion with reduced or uneven microcirculatory blood flow that is inadequate to meet tissue needs. Persistant perfusion deficiency leads to an imbalance between oxygen supply and demand, and functional impairment of cells, tissues, and organs.

Hypoperfusion

Reduction or maldistribution of microcirculatory blood flow may be associated with cardiogenic, hypovolemic, or distributive (vasogenic) shock.

Cardiogenic Shock

Cardiogenic shock results from the inadequate ability of the heart muscle to pump blood. Impaired pump function may result from myocardial damage or from obstruction to blood flow somewhere in the cardiovascular system.

Cause. The most common cause of myocardial damage is coronary artery disease with resultant myocardial infarction (see Clinical Findings 5–3). Cardiogenic shock occurs when a significant portion of the left ventricular myocardium (>40%) has been destroyed. Other causes of myocardial damage include myocarditis, cardiomyopathies, and metabolic disorders such as acidosis, hypoxemia, hypocalcemia, and hypoglycemia. Causes of obstruction to blood flow include cardiac tamponade (see Chapter 5) and pulmonary embolism (see Clinical Findings 4–7).

Hemodynamic Parameters. In cardiogenic shock, decreased contractility reduces systolic emptying, which decreases the ejection fraction and the stroke volume. The decreased ejection fraction increases the filling pressures of the left ventricle and the left atria. The increased filling pressures are transmitted back to the pulmonary circulation, leading to pulmonary edema (see Fig. 5–15).

The decreased stroke volume decreases the cardiac output, which leads to hypotension and activation of the compensatory mechanisms (see Fig. 5–15). Compensatory tachycardia shortens diastole, and the filling of the coronary arteries is compromised, compounding myocardial ischemia and increasing the area of ventricular destruction (myocardial necrosis). Increased afterload (compensatory vasoconstriction) increases the systemic vascular resistance, which increases myocardial workload and oxygen demand and further decreases the cardiac output (see Fig. 14–2 for related information on hemodynamic parameters associated with cardiogenic shock and Table 14–2 for related information on hemodynamic parameters and formulas for calculation).

Oxygen Delivery and Oxygen Consumption. Decreased cardiac output leads to decreased tissue perfusion relative to tissue needs. The total amount of oxygen being used by the tissues, or oxygen consumption ($\dot{V}o_2$), is decreased because of decreased oxygen delivery (Do_2). Mixed venous oxygen saturation ($S\bar{v}o_2$) is also decreased because of a decrease in CO and increased oxygen extraction by the tissues (see Chapter 14 and Table 14–1 for related information on mixed venous oxygen saturation and oxygen delivery, extraction, and consumption parameters and formulas for calculation).

Hypovolemic Shock

Hypovolemic shock results from an inadequate intravascular volume. The depleted intravascular volume may result from either internal or external fluid losses.

Causes. Internal losses include internal hemorrhage, leakage and pooling of fluid in the interstitial space, and fracture of long bones. External losses include hemorrhage (the most common cause of hypovolemic shock), burns, osmolar diuresis, vomiting, diarrhea, and dehydration.

Hemodynamic Parameters. In hypovolemic shock, decreased venous return causes decreased ventricular filling pressures, which result in decreased stroke volume, cardiac output, and tissue perfusion (see Fig. 14–2 for related information on hemodynamic parameters associated with hypovolemic shock and Table 14–2 for related information on hemodynamic parameters and formulas for calculation). Hypovolemic shock may occur abruptly or evolve through three stages.

Stages of Hypovolemic Shock. In stage I, there is a volume deficit of 10%, or approximately 500 ml. Compensatory mechanisms such as sympathetic vasoconstriction and tachycardia, activation of the renin-angiotensin cascade, increased secretion of aldosterone and antidiuretic hormone, and fluid shifts from the interstitial to the vascular space are generally able to maintain cardiac output and arterial pressure. Stage II occurs with a volume deficit of 15% to 25%. Marked decreases in cardiac output and arterial pressure occur despite tachycardia and intense arterial vasoconstriction and venoconstriction. Stage III occurs with a volume deficit greater than 25%. Compensatory mechanisms are fully mobilized and may or may not be able to maintain adequate perfusion.

Oxygen Delivery and Oxygen Consumption. Persistant hypovolemia leads to decreased tissue perfusion relative to tissue needs. $\dot{V}O_2$ is decreased because of decreased DO_2 related to hypovolemia and decreased cardiac output. $S\bar{v}O_2$ is also decreased because of decreased DO_2 and increased oxygen extraction by the tissues (see Chapter 14 and Table 14–1 for related information on $S\bar{v}O_2$ and oxygen delivery, extraction, and consumption parameters and formulas for calculation).

Distributive Shock

Distributive, or vasogenic, shock is due to the abnormal distribution of intravascular volume. Distributive shock may be divided into three types.

Neurogenic Shock. Neurogenic shock results from massive vasodilation related to the loss of sympathetic tone. This type of shock is generally transitory and is usually associated with injury and disorders of the spinal cord, including high-level spinal cord injury (see Clinical Findings 6–7), spinal anesthesia, vasomotor center depression (drug overdose, severe pain, or emotional stress), and ganglionic and adrenergic blocking drugs, which may impair nerve impulse transmission and decrease sympathetic tone.

Hemodynamic Parameters. In neurogenic shock, massive unopposed vasodilation results in dilated arterioles, decreased peripheral vascular resistance, and dilated veins and venules. Decreased venous return causes decreased ventricular filling pressures, which result in decreased stroke volume, cardiac output, and peripheral blood flow (see Fig. 14–2 for related information on hemodynamic parameters associated with neurogenic shock).

Anaphylactic Shock. Anaphylactic shock results from massive vasodilation and increased capillary permeability related to a severe allergic reaction. Possible allergens include drugs, contrast media, insect bites, and food.

In anaphylactic shock, the antigen is attacked by antibodies when it enters the body. The antigen-antibody reaction stimulates the release of chemical mediators such as histamine, bradykinin, serotonin, platelet-activating factor, prostaglandins, and leukotrienes from basophils, mast cells, and eosinophils. These chemical mediators act on blood vessels to produce vasodilation and increased capillary permeability.

Hemodynamic Parameters. Fluid shift from the blood vessels into the interstitium leads to decreased circulating blood volume, which decreases ventricular filling pressures. This results in decreased stroke volume, cardiac output, and peripheral blood flow (see Fig. 14–2 for related information on hemodynamic parameters associated with anaphylactic shock).

Septic Shock. Septic shock results from the maldistribution of blood flow due to an overwhelming systemic infection. Various chemical mediators released during the body's inflammatory response contribute to the pathogenesis (see Fig. 12–2).

SIRS, Sepsis, and Septic Shock. An infection is defined as an inflammatory response to the presence of microorganisms or the invasion of normally sterile host tissue by those organisms. The systemic

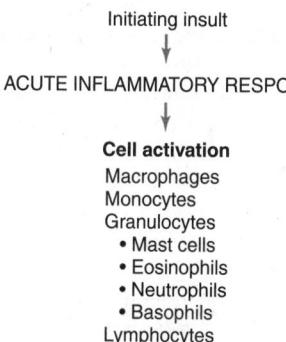

Initiating insult
↓
ACUTE INFLAMMATORY RESPONSE
↓
Cell activation
Macrophages
Monocytes
Granulocytes
• Mast cells
• Eosinophils
• Neutrophils
• Basophils
Lymphocytes
• T cells
• B cells
↕
**Chemical mediators that intensify the inflammatory
response in sepsis include but are not limited to**
Endotoxin
Oxygen-free radicals
Proteases
Cytokines
• TNF
• IL-1
• IL-2
Platelet-activating factor
Arachidonic acid cascade
• Leukotrienes
• Prostaglandins
• Thromboxane
• Prostacyclin
Complement cascade
Coagulation cascade
Bradykinin
Myocardial depressant factor
β-endorphin

FIGURE 12–2
Cells and mediators that can intensify the inflammatory response in sepsis.

inflammatory response syndrome (SIRS) is defined as the systemic response to a variety of clinical insults, including infection, trauma, and burns. Sepsis is defined as SIRS plus infection. Severe sepsis is associated with hypoperfusion, hypotension, and organ dysfunction. Septic shock is associated with persistant hypoperfusion, hypotension, and organ failure.

Causes of Septic Shock. Microorganisms that may cause septic shock include gram-negative bacteria, gram-positive bacteria, viruses, fungi, and rickettsiae. Gram-negative organisms are the most common cause of septic episodes in the critically ill adult. Gram-negative bacteria include *Escherichia coli, Klebsiella pneumoniae, Enterobacter aerogenes, Serratia marcescens, Proteus* species, *Pseudomonas aeruginosa,* and *Neisseria meningitidis.* Endotoxins found within gram-negative bacteria cell walls are liberated during bacterial cell lysis and initiate a chain of events involving immunologic cells and chemical mediators (see Fig. 12–2).

Pathophysiology. Activation of macrophages may directly or indirectly release toxic oxygen-free radicals and proteolytic enzymes, and the cytokines tumor necrosis factor (TNF), interleukin-1 (IL-1), and interleukin-2 (IL-2). Oxygen-free radicals and proteolytic enzymes are thought to destroy cells, particularly pulmonary endothelium and red blood cells. TNF, also called cachexin, plays a role in numerous reactions and interactions. The collective responses include cachexia associated with an increased metabolic rate, anorexia, and the inability of the body to metabolize and store fats, pyrogenic effects causing fever, and the stimulation of the production of platelet-activating factor, IL-1, and prostaglandin.

The release of platelet-activating factor results in sequestration of platelets, vasodilation, increased capillary permeability, and the promotion of diffuse intravascular coagulation. IL-1 stimulates the movement of WBCs toward injured, ischemic, or infected cells and may alter metabolism by provoking muscle breakdown, causing fever, and increasing the basal metabolic rate (similar to TNF). IL-1 also stimulates the release of IL-2 and arachidonic acid metabolites.

IL-2 is thought to contribute to the decreased blood pressure, decreased SVR, decreased ejection fraction, increased cardiac output, and increased heart rate seen during sepsis. Arachidonic acid metabolites include leukotrienes and prostaglandin products such as prostacyclin, and thromboxane. Leukotrienes are associated with increased capillary permeability, bronchoconstriction, and the activation of more neutrophils.

Prostacyclin is a potent vasodilator and has an anti-platelet-aggregating effect that attempts to balance the effects of other chemical mediators during the inflammatory response. However, during an overwhelming inflammatory response, thromboxane, which is a potent vasoconstrictor and has a platelet-aggregating effect, dominates and contributes to the maldistribution of blood flow and tissue hypoperfusion.

Activation of the complement system results in the release of C5a, which stimulates neutrophil aggregation and the release of toxic oxygen-free radicals, resulting in endothelial destruction and tissue necrosis. Injury to the endothelium, as well as the chemical mediators, stimulates the release of Hageman factor and tissue thromboplastin and leads to fibrin clot formation, activation of the coagulation cascade, fibrinolysis, and the formation of microemboli. Activation of the complement system also results in the release of C3a, which binds to lymphokines secreted by the suppressor T lymphocytes and decreases the amount of antibodies produced.

In addition, activation of the complement system stimulates the kinin system and the release of bradykinin. Bradykinin contributes to volume depletion through vasodilation and increased capillary permeability. Histamine is released by the mast cells and adds to the capillary leak. Myocardial depressant factor is released from ischemic pancreatic cells and causes decreased myocardial contractility. Maldistribution of blood flow, vasodilation, and cellular alterations precipitate the release of beta-endorphins which contribute to vasodilation, and decreased cardiac contractility.

Physical Findings Early in the Septic Syndrome. In the initial stages of the septic syndrome, vasoactive mediators create a flushed appearance due to vasodilation. The pulses may be full and bounding and the skin may be warm. The core body temperature is generally increased (may be $>38°$ C) due to activation of WBCs (WBC may be $>12,000/mm^3$) and the release of pyrogens. However, elderly patients and patients who have lost the skin's thermoregulatory function such as burn injuries may have sepsis in the absence of fever (temperature $<35°$ C). As sepsis progresses, leukopenia (WBC $<4000/mm^3$) may be present in the immunocompromised patient.

Hemodynamic Parameters in the Septic Syndrome. The initial cardiovascular changes in the septic syndrome include a high cardiac index, a low SVR, and a widened pulse pressure. Profound vasodilation results in maldistribution of blood flow so that some tissues are underperfused and some are overperfused. The maldistribution of blood flow and formation of microemboli interfere with the tissues ability to extract oxygen and the $S\overline{v}O_2$ may be elevated (see Chapter 14 for related information on $S\overline{v}O_2$ and oxygen delivery, extraction, and consumption parameters and formulas for calculation). Myocardial depression contributes to a reduced ejection fraction which usually remains decreased even though the cardiac output may remain high. Increased capillary permeability allows large amounts of fluid to leak into the interstitium and pooling of fluid leads to a decreased venous return and a decreased PCWP (see Fig. 14–2 for related information on hemodynamic parameters associated with the septic syndrome).

Hemodynamic Parameters Associated with Septic Shock. Persistent hypoperfusion and hypotension may precipitate septic shock (variables include the causative organism, the patient's defense system, and the presence of underlying illnesses). Hemodynamic parameters include decreased cardiac output related to severe myocardial depression, increased SVR related to sympathetic nervous system stimulation, and profound hypotension related to the decreased myocardial contractility and increased afterload (see Fig. 14–2 for related information on hemodynamic parameters associated with septic shock, and Table 14–2 for related information on hemodynamic parameters and formulas for calculation).

Cellular Impairment and Organ Failure in Shock

In all forms of shock, persistant hypoperfusion reduces oxygen delivery to the cells. Cells require oxygen to convert adenosine diphosphate to adenosine triphosphate (ATP) to be used by the body for energy to carry out its many functions.

In the absence of oxygen, cells revert to anaerobic metabolism. Large amounts of pyruvic acid are produced, which is converted to lactic acid, the end product of anaerobic metabolism. Lactic acid accumulates within the cell, causing acidosis. As the cellular pH falls, enzymes are released from the lysosome within the cell that destroy the cell.

In hypoxic, acidotic capillary beds, macrophages, endothelial cells, and leukocytes release mediators of the systemic inflammatory response syndrome, including but not limited to endotoxins, oxygen-free radicals, cytokines, kinins, and histamine. These mediators do not initiate hemodynamic alterations, but rather intensify systemic inflammatory responses that may worsen shock and precipitate organ failure.

Increased capillary permeability allows protein to leak into the tissue and decreases the plasma colloid osmotic pressure. In the lung, acute injury leads to pulmonary interstitial edema, intra-alveolar edema, refractory hypoxemia, and the clinical picture of ARDS (see Clinical Findings 4–1).

Decreased circulating blood volume may potentiate renal hypoperfusion and acute tubular necrosis (see Clinical Findings 8–1). Ischemia to the gut damages the protective mucous layer and permits bacteria and toxins to move into the peritoneal cavity and portal circulation. The Kupffer cells of the liver may become overwhelmed, taxing an already failing organ (see Clinical Findings 7–2). Increased blood viscosity, sluggish blood flow, and microemboli increase the risk for the development of DIC (see Clinical Findings 10–1).

Assessment

The clinical manifestations of shock often do not reflect the severity of the underlying perfusion deficit (see Clinical Findings 12–3). Regardless of the type of shock, microcirculatory hypoperfusion begins at the onset of injury or illness, not with the onset of hypotension.

POINTS TO REMEMBER

▶ Septic shock is the most common cause of death in critical care units in the United States.

▶ The increased incidence of septic shock has been attributed to a number of factors, including

  – Invasive devices and procedures such as pulmonary artery catheters, endotracheal tubes, and urinary catheters which disrupt normal host defense mechanisms as well as allow microorganisms to enter the body

  – Growing numbers of immunosuppressed patients, including the elderly population, who may also have one or more chronic illnesses

  – Increased survival of patients prone to sepsis, such as multiple trauma and burn victims

  – Cytotoxic and immunosuppressive therapies, including antibiotics and corticosteroids, and increased numbers of antibiotic-resistant microorganisms

▶ Because of the critically ill adult's vulnerability for the development of SIRS, sepsis, and septic shock, a thorough nursing history (see Table 1–1 and Clinical Findings 12–1 and 12–2) is crucial to identify patients at risk.

▶ Because clinical manifestations occur late in the process of the shock state, a thorough nursing history (see Tables 1–1, 4–1, 5–1, 6–1, 7–1, and 8–1 and Clinical Findings 12–1 and 12–2) is crucial to identify patients at risk for developing all forms of shock, including cardiogenic, hypovolemic, and distributive types of shock.

▶ In addition to the initial and baseline assessments (see Table 2–1), focused assessments of all organ systems (see Tables 2–1, 4–1, 5–1, 6–1, 7–1, 8–1, and 11–1) should be completed as often as each patient's condition dictates to detect or anticipate and prevent the development of reduced or uneven microcirculatory blood flow, hypoperfusion, and shock.

▶ Ongoing assessment incorporates the evaluation of responses to diagnostic procedures and therapeutic interventions aimed at the early detection of hypoperfusion and correction of the underlying cause; it includes collaboration with other members of the health team to prevent further deterioration and multiple organ dysfunction (the progressive failure of two or more organ systems).

Clinical Findings 12–3   *The Stages of Shock*

Stages of Shock	Clinical Findings
Progression through the stages of shock varies with the individual's response to the shock state and interruption with therapeutic correction	Findings vary with the individual's response to the shock state
1. *Initial stage*	
• The initiating disorder such as myocardial infarction, gastrointestinal hemorrhage, sepsis, burns, or trauma results in an episode or episodes of reduced or uneven microcirculatory blood flow and decreased delivery	1. *Initial stage:* At this point, there are usually no clinical findings that reflect the underlying shock physiology

Stages of Shock	**Clinical Findings**

of oxygen and nutrients to
the cells
- Hypoperfusion initiates altered cellular metabolism

2. *Compensatory stage:*
Compensatory mechanisms are
activated to restore the cardiac
output and tissue perfusion

- Decreased cardiac output
(CO) decreases the mean arterial pressure (MAP)
- Decreased MAP triggers the
baroreceptor reflex
- The sympathetic nervous
system (SNS) is stimulated,
and epinephrine and norepinephrine are released by the
adrenal medulla
- β_1 Receptors in the heart respond by increasing myocardial contractility and heart
rate to increase CO
- β_2 Receptors respond by dilating coronary arteries to
meet the increased oxygen
demands of the myocardium
- β_2 Stimulation in the lung
results in bronchodilation
- α-Receptor stimulation
causes vasoconstriction, and
fluid flow through the capillary bed is decreased
- Reduction in capillary hydrostatic pressure causes fluid
to shift out of the interstitial
spaces into the intravascular
space in an effort to increase venous return and CO

2. *Compensatory stage*

- Blood pressure may be normal and with or without a
narrowed pulse pressure

- Sinus tachycardia may exceed 100 bpm

- Skin may be pale or cyanotic

Stages of Shock	Clinical Findings
• Activity of the sweat glands is increased	• Cool and clammy skin
• The radial muscle of the iris contracts	• Dilated pupils
• Blood is shunted from the gastrointestinal (GI) tract including the gut, pancreas, and liver to increase the blood flow to the heart and the brain	• Hypoactive bowel sounds
• The liver breaks down glycogen to increase the amount of glucose available for energy production	• Hyperglycemia
• Decreased renal perfusion and renal vasoconstriction stimulate the renin-angiotensin cascade and the release of aldosterone	• Decreased urinary output (<30 ml/h)
• Sodium and water are reabsorbed in an effort to increase venous return	
• Increased levels of serum sodium increase the serum osmolality	• Hypernatremia
• Osmoreceptors in the hypothalamus respond by stimulating the posterior pituitary gland to release antidiuretic hormone (ADH) and water retention is increased	• Thirst
• Decreased pulmonary blood flow results in ventilation-perfusion mismatch in the lung and decreased gas exchange between the alveoli and capillaries	• Hypoxemia • Restlessness, excitability, confusion, agitation, or lethargy may be present

Stages of Shock	Clinical Findings
• Chemoreceptors respond to the decreased arterial oxygen tension and stimulate the respiratory center in the brain	• Rapid and deep respirations
• In the patient with healthy lungs, large amounts of carbon dioxide may be exhaled	• Respiratory alkalosis
3. *Progressive stage:* Compensatory mechanisms fail to maintain tissue perfusion and without intervention adversely affect organ system function	3. *Progressive stage*
• Persistant hypoperfusion and vasoconstriction lead to inadequate O_2 delivery to the cells	• Decreased blood pressure (<80–90 mm Hg systolic) with a narrow pulse pressure
	• Weak, rapid, and thready peripheral pulses
	• Cyanotic extremities, particularly distal areas such as fingers, toes, tip of the nose, and tips of the ears
• The cells increase anaerobic metabolism	
• Lactate levels increase, and the pH falls	• Metabolic acidosis
• The decreased amount of ATP causes the sodium-potassium pump to fail	• Severe muscle weakness and fatigue
• Potassium moves out of the cell, and sodium and water move into the cell, causing the cell to swell	
• Alteration of sodium and potassium concentrations affects the membrane potential and, depolarization and repolarization become prolonged	• Electrolyte imbalances

Stages of Shock	Clinical Findings
• Precapillary sphincters relax, but postcapillary sphincters remain constricted • In hypoxic and acidotic capillary beds, cells release chemical mediators that cause unequal distribution of blood flow and increased capillary permeability • The net movement of fluid is out of the intravascular space and into the interstitium • Ischemia and acidosis decrease myocardial contractility, and cellular hypoxia is further potentiated • Sluggish blood flow results in the inadequate removal of waste products, and the accumulation of microemboli (DIC)	• Peripheral edema • Pulmonary crackles and wheezes • Dysrhythmias • Tachycardia may be >150 bpm and irregular • Increased creatine phosphokinase (CPK) • Bruising and external or occult bleeding from body orifices, puncture sites, and drainage tubings • Increased partial thromboplastin time (PTT), prothrombin time (PT), and fibrin split products (FSP) • Decreased platelet count and fibrinogen level
• Decreased cerebral perfusion alters the level of consciousness • Decreased renal perfusion causes acute tubular necrosis • Prolonged GI hypoperfusion causes ischemia and ulceration of the luminal surface of the stomach and intestines	• Progressive decrease in response to verbal and painful stimuli • Decreased urine output (<20 ml/h) and specific gravity • Increase BUN and creatinine • Absent bowel sounds

Stages of Shock	Clinical Findings
and increases the risk for bacterial invasion or GI hemorrhage	
• Persistant hypoperfusion of the liver causes hepatic failure as the liver becomes unable to perform its many functions	• Jaundice • Increased lactate dehydrogenase (LDH), aspartate aminotransferase (AST, SGOT), alanine aminotransferase (ALT, SGPT)
• Poorly perfused pancreatic cells release enzymes such as myocardial depressant factor, which further decreases myocardial contractility	• Increased amylase and lipase
• Persistent reduction in pulmonary capillary blood flow further impairs gas exchange, and alveolar cells become ischemic	• Refractory hypoxemia • Hypercapnia
• Surfactant production is decreased, and alveoli collapse causing large areas of atelectasis	• Diminished or absent breath sounds over atelectic areas
• Increased pulmonary capillary permeability causes interstial and intra-alveolar edema (ARDS)	• Stiff, wet lungs, refractory hypoxemia, metabolic, and respiratory acidosis
4. *Refractory stage:* The ability of the patient to respond to therapeutic intervention is severely compromised; progression to multiple organ failure is inevitble	4. *Refractory stage:* The failure of multiple organ systems usually results in death

III

Common Laboratory Studies and Bedside Monitoring Techniques

13

Common Laboratory Studies

RESPIRATORY FUNCTION
Pulmonary Function Studies

Pulmonary function studies assist in evaluating the mechanical efficiency of the respiratory system. These studies evaluate lung mechanics by measuring the volume of gas moved in and out during respiration (see Fig. 13–1). The critically ill adult may not be able to participate in many of these tests; therefore only selected tests may be used.

Results of pulmonary function studies can be used to differentiate between obstructive and restrictive respiratory disorders (see Chapter 4), quantify the severity of respiratory disorders such as adult respiratory distress syndrome (ARDS; see Clinical Findings 4–1), identify patients at risk for postoperative respiratory failure, assist in weaning from mechanical ventilation, and monitor the response of the critically ill adult with a respiratory disorder to treatment. Frequently performed pulmonary function studies include measurements of compliance, lung volumes, and lung capacities (see Table 13–1).

POINTS TO REMEMBER

▶ No single measurement can define pulmonary status.
▶ Normals for these studies are predicted on the basis of age, height, weight, sex, activity, and barometric pressure.
▶ Volumes and lung capacities may decrease with increased pressure on the diaphragm from displaced abdominal contents related to factors such as horizontal positioning, ascites, pregnancy, and obesity.

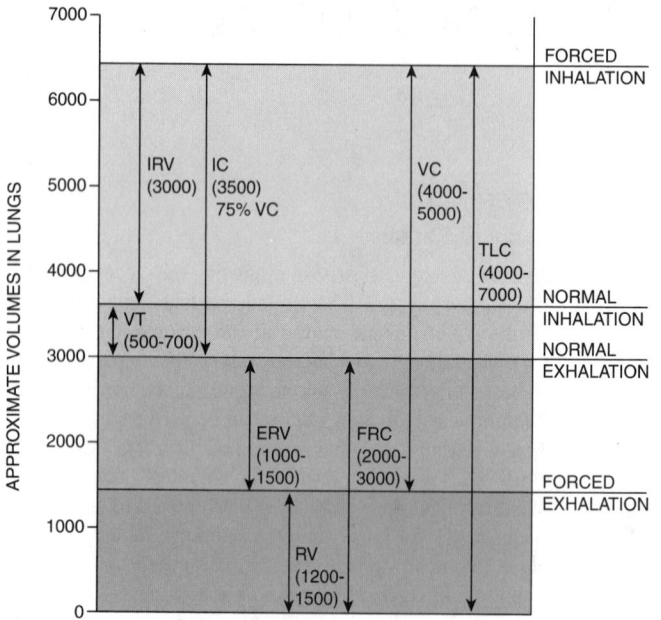

FIGURE 13–1
Pulmonary function.

TABLE 13-1 Pulmonary Function Studies

Description of Test and Rationale	Interpretation of Results	Geriatric Considerations
Compliance		
Description		
Compliance is the expansibility of the lungs and chest wall	Increased in emphysema because of loss of elastic recoil of the lung	Lung compliance increases with age because of loss of elastic recoil of the lung and degeneration of respiratory muscles
Compliance is measured by the relationship between pressure and volume: the less the compliance, the greater the pressure required to deliver a given tidal volume (dynamic compliance) and to hold the lungs at end-inspiration after a set tidal volume has been delivered (static compliance)	Decreased in conditions that increase the resistance of the chest wall such as structural deformities, musculoskeletal disorders, tight dressings, pregnancy, obesity, and chest injuries	However, because changes in thoracic vertebrae and intervertebral discs (ossification of rib cartilage and reduced mobility of the ribs) restrict expansion of the chest wall, overall compliance decreases, requiring increased muscle work to move air, especially with exertion or minimal respiratory or cardiovascular insults
Dynamic compliance is normally measured in the critically ill adult on mechanical ventilation by dividing the tidal volume by (the peak inspiratory pressure [PIP] — the positive end-expiratory pressure [PEEP]); **(35–55 ml/cm H$_2$O)**	Decreased in conditions that stiffen the lung and increase the pressure required to open the alveoli such as pulmonary edema, ARDS, pneumonia, and atelectasis	
Static compliance may be measured by dividing the tidal volume by (the plateau pressure — PEEP); **(50–100 ml/cm H$_2$O)**		

Table continued on following page

617

TABLE 13-1 Pulmonary Function Studies *Continued*

Description of Test and Rationale	Interpretation of Results	Geriatric Considerations
Rationale Results may be used to assist in determining which component (airways, lungs, or chest wall) is contributing to changes in compliance, the amount of PEEP required, and as an indicator for weaning from mechanical ventilation		
Tidal Volume (VT) ***Description*** Tidal volume is the amount of air inhaled and exhaled with a normal breath **(6–7 ml/kg, or 500–700 ml)**	Decreased with patient fatigue, depression of the respiratory center, and restrictive lung disease	Variable May increase slightly with normal aging because of increases in anatomical dead space from enlarged airways May decrease because of decreased chest wall compliance
Rationale Value used with other parameters to determine the need for mechanical ventilation as well as an indicator for weaning from it		

Inspiratory Reserve Volume (IRV)

Description

IRV is the volume of air that can be inhaled after a normal inspiration **(about 3000 ml)**

Rationale

Value used to calculate inspiratory capacity (IC)

Not clinically significant alone

Decreases with normal aging because of a stiff chest wall and decreased respiratory muscle strength

Expiratory Reserve Volume (ERV)

Description

ERV is the volume of air that can be exhaled after a normal expiration **(1000–1500 ml)**

Rationale

Value is used to calculate the vital capacity (VC)

Not clinically significant alone

Decreases with normal aging because of a stiff chest wall and decreased respiratory muscle strength

Residual Volume (RV)

Description

RV is the amount of air that remains in the lungs after full exhalation **(average 1200 ml)**

Increased in obstructive lung disease (air trapping)

Decreased in restrictive lung disease (limited lung expansion)

Increases with normal aging probably because of elastic recoil, alveolar enlargement, and collapse of the alveoli before emptying, which results in air trapping

Table continued on following page

619

TABLE 13–1 Pulmonary Function Studies *Continued*

Description of Test and Rationale	Interpretation of Results	Geriatric Considerations
Inspiratory Capacity (IC) *Description* IC is the maximum volume of air that can be inhaled after exhalation (**about 3500 ml**) VT + IRV (**75% of VC**)	Decreased in restrictive lung disease	Decreases with normal aging because of stiff chest wall and decreased respiratory muscle strength
Functional Residual Capacity (FRC) *Description* FRC is the volume of air left in the lungs after normal exhalation (**2000–3000 ml**) ERV + RV (maintains a constant supply of air in the lungs for ventilatory needs)	Increased with overdistention of the lungs from chronic obstructive pulmonary disease (COPD); contributes to the increased muscular work of breathing because of the increase in thoracic size Decreased in restrictive lung disorders that occlude the alveoli and contribute to hypoxemia, such as pneumonia, atelectasis, pulmonary edema, and ARDS	Increases with age because of loss of elastic lung recoil

Total Lung Capacity (TLC)

Description

TLC is the total amount of air in the lungs **(4000–7000 ml)**

FRC + IC

Increased in obstructive lung disease (air trapping)

Decreased in restrictive lung disease (limited lung expansion or area for gas exchange)

Remains the same or increases slightly with age

Vital Capacity (VC)

Description

VC is the amount of air that can be forcefully exhaled after a maximum inhalation **(4000–5000 ml)**

IC + ERV (ability to take a deep breath)

Rationale

Value used as an indicator for readiness to wean from ventilator

Decrease may be due to depression of the respiratory center, obstructive lung disease, or restrictive lung disease

Decreased with the normal aging process because of a stiff chest wall and diminished respiratory muscle strength

Spontaneous Peak Inspiratory Pressure (PIP)

Description

PIP is the amount of negative pressure required to inhale an adequate amount of gas on inspiration **(minimally -20 cm H_2O)**

Rationale

Value used as an indicator for weaning from mechanical ventilation

Decreases may be due to deconditioned or malnourished respiratory muscles or neuromuscular disease

Arterial Blood Gas Studies

Arterial blood gas studies may be used to diagnose acid-base disorders, determine the oxygen content of the blood, and assess the efficiency of gas exchange.

Acid-Base Balance

pH. The pH reflects the balance between the partial pressure of carbon dioxide ($PaCO_2$) and the concentration of bicarbonate (HCO_3^-) in the blood:

- Normal pH = 7.35–7.45
- pH >7.45 = alkalosis (decreased hydrogen ion concentration in the blood)
- pH <7.35 = acidosis (increased hydrogen ion concentration in the blood)

$PaCO_2$. The $PaCO_2$ reflects the ability of the ventilatory control system to maintain a normal pH. As carbon dioxide levels increase, chemoreceptors in the brain stem and the carotid bifurcation in the neck are stimulated to increase the rate and depth of respirations and blow off CO_2. As carbon dioxide levels fall, the chemoreceptors are inhibited, and CO_2 is retained. The respiratory system responds quickly to acid-base changes.

- Normal $PaCO_2$ = 35–45 mm Hg
- $PaCO_2$ >45 mm Hg = acidosis
- $PaCO_2$ <35 mm Hg = alkalosis

HCO_3^-. The HCO_3^- reflects the ability of the kidneys to maintain a normal pH. The renal system responds to acid-base imbalances primarily by the reabsorption of bicarbonate and secretion of hydrogen ions in the presence of acidosis and the inhibition of bicarbonate reabsorption in the presence of alkalosis. The renal system is much slower to respond to acid-base changes.

- Normal HCO_3^- = 22–26 mEq/L
- HCO_3^- >26 mEq/L = alkalosis
- HCO_3^- <22 mEq/L = acidosis

Interpretation of Acid-Base Disorders (see Fig. 13–2)

If the $PaCO_2$ and pH are both acidotic, the primary disorder is respiratory acidosis (an excess of carbonic acid in the extracellular fluid).

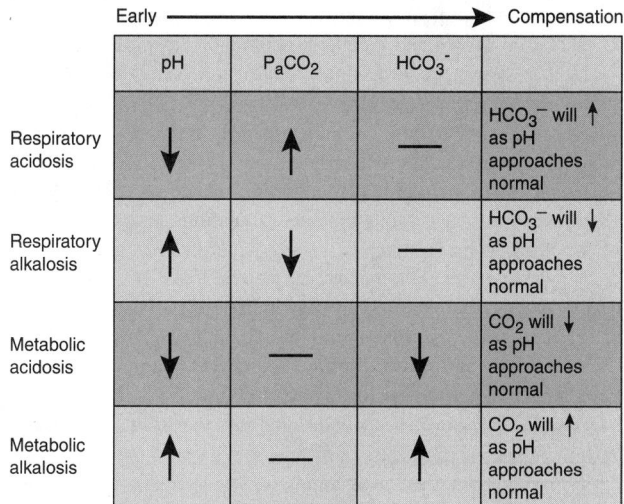

	pH	P_aCO_2	HCO_3^-	
Respiratory acidosis	↓	↑	—	HCO_3^- will ↑ as pH approaches normal
Respiratory alkalosis	↑	↓	—	HCO_3^- will ↓ as pH approaches normal
Metabolic acidosis	↓	—	↓	CO_2 will ↓ as pH approaches normal
Metabolic alkalosis	↑	—	↑	CO_2 will ↑ as pH approaches normal

FIGURE 13–2

Interpretation of acid-base balance.

- Causes may include hypoventilation related to obstructive lung disease, central nervous system depression (anesthesia, narcotics, sedatives, drug toxicity), neuromuscular disease, head trauma, splinting, pneumothorax, flail chest, obesity, ascites, and pregnancy.
- Associated clinical findings may include dyspnea, hypoventilation, fatigue, weakness, headache, apprehension, restlessness, confusion, drowsiness, uncoordination, coma, and warm, flushed skin.

If the HCO_3^- and pH are both acidotic, the primary disorder is metabolic acidosis (a deficit of bicarbonate in the extracellular fluid).

- Causes may include an increase in acid retention or production, or a loss of base from the body related to factors such as shock, burns, acute myocardial infarction, lactic acidosis, diabetic ketoacidosis, renal failure, hypoaldosteronism, severe diarrhea, malnutrition, salicylate intoxication, and potassium-sparing diuretics.

- Associated clinical findings may include headache, fatigue, anorexia, nausea and vomiting, Kussmaul's respirations, flushed skin, restlessness, drowsiness, confusion, seizures, coma, hypotension, and dysrhythmias.

If the $PaCO_2$ and pH are both alkalotic, the primary disorder is respiratory alkalosis (a deficit of carbonic acid in the extracellular fluid).

- Causes may include hyperventilation related to restrictive lung disease, central nervous system stimulation, anxiety, fever, thyrotoxicosis, brain injury or lesions, hepatic coma, gram-negative sepsis, and excessive mechanical ventilation.
- Associated clinical findings may include hyperventilation, dizziness, syncope, confusion, anxiety, feeling of panic, dry mouth, sweating, parathesis of extremities, muscle cramps, convulsions, tetany, coma, hypotension, and dysrhythmias.

If the HCO_3^- and pH are both alkalotic, the primary disorder is metabolic alkalosis (an excess of bicarbonate in the extracellular fluid).

- Causes may include an accumulation of excess base or a loss of hydrogen from the body, related to factors such as diuretic therapy, gastric suction, severe vomiting, peptic ulcer, hypokalemia, hypercalcemia, excessive administration of antacids, laxative abuse, hepatic failure, corticosteroids, hyperaldosteronism, Cushing's disease, and cystic fibrosis.
- Associated clinical findings may include nausea and vomiting, diarrhea, hypoventilation, irritability, muscle cramps, tetany, seizures, confusion, stupor, and coma.

Compensation. As compensation occurs, the pH returns to normal but leans to the side of the primary defect. Watch the value that *does not* match the pH. If this value is changing in the opposite direction of the acid-base imbalance, then compensation is occurring. Compensation is partial until the pH returns to normal limits.

Base Excess. The base excess is frequently assessed with the HCO_3^- value to give a more accurate reflection of the metabolic causes of acid-base imbalances:

- Normal value = -2 to $+2$ mEq/L or -2 to $+2$ mmol/L.
- A base deficit, or negative balance < -2, reflects metabolic acidosis.
- A base excess, or positive balance $> +2$, reflects metabolic alkalosis.

Oxygen Content

The PaO_2 and SaO_2, along with hemoglobin (Hgb), determine the oxygen content of arterial blood (CaO_2).

PaO_2. The PaO_2 is a measure of the partial pressure of oxygen dissolved in arterial blood. Normal value = 80–100 mm Hg.

SaO_2. The SaO_2 is the percentage of hemoglobin saturated with oxygen. Normal value = 95%–100%.

CaO_2. $CaO_2 = (1.34 \times Hgb \times SaO_2) + (0.003 \times PaO_2)$. Each gram of hemoglobin is capable of binding with 1.34 ml of oxygen. The oxygen solubility coefficient, 0.0003, is used to determine the contribution of the oxygen dissolved in plasma. Normal value = 20%.

Oxyhemoglobin. Oxygen is transported in the blood bound to hemoglobin (oxyhemoglobin). Alterations in the PaO_2 influence the saturation of hemoglobin with oxygen:

- Hgb has a high affinity for oxygen in the presence of a high PaO_2, such as in the pulmonary capillaries or the alveoli.
- Hgb has a low affinity for oxygen in the presence of low pressures, such as in the tissue capillaries where oxygen is released to the tissues.

This relationship is expressed in the oxyhemoglobin dissociation curve (see Fig. 13–3):

- Decreases in the PaO_2 may have a minor effect on arterial oxygenation if the accompanying change in the SaO_2 is small: For example, at PaO_2 levels above 60 mm Hg, the SaO_2 remains about 90%.
- However, when the PaO_2 drops below 60 mm Hg, the effect on arterial oxygenation may be profound. The hemoglobin starts rapidly unloading oxygen to make more oxygen available to the tissues and the SaO_2 drops dramatically.
- A prolonged SaO_2 level below 70% may greatly endanger the critically ill adult's balance between oxygen supply and oxygen demand (see Chapter 14, Respiratory Monitoring).

Additional conditions affecting the affinity of hemoglobin for oxygen are (see Fig. 13–4)

- Fever and acidosis: The affinity of hemoglobin for oxygen is decreased, and more oxygen is released to the tissues (right shift).

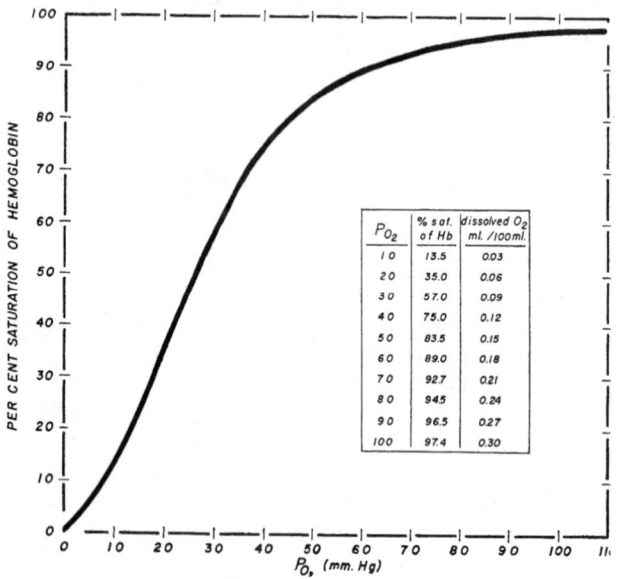

P_{O_2}	% sat. of Hb	dissolved O_2 ml./100ml.
10	13.5	0.03
20	35.0	0.06
30	57.0	0.09
40	75.0	0.12
50	83.5	0.15
60	89.0	0.18
70	92.7	0.21
80	94.5	0.24
90	96.5	0.27
100	97.4	0.30

FIGURE 13–3

Oxyhemoglobin dissociation curve at temperature 38° C, pH 7.40. (From Clockesy, J. M. Breu, C., Cardin S., Whittaker, A. A., & Rudy, E. B. [Eds.]. [1996]. *Critical care nursing* [2nd ed., p. 577]. Philadelphia: W. B. Saunders.)

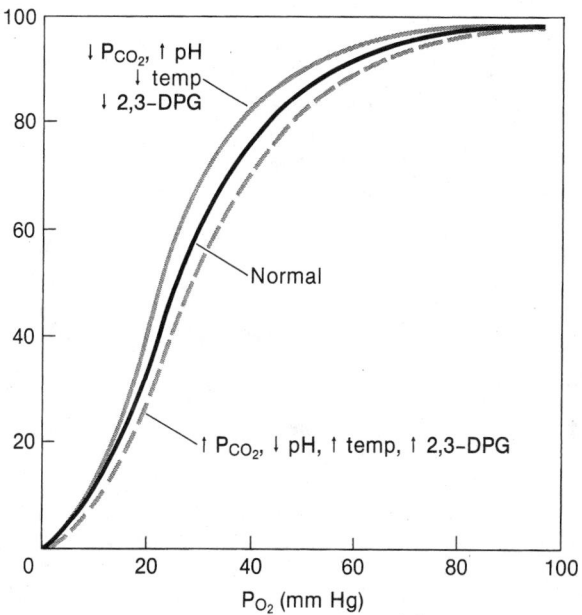

FIGURE 13-4

The effects of changes in P_{CO_2}, pH, temperature, and 2,3-diphosphoglyc-erate (2,3-DPG) on oxygen binding to hemoglobin. An increase in partial pressure of CO_2, decrease in pH, increase in temperature, or increase in 2,3-DPG produce a shift to the right of the hemoglobin oxygen dissocia-tion curve. The hemoglobin-oxygen dissociation curve is shifted to the left by a fall in carbon dioxide, increase in pH, decrease in temperature, or de-crease in concentration of 2,3-DPG. (From Clockesy, J. M., Breu, C., Cardin S., Whittaker, A. A., & Rudy, E. B. [Eds.]. [1996]. *Critical care nursing* [2nd ed., p. 577]. Philadelphia: W. B. Saunders; modified from Berne, R. M., & Levy, M. N. [1988]. *Physiology* [2nd ed., p. 610]. St. Louis: C. V. Mosby.)

- Hypothermia and alkalosis: The affinity of hemoglobin for oxygen is increased, and less oxygen is released to the tissues (left shift).

Efficiency of Gas Exchange

Paco$_2$. The Paco$_2$ reflects alveolar ventilation:
- Paco$_2$ >40 mm Hg reflects alveolar hypoventilation
- Paco$_2$ <40 mm Hg reflects alveolar hyperventilation
- Analysis of end-tidal carbon dioxide (capnography) can provide an approximate Paco$_2$ value (see Chapter 14 and Fig. 14–1 for related information on capnography)

Pao$_2$. The Pao$_2$ may be used to assist in measuring or estimating intrapulmonary shunting ($\dot{Q}s/\dot{Q}t$), which is the amount of venous blood that passes through the lungs without becoming adequately oxygenated ($\dot{Q}$ is equal to pulmonary blood flow, *s* is equal to shunted flow, and *t* is equal to total flow). Normally the intrapulmonary shunt is less than 5% of the total pulmonary blood flow.

An increased intrapulmonary shunt increases the work of breathing as well as the workload on the heart. Severe intrapulmonary shunts may require mechanical ventilation to improve arterial oxygenation.

Various methods may be used to estimate intrapulmonary shunting, including the alveolar-arterial gradient, the arterial/alveolar ratio, and the Pao$_2$/Fio$_2$ ratio:

Alveolar-Arterial (A-a) or A-a PO$_2$ Gradient. Estimates the $\dot{Q}s/\dot{Q}t$ by measuring the difference between the Po$_2$ of alveolar gas (Pao$_2$) and the Po$_2$ of arterial blood (if gas exchange is taking place, the difference between the two should be minimal):
- Pao$_2$ − Pao$_2$
- Normal value = 0–20 mm Hg
- The value increases with advancing age and with an increase in the concentration of inspired oxygen
- The Pao$_2$ may be calculated with the following equation:

$$PAo_2 = Fio_2 \, (PB - PH_2O) - Paco_2/RQ$$

where Fio$_2$ represents the fraction of inspired oxygen, PB represents the barometric pressure (760 mm Hg), PH$_2$O represents water vapor pressure (47 mm Hg), Paco$_2$ represents the arterial PCO$_2$, and RQ represents the respiratory quotient (0.8)

Pao$_2$/Pao$_2$, or a/A Po$_2$ Ratio. Estimates the $\dot{Q}s/\dot{Q}t$ by measuring the percentage of Pao$_2$ that Pao$_2$ represents
- Normal value >60%.
- The lower the value, the more severe the shunt.
- The value is not affected by the Fio$_2$: therefore the a/A Po$_2$ ratio may provide more accuracy in reflecting the efficiency of gas exchange than the A-a Po$_2$ gradient.

Pao$_2$/Fio$_2$ Ratio. Estimates the $\dot{Q}s/\dot{Q}t$ by measuring the amount of gas delivered to the large airways and whether the gas was able to diffuse into the blood:
- Normal value: >300.
- Values of <200 reflect intrapulmonary shunting.
- The lower the value, the more severe the shunt.

Serum Lactate

Lactate acid levels may be used to assist in the evaluation of tissue oxygenation. In the absence of oxygen, cells revert to anaerobic metabolism, and lactic acid is produced. A rising lactate level may indicate significant tissue oxygen deficits and a need to examine oxygen delivery and consumption parameters (see Table 14–1). Normal value = 1–2 mEq/L or 1–2 mmol/L.

CARDIOVASCULAR FUNCTION
Serum Lipoproteins

Lipoproteins are generally measured to assess the risk of coronary artery disease (CAD). The term *lipoprotein* refers to lipids bound to protein. The main lipoproteins are phospholipids, cholesterol, and triglycerides (see Table 13–2).

POINTS TO REMEMBER

▶ Normal reference values for these tests are often predicted on the basis of age and sex and may vary slightly with different laboratories.

▶ In addition to CAD, serum lipoproteins may be elevated in disorders such as familial hyperlipoproteinemia, hypothyroidism, diabetes mellitus, alcoholism, liver disease, pancreatitis, and renal disease (nephrotic syndrome).

TABLE 13-2 Serum Lipoproteins

Lipoprotein and Normal Value	Clinical Significance
Cholesterol, total: 120–200 mg/dl	Levels >200 mg/dl are thought to increase the risk of CAD as hypercholesterolemia contributes to plaque formation in the coronary arteries
Low-density lipoprotein (LDL) (primarily cholesterol and protein): 60–160 mg/dl	Levels >160 mg/dl are thought to increase the risk of atherosclerosis and CAD Levels <130 mg/dl are considered low risk
High-density lipoprotein (HDL) (primarily phospholipids and protein): 29–77 mg/dl	HDLs carry lipids away from body tissues and back to the liver for destruction (decrease plaque deposits in vessels) Levels >44–45 mg/dl for a male and >55 mg/dl for a female are thought to decrease the risk of CAD
Triglycerides: 10–190 mg/dl	Elevated levels of triglycerides contribute to arterial disease and frequently accompany high cholesterol levels (increase the level of very low-density lipoproteins)

▶ Decreased levels of serum lipoproteins may be associated with disorders such as hyperthyroidism, liver disease, malabsorption, and malnutrition.

▶ Clinical findings associated with elevated levels of serum lipoproteins may include xanthelasma (plaques of cholesterol seen on the nasal portion of the upper or lower eyelid as flat, slightly raised, irregularly shaped, yellow-colored lesions), corneal arcus in the young adult (a thin, grayish-white arc or circle at the edge of the cornea), hypertension, and obesity.

Cardiac Isoenzymes

Creatine kinase (CK) is an enzyme found in the heart, skeletal muscle, and brain tissue. It is subdivided into the isoenzymes MM found in the skeletal muscle, BB found in the brain, and MB found in the heart muscle.

Within hours of myocardial injury, the total CK will rise. An elevation of CK-MB greater than 6% of the total CK is highly diagnostic of a myocardial infarction and may be accurate enough to be used without other isoenzymes in the patient presenting with early chest pain (see Table 13–3).

Lactate dehydrogenase (LDH) is an enzyme found in the skeletal muscle, heart, liver, kidney, red blood cells, lung, and brain. It is subdivided into the isoenzymes LDH1 found in the heart and red blood cells; LDH2 found in the reticuloendothelial cells and kidney; LDH3 found in the lungs, lymphatics, and spleen; LDH4 found in the kidney, placenta, and liver; and LDH5 found in the kidney, liver, and skeletal muscle.

LDH rises more slowly following injury. Normally, LDH1 is less than LDH2. With myocardial injury, an elevation of LDH1 greater than an elevation of LDH2 is called a "flipped" LDH and is highly indicative of a myocardial infarction. A flipped LDH may be useful for diagnosing infarction when patients present to the hospital late (see Table 13–3).

TABLE 13–3 Cardiac Isoenzymes

Isoenzyme and Normal Value	Onset	Peak and Duration
CK		
• Male: 20–170 U/L	Within 4–6 hours	Peak: 18–24 hours
• Female: 10–135 U/L		Duration: 2–3 days
• CK-MB 0–6% of total CK	Within 4–6 hours	Peak: 12–24 hours
		Duration: 12–48 hours
LDH	24–48 hours	Peak: 3–4 days
• 60–120 U/L		Duration: 10–14 days
• LDH1 14%–26% of total LDH	12–24 hours	Peak: 48 hours
		Duration: variable
• LDH2 29%–39% of total LDH	12–24 hours	Peak: 48 hours
		Duration: variable

NEUROMUSCULAR FUNCTION
Cerebrospinal Fluid Analysis

Cerebrospinal fluid (CSF) is a clear, colorless, odorless, liquid that continuously circulates in the spaces surrounding the brain and spinal cord. Normally, CSF contains no red cells, few white cells, and little protein. Glucose levels vary with the serum glucose (approximately 60% of that value). Electrolyte values are the same or less than serum electrolyte values except for chloride, which is higher.

CSF functions to cushion the brain and spinal cord, carry nutrients and waste products, and assist in regulating intracranial pressure. In the critically ill adult, CSF is most commonly sampled via lumbar puncture (LP) to

- Assist in determining the cause of coma, such as metabolic or cerebral disorders, trauma, or drug intoxication
- Assist in diagnosing subarachnoid or intracranial hemorrhage, tumors, viral and bacterial infections such as meningitis and encephalitis, brain abscess, and demyelinating diseases such as Guillain-Barré syndrome
- Measure CSF pressure

POINTS TO REMEMBER

▶ A lumbar puncture should be performed with extreme caution in the presence of increased intracranial pressure, because withdrawl of CSF can precipitate brain herniation.

▶ Serum electrolytes and glucose levels should be measured simultaneously with CSF for comparison.

▶ CSF is absorbed by the venous system, and CSF pressure is related to jugular venous pressure (CSF pressure will be increased with heart failure and decreased with circulatory collapse).

▶ CSF values should be correlated with clinical findings of neuromuscular disorders, since some findings may not reflect the underlying disorder. For example, the CSF may remain clear in the presence of intracranial hemorrhage.

CSF Analysis

1. *Color*
   - Normally clear
   - Blood evenly distributed in all three tubes may indicate subarachnoid hemorrhage (the color in the third tube will be lighter if the blood is related to a traumatic tap)

- Yellow pigment may indicate previous bleeding (subarachnoid hemorrhage), meningitis, encephalitis, tumor, or demyelinating disease

2. *Pressure*
   - Normally 75–175 mm H_2O
   - Increased levels may indicate intracranial hemorrhage, hematoma, tissue edema, tumor, abscess, meningitis, or encephalitis
   - Decreased levels may indicate spinal cord tumor (obstructing CSF flow), dehydration, hypovolemia, or diabetic coma

3. *Protein*
   - Normally 15–45 mg/dl
   - Increased levels may indicate meningitis, poliomyelitis, brain abscess, multiple sclerosis, Guillain-Barré syndrome, brain tumor, or subarachnoid hemorrhage

4. *Chloride*
   - Normally 118–132 mEq/L
   - Decreased levels may indicate tuberculous meningitis or bacterial meningitis

5. *Glucose*
   - Normally 40–80 mg/dl
   - Increased levels may indicate cerebral trauma, hypothalmic lesions, or hyperglycemia
   - Decreased levels may indicate tuberculous meningitis, lymphomas, leukemias, subarachnoid hemorrhage, inflammatory disorders, or hypoglycemia

6. *Cell count* (lymphocytes)
   - Normally 0–5/mm³
   - Increased levels may be related to factors such as viral infections, poliomyelitis, multiple sclerosis, abscess, brain tumor, subarachnoid hemorrhage, tuberculous meningitis, bacterial meningitis, and Guillain-Barré syndrome
   - WBC differential may be done to identify the types of leukocytes. For example, increased neutrophils may be related to bacterial meningitis or encephalomyelitis; increased lymphocytes may be related to meningitis, parasitic infection, cerebral abscess, tumor, or infarction; increased eosinophils may be related to parasitic or fungal infections or an allergic reaction within the central nervous system; and increased malignant cells may be related to lymphomas, leukemia, medulloblastoma, or metastatic carcinoma.

GASTROINTESTINAL FUNCTION

Several laboratory studies may be used to assist in the diagnosis of gastrointestinal disorders. In general, these studies measure the metabolic functions of the liver, exocrine function of the pancreas, the effects of cholestasis in the liver or biliary system, and the presence of organ damage or necrosis (see Table 13–4).

TABLE 13–4 Laboratory Studies Used to Assist in the Diagnosis of Gastrointestinal Disorders

Description of Test and Reference Value	Clinical Significance
Total Serum Protein An indicator of the concentration of all plasma proteins except fibrinogen Normal value: 6.4–8.2 g/dl	Total protein may be increased with dehydration, vomiting, diarrhea, and multiple myeloma Total protein may be decreased with chronic liver disease, malnutrition, starvation, cancer of the GI tract, Hodgkin's disease, nephrotic syndrome, ulcerative colitis, Crohn's disease, intestinal fistulas, blood dyscrasias, hemorrhage, severe burns, and water intoxication
Albumin Albumin is a plasma protein synthesized by the liver that is essential for maintaining plasma colloid oncotic pressure Acts as a reserve nitrogen source for tissue growth and healing Acts as a transport vehicle for many substances, such as lipids, bilirubin, fat-soluble vitamins, hormones, minerals, and medications Normal value: 3.5–5 g/dl	Albumin may be increased with dehydration or multiple myeloma Albumin may be decreased with hepatic disease, malnutrition, chronic alcoholism, hyperthyroidism, peptic ulcer, collagen diseases, infection, fever, heart failure, nephrotic syndrome, and severe burns Decreased levels of albumin may result in fluid shifts from the vessels to the tissue and lead to edema

TABLE 13–4 Laboratory Studies Used to Assist in the Diagnosis of Gastrointestinal Disorders *Continued*

Description of Test and Reference Value	Clinical Significance
Globulin	
α- and β-Globulins are plasma proteins synthesized by the liver	α- and β-Globulin synthesis may increase, decrease, or remain normal with hepatic disease
α-Globulins primarily act as enzymes such as α_1-globulin (antitrypsin), which inactivates trypsin in the blood, and the α_2-globulin haptoglobin, which binds hemoglobin released from the lysis of erythrocytes, and the α_2-globulin macroglobulin, which is a protease inhibitor	An increase in the total level of globulins is usually related to an increased production of γ-globulins by the reticuloendothelial system, reflecting an immune response to hepatic disease such as cirrhosis or chronic active hepatitis, but may also reflect infection, inflammation, neoplasms, and collagen diseases such as rheumatoid arthritis and systemic lupus erythematosus.
Normal value α_1-globulin: 0.1–0.3 g/dl α_2-globulin: 0.6–1 g/dl	An increase in α_1-globulins may be related to inflammatory or neoplastic disease
β_1-Globulins transport substances such as iron from intracellular storage to the bone marrow	An increase in α_2-globulins may be related to nephrotic syndrome, rheumatic fever, neoplasm, or acute infection
β_2-Globulins include the low-density lipoprotein that transports cholesterol to the cells, as well as fibrinogen and complement factors	An increase in β-globulins may be related to hyperlipoproteinemia or multiple myeloma
Normal value β-globulins: 0.7–1.1 g/dl	A decrease in the total number of globulins may be related to cytotoxic or immunosuppressive medication, lymphocytic leukemia, lymphosarcoma, or immunodeficiency syndrome
γ-Globulin is made by the reticuloendothelial system	Decreased α_1-globulin may be related to hereditary α_1-antitrypsin deficiency
γ-Globulins (IgG, IgA, IgD, IgE, and IgM) generally act as immunologic agents	Decreased α_2-globulins may be related to hemolysis or hepatocellular damage
	Decreased β-globulins may be related to hypolipoproteinemia

Table continued on following page

TABLE 13–4 Laboratory Studies Used to Assist in the Diagnosis of Gastrointestinal Disorders *Continued*

Description of Test and Reference Value	Clinical Significance
Normal value: γ-globulins: 0.8–1.6 g/dl	

Ammonia

| Ammonia is a by-product of protein metabolism and is converted to urea in the liver
Normal value: 15–45 μg/dl | Elevated levels of ammonia are generally related to hepatic failure and the decreased ability of the liver to convert ammonia to urea, or an impairment of the portal vein circulation that prevents ammonia from reaching the liver
High levels of ammonia may cause hepatic encephalopathy and alterations in the level of consciousness. |

Bilirubin

| Bilirubin is formed from the destruction of RBCs and the breakdown of hemoglobin
The heme portion of hemoglobin is converted to bilirubin (unconjugated or indirect) and transported in the plasma to the liver to be conjugated (direct form)
This yellow pigment is then excreted in the bile
Normal values
  Total 0.1–1.2 mg/dl
  Direct 0.1–0.3 mg/dl
  Indirect 0.1–1 mg/dl | Elevated direct bilirubin levels are usually related to hepatocellular damage or biliary tree obstructions such as stones or tumors (cancer of the head of the pancreas)
Elevated indirect levels of bilirubin are usually related to hemolysis (increased destruction of red blood cells) associated with factors such as traumatic tissue injury, blood transfusion incompatibility, or medications
Increased levels of bilirubin may cause jaundice of the sclera, skin, and mucous membranes |

TABLE 13–4 Laboratory Studies Used to Assist in the Diagnosis of Gastrointestinal Disorders *Continued*

Description of Test and Reference Value	Clinical Significance

Alanine Aminotransferase (ALT; Formerly Serum Glutamic-Pyruvic Transaminase [SGPT])

ALT is an enzyme found in liver cells ALT is released into the blood with hepatocellular destruction Normal value: 10–35 U/L at 37° C	High levels of ALT may be related to acute viral hepatitis or severe hepatotoxicity (drug or chemical) causing necrosis of the liver Moderate increases in ALT may be related to cirrhosis of the liver, acute alcohol intoxication, cancer of the liver, or heart failure Slight increases in ALT may be related to acute myocardial infarction Elevations may be accompanied by jaundice

Aspartate Aminotransferase (AST; Formerly Serum Glutamic-Oxaloacetic Transaminase [SGOT])

AST is an enzyme found primarily in the heart muscle and the liver (small amounts may be found in the skeletal muscle, kidneys, and pancreas); Normal value: 8–20 U/L	Increased levels of AST are related to the release of the enzyme into the blood with the destruction of cells In an acute myocardial infarction (MI) the level rises in 6–10 hours and peaks in 24–48 hours, returning to normal in 4–6 days In liver failure the level increases to 10 times or more above normal and remains elevated for a longer period of time Intramuscular injections can cause a transient elevation Elevations related to acute MI may be accompanied by chest pain and other symptoms of heart disease

Table continued on following page

TABLE 13–4 **Laboratory Studies Used to Assist in the Diagnosis of Gastrointestinal Disorders** *Continued*	
Description of Test and Reference Value	**Clinical Significance**
	Elevations related to liver disease may be accompanied by jaundice and other symptoms of liver failure
Alkaline Phosphatase (ALP)	
ALP is an enzyme found primarily in the liver and the bone, but it may also be produced in the intestine, kidney, and placenta	ALP may be increased related to obstructive biliary disease, hepatocellular cirrhosis, hepatitis, and cancer of the liver related to a decreased excretion in the bile
Isoenzymes ALP_1 (liver origin) and ALP_2 (bone origin) are more specific in distinguishing organ involvement	Elevations associated with liver disease may be accompanied by physical findings of hepatic failure
Normal value: 32–92 U/L	
Serum Amylase	
Amylase is an enzyme released from the pancreas, salivary gland, and liver	Elevations may be twice normal (>200 units) in acute pancreatitis
Normal value: 25–125 U/L	The level increases within 2–12 hours after onset of pancreatitis and returns to normal in 2–4 days
	Increased values may also be associated with numerous other disorders such as gastric disease and surgery, gallbladder disease and surgery, pancreatic cancer, renal failure, burns, trauma, pregnancy, and acute alcohol intoxication
	Decreased values may be associated with advanced chronic pancreatitis, chronic alcoholism, and necrosis of the liver

TABLE 13–4 Laboratory Studies Used to Assist in the Diagnosis of Gastrointestinal Disorders *Continued*

Description of Test and Reference Value	Clinical Significance
Urine Amylase As above; Normal value: 4–30 IU/2 h	Helpful in assisting with the diagnosis of acute pancreatitis, as levels may remain elevated for up to 2 weeks after an acute episode
Serum Lipase Lipase is an enzyme secreted by the pancreas to aid in the digestion of fats in the duodenum Normal value: <200 U/L	Assists in the diagnosis of pancreatitis, as levels increase within 2–12 hours after onset and remain elevated for up to 14 days Increases may also be associated with gastric disease, pancreatic cancer, and renal failure

RENAL FUNCTION
Electrolytes

Electrolyte balance is maintained by intake, absorption, distribution in extracellular (EC) and intracellular (IC) compartments, and excretion. Disruption in one or more of these regulatory mechanisms may lead to an electrolyte imbalance (reference values may vary slightly with different laboratories).

Sodium (135–145 mEq/L)

Sodium is the primary EC cation. In addition to contributing to osmolality and the regulation of fluid in the body compartments, sodium plays a role in the generation of sympathetic transmission in the nervous system, the conduction of electrical impulses to muscle fibers, and in the chemical reaction with chloride and bicarbonate in the regulation of acid-base balance.

The kidney regulates the balance of sodium in response to extracellular fluid (ECF) volume. When the ECF volume drops, the renin-angiotensin-aldosterone system and the thirst-ADH mechanism are activated to conserve sodium and water. Conversely, with an expansion of the ECF volume, atrial natriuretic peptide (ANP) is secreted from cells in the atria in response to atrial stretch, and sodium is excreted in the urine (natriuresis) accompanied by water.

ECF Volume Deficit. An ECF volume deficit occurs with the removal of ECF from the body in conditions such as gastric losses, burns, and hemorrhage. Third-space accumulation may also cause an ECF volume deficit. In an uncomplicated ECF volume deficit, the composition of the ECF may remain normal, but the amount of sodium and water may be greatly decreased. Clinical findings such as weight loss, postural hypotension, flat neck veins in the horizontal position, dizzinesss, oliguria, sunken eyeballs, dry mucous membranes, and skin tenting over the sternum primarily reflect dehydration and hypovolemia.

ECF Volume Excess. An ECF volume excess occurs when the ECF is abnormally increased in conditions such as heart failure, cirrhosis, renal disease, Cushing's disease, and primary hyperaldosteronism. In an uncomplicated ECF volume expansion, the composition of the ECF may remain normal, but the amount of sodium and water may be greatly increased. Clinical findings such as weight gain, edema, bounding pulses, distended neck veins in the upright position, dyspnea, orthopnea, crackles, and possibly frothy sputum primarily reflect fluid overload and hypervolemia.

Hypernatremia. Hypernatremia is characterized by too little water for the amount of sodium present in the ECF. Hypernatremia may occur with a gain in sodium in excess of water, a loss of water in excess of sodium, inadequate replacement of water in an ECF volume deficit, or insufficient oral intake of water (see Table 13–5).

Hypernatremia increases the osmolality of the ECF. The hyperosmolality causes water to move out of the cell into the ECF, resulting in IC dehydration and expansion of the ECF volume. Clinical findings primarily reflect the neuromuscular excitability associated with the increased plasma osmolality and central nervous system dehydration (see Table 13–5). Additional findings may reflect an alteration in the ECF volume (see ECF Volume Deficit and ECF Volume Excess above).

TABLE 13–5   Clinical Findings Associated with Electrolyte Imbalances

History	Assessment Findings

Hypernatremia (Na >145 mEq/L)

Recognize patients at risk

1. A gain in Na in excess of H_2O related to factors such as
   - Inappropriate administration of $NaHCO_3^-$ or NaCl
   - Hypertonic dialysis
   - Primary hyperaldosteronism
   - Cushing's syndrome
   - Excessive use of corticosteroid therapy
2. A loss in water in excess of Na related to factors such as
   - An increased loss of water from the lungs associated with hyperventilation, fever (increased respirations), respiratory infection, or ventilated patients with insufficient humidification
   - An increased loss of water from the kidneys associated with diabetes mellitus (DM) (osmotic diuresis secondary to hyperglycemia), or diabetes insipidus (DI) (insufficient ADH secretion)
3. Inadequate replacement of water associated with factors such as
   - Burns, profuse sweating, diarrhea, vomiting, or other GI losses
   - Concentrated tube feeds without supplemental water

Neuromuscular findings related to the increased osmolality of the ECF and central nervous system dehydration may include

- Alterations in mental status progressing from confusion, restlessness, irritability, and lethargy to coma
- Alterations in sensory and motor function progressing from tremors to seizures

In general, findings related to alterations in the ECF volume will vary with the underlying pathophysiological disorder(s) and the renal function of the critically ill adult (see ECF Volume Deficit and ECF Volume Excess)

Table continued on following page

**TABLE 13–5 Clinical Findings Associated with Electrolyte
                        Imbalances** *Continued*

History	Assessment Findings

---

4. Insufficient oral intake of water in
   the critically ill adult may be related to factors such as
   - Immobility (no access to water)
   - Inability to swallow or to ex-
     press or respond to thirst (confu-
     sion, unconsciousness, artificial
     airways, or prolonged nausea)

Hyponatremia (Na <135 mEq/L)

A. Recognize patients at risk for a
   dilutional imbalance
   1. A gain in H_2O in excess of Na
      related to factors such as
      - Overhydration with hypo-
        tonic solutions such as tap
        water in individuals with ex-
        treme thirst, or excessive ad-
        ministration of D_5W in the
        hospitalized patient
      - Endocrine disorders such as
        SIADH (increased secretion
        of ADH causes water reten-
        tion and volume expansion)
      - Pain, anxiety (increased
        stress response activates the
        renin-angiotensin-aldo-
        sterone mechanism)
   2. An increase in total body water
      with a smaller increase in
      sodium related to factors such
      as cirrhosis, heart failure, or
      renal failure

Neuromuscular findings related to the
   decreased osmolality of the ECF
   and brain swelling may include
   - Alterations in mental status pro-
     gressing from complaints of
     headache, malaise, and lethargy
     to confusion and coma
   - Alterations in sensory and motor
     function progressing from dizzi-
     ness and muscle twitching to
     seizures
Gastrointestinal findings related to
   the hypoosmolar imbalance may
   include
   - Abdominal cramps
   - Nausea and vomiting
In general, findings related to a dilu-
   tional imbalance may reflect an in-
   crease in the ECF volume (see ECF
   Volume Excess)

TABLE 13–5 Clinical Findings Associated with Electrolyte Imbalances *Continued*

History	Assessment Findings
B. Recognize patients at risk for a depletional imbalance	In general, findings related to a depletional imbalance may reflect a loss of ECF volume (see ECF Volume Deficit)
1. A loss of Na in excess of water related to factors such as	
• Salt wasting associated with acute or chronic renal failure	
• Excesive use of diuretics	
• Adrenal insufficiency	
2. Inadequate replacement of salt associated with factors such as hemorrhage, severe burns, massive diaphoresis, and GI losses such as diarrhea, vomiting, gastric suction, and fistula drainage	
3. Insufficient oral intake of sodium related to factors such as ingestion of hypoosmotic solutions as a replacement for fluid losses	

Hyperchloremia (Cl >105 mEq/L)
Recognize patients at risk
- Hypernatremia
- Metabolic acidosis
- Dehydration
- Acute renal failure
- Prolonged diarrhea
- Diabetes insipidus
- Hyperparathyroidism
- Adrenocortical hyperfunction
- Excessive replacement in IV solutions

In general, findings are similar to the clinical presentations of hypernatremia and metabolic acidosis and may include
- Alterations in neuromuscular function progressing from weakness and lethargy to stupor and coma
- Hyperventilation (deep and rapid respirations)

Hypochloremia (Cl <95 mEq/L)
Recognize patients at risk
- Hyponatremia

In general, findings are similar to the clinical presentations of hypona-

Table continued on following page

TABLE 13–5 Clinical Findings Associated with Electrolyte Imbalances *Continued*

History	Assessment Findings
• Metabolic alkalosis • Prolonged vomiting • Nasogastric drainage • Salt-wasting renal disease • Chronic renal failure • Heart failure • SIADH	tremia and metabolic alkalosis and may include • Alterations in neuromuscular function progressing from twitching and tremors associated with muscular hypertonicity (tetany) to seizures • Hypoventilation (slow and shallow respirations)

Hyperkalemia (K >5.0 mEq/L)
Recognize patients at risk
1. Decreased renal excretion of K related to factors such as
   • Oliguric renal failure (most common cause of hyperkalemia)
   • Decreased circulating blood volume
   • Adrenal insufficiency
   • Potassium-sparing diuretics
2. Shift of K from the ICF to the ECF related to factors such as
   • Cell damage secondary to massive trauma, severe burns, or extensive surgery
   • Metabolic acidosis
   • Insulin deficit
   • Hyperglycemia (increases the osmolality of the ECF, causing fluid and K to move out of the cell)
   • Digitalis toxicity (inhibits the Na^+-K^+-ATPase pump, which is responsible for maintaining high levels of IC K and high levels of EC Na)

Neuromuscular findings related to hypopolarization of the skeletal muscles may include muscle weakness progressing to loss of muscle tone and then flaccid paralysis (begins first in the lower extremities)
Gastrointestinal findings related to hypopolarization of the smooth muscle cells may include cramping and diarrhea
Cardiac findings related to a decreased duration, rate, and rise of cardiac action potentials, and decreased conduction velocity in the heart may include
• ECG changes progressing from a shortened QT interval with a tall, narrow T wave to a prolonged PR interval, widened QRS complex, and depressed ST segment, and then cardiac asystole
• Bradydysrhythmias and changes in conduction that may cause ventricular irritability and fibrillation

---

TABLE 13–5 **Clinical Findings Associated with Electrolyte Imbalances** *Continued*

History	Assessment Findings

- β-Blockers
- Cytotoxic drugs

3. Increased intake of K related to factors such as
   - Excessive IV infusion
   - Large transfusion of stored blood

Hypokalemia (K <3.5 mEq/L)
Recognize patients at risk

1. Increased loss of body K related to factors such as
   - GI losses, including vomiting, gastric suction, intestinal drainage, fistulas, diarrhea, and laxative abuse
   - Renal losses including diuretics, hyperaldosteronism, Cushing's syndrome, and osmotic diuresis
   - Excessive diaphoresis
   - Dialysis
2. Shift of K from the ECF to the ICF related to factors such as
   - Metabolic alkalosis
   - Insulin excess
   - Increased β-adrenergic activity
3. Decreased intake of K related to factors such as
   - Anorexia, starvation, and crash diets
   - Malnutrition (the elderly and the alcoholic patient are particularly at risk)
   - Lack of IV replacement therapy

Neuromuscular findings related to hyperpolarized skeletal muscle cells may include bilateral muscle weakness progressing to ascending flaccid paralysis, which may involve the respiratory muscles and lead to respiratory arrest (the muscles become less reactive to stimuli)

Gastrointestinal findings related to atony of smooth muscle cells may include anorexia, nausea, vomiting, paralytic ileus, abdominal distention, constipation, and diminished bowel sounds

Cardiac findings related to delayed ventricular repolarization, a shortened absolute refractory period, and a prolonged relative refractory period may include
- ECG changes, including a prolonged QT interval, a depressed ST segment with a flat or inverted T wave, and U waves (hypokalemia enhances the effects of digitalis preparations)

Table continued on following page

TABLE 13-5 Clinical Findings Associated with Electrolyte Imbalances *Continued*

History	Assessment Findings
	• Dysrhythmias such as sinus brady-cardia, premature atrial contractions, premature ventricular contractions, atrioventricular block, and paroxysmal atrial tachycardia
Hypercalcemia (Ca >10.2 mg/dl) Recognize patients at risk 1. Increased absorption from the GI tract: Excessive intake of milk products, antacids, or vitamin D 2. Increased absorption from the bone • Hyperparathyroidism • Numerous malignancies with bone metastases, including breast, lung, cervical, prostate, multiple myeloma, lymphoma and renal primary sites • Prolonged immobilization particularly in the critically ill adult with multiple trauma, severe fractures, or spinal cord injury 3. Decreased renal excretion: Thiazide diuretics	Neuromuscular findings related to decreased neuromuscular excitability (elevation of the threshold potential of excitable cells) may include • Alterations in mental status such as lethargy, fatigue, drowsiness, disorientation, loss of memory, and confusion • Alterations in sensory and motor function, such as muscle weakness and flaccidity • Diminished deep tendon reflexes Gastrointestinal findings related to decreased smooth muscle tone and hypoactivity of the bowel may include anorexia, nausea, vomiting, and constipation Cardiac findings related to a shortened plateau phase of the action potential, delayed atrioventricular conduction, and increased myocardial contractility may include • ECG changes such as a shortened QT segment, shortened ST interval, and depressed T wave (hypercalcemia may increase the patient's susceptibility to digitalis toxicity)

TABLE 13–5 Clinical Findings Associated with Electrolyte Imbalances *Continued*

History	Assessment Findings
	• Dysrhythmias such as heart blocks and cardiac standstill
	Cardiac findings related to increased peripheral vascular resistance may include hypertension
	Genitourinary findings may include
	• Flank pain related to renal calculi
	• Oliguria related to obstruction of renal tubule or outflow tract by calculi
	• Polyuria related to osmotic diuresis
Hypocalcemia (Ca <8.2 mg/dl)	
Recognize patients at risk	Neuromuscular findings related to neuromuscular irritability (decreased threshold potential of excitable cells) may include
1. Decreased levels of PTH	
• Trauma to, or removal of, the parathyroid gland	• Alterations in mental status such as anxiety, restlessness, and confusion
• Hypomagnesemia (common in the critically ill adult related to inadequate magnesium replacement in total parenteral nutrition [TPN] solutions)	• Alterations in sensory and motor function such as circumoral or digital paresthesias, muscle cramping, muscle spasms of hands and feet (carpopedal spasm), tetany, seizures, and laryngospasm (laryngeal stridor and respiratory muscle spasm may cause airway obstruction and respiratory arrest)
2. Abnormalities in vitamin D metabolism in the critically ill adult: NPO, clear liquid diet, gastric surgeries, and disturbances in the conversion of vitamin D to the active form associated with disorders such as hepatic or renal failure	
3. Pancreatitis	• Hyperactive deep tendon reflexes
• Ca binds to fatty acids in soft tissue spaces	
• Steatorrhea	

Table continued on following page

TABLE 13–5   **Clinical Findings Associated with Electrolyte Imbalances** *Continued*

History	Assessment Findings

4. Blood transfusions: Ca binds with the citrate solution used to store blood (worse in liver failure, as liver disease decreases the metabolism of citrate)
 	
5. Hyperphosphatemia: Damage to muscle cells (rhabdomyolysis) causes reciprocal effect
 	
6. Nutritional effects
   • Decreased intake of dairy products and leafy green vegetables
   • Malabsorption of fat and fat-soluble vitamin D
	• Positive Chvostek's sign (twitch of nose or lip in response to tapping of the facial nerve just below the temple)
	• Positive Trousseau's sign (contraction of hand or fingers in response to blood pressure cuff inflation >3 minutes)
	Cardiac findings related to prolongation of the cardiac action potential, impaired atrioventricular and intraventricular conduction, and decreased contractility may include
	   • ECG changes, including a prolonged QT interval (increased susceptibility to the development of torsades de pointe)
	   • Dysrhythmias such as heart blocks and ventricular irritability
	Cardiac findings related to decreased contractility and decreased peripheral vacular resistance may include hypotension

Hyperphosphatemia (P >4.5 mg/dl)
Recognize patients at risk
1. Decreased renal excretion of P related to factors such as
   • Acute or chronic renal failure with a large loss of glomerular filtration
   • Hypoparathyroidism
2. Cell breakdown related to factors such as
	In general, the clinical findings associated with hyperphosphatemia reflect the concurrent hypocalcemia (see hypocalcemia)

**TABLE 13–5 Clinical Findings Associated with Electrolyte
Imbalances** *Continued*

History	Assessment Findings

- Metastatic tumors treated with chemotherapy (cell lysis)
- Crush injuries
- Rhabdomyolysis

3. Increased absorption related to factors such as
  - Chronic use of phosphate-containing enemas or laxatives
  - Excessive phosphate supplementation

Hypophosphatemia (P <2.5 mg/dl)
Recognize patients at risk

1. Increased renal excretion of P related to factors such as
  - Hyperparathyroidism
  - Some diuretics
  - Osmotic diuresis
  - Metabolic acidosis
2. Cellular redistribution of P from the EC to the IC compartment related to factors such as
  - Respiratory alkalosis (cell uses phosphorous for increased glucose metabolism)
  - Glucose infusion and insulin administration drive P into skeletal muscle and liver cells
  - Total parenteral nutrition without P
3. Intestinal malabsorption may be related to factors such as
  - Magnesium- and aluminum-containing antacids (bind with P)

All tissue cells are at risk for reduced oxygen delivery and tissue hypoxia related to a reduction in the formation of 2,3-DPG and a shift of the oxyhemoglobin dissociation curve to the left

All cellular functions may be decreased related to the reduction in ATP, the major source of energy for many cells

Neuromuscular findings may include

- Alterations in mental status such as malaise, confusion, stupor, and coma
- Alterations in sensory and motor function such as paresthesias, muscle pain, muscle weakness including respiratory muscles (potential for respiratory failure), and rhabdomyolysis
- Diminished deep tendon reflexes

Table continued on following page

TABLE 13–5 Clinical Findings Associated with Electrolyte Imbalances *Continued*

History	Assessment Findings

• Vitamin D deficiency decreases P absorption and retards the movement of P from the bone to the ECF
• Chronic alcohol abuse
• Chronic diarrhea
• Malabsorption syndromes
• Vomiting
• Starvation
	Cardiac findings may include
	  • Decreased cardiac contractility and stroke work index
	  • Increased left ventricular end-diastolic pressure (congestive cardiomyopathy may result)
	Hematopoietic findings may include
	  • Decreased leukocyte phagocytosis and impaired resistance to infection
	  • Thrombocytopenia
	  • Hemolysis (red blood cell fragility)
	  • Decreased platelet survival
	Bone pain and pathological fractures may be present, related to resorption of phosphorus from the bone

Hypermagnesemia (Mg >2.5 mEq/L)
Recognize patients at risk
1. Decreased renal excretion may be related to factors such as
  • Acute or chronic renal failure
  • Adrenal insufficiency
2. Redistribution from the IC to the EC compartment related to factors such as
  • Massive tissue injury or surgery
  • Rhabdomyolysis
3. Increased intestinal absorption may be related to factors such as
  • Excessive intake of magnesium-containing antacids
  • Increased magnesium in dialysate
	Neuromuscular findings related to depressed skeletal muscle and nerve function may include
	  • Alterations in mental status such as lethargy and drowsiness
	  • Alterations in sensory and motor function such as muscle weakness (including respiratory muscles and the potential for respiratory depression), and flaccid paralysis
	  • Diminished deep tendon reflexes
	Cardiac findings related to decreased cardiac conduction and depression of membrane excitability may include

TABLE 13-5 Clinical Findings Associated with Electrolyte Imbalances *Continued*

History	Assessment Findings
• Total parenteral nutrition • Magnesium-containing laxatives or enemas	• ECG changes such as prolonged PR and QRS intervals and increased QT interval • Dysrhythmias such as bradycardia, complete heart block, and cardiac arrest Cardiac findings related to peripheral vasodilation may include • Hypotension • Flushing • Diaphoresis

Hypomagnesemia (Mg <1.5 mEq/L)
Recognize patients at risk
1. Increased renal excretion may be related to
  • Loop or thiazide diuretics
  • Osmotic diuresis with diabetic ketoacidosis (DKA)
  • Diuretic phase of recovery from acute renal failure can cause Mg wasting
  • Hyperaldosteronism
  • Hyperparathyroidism
2. Cellular redistribution of Mg related to factors such as acute hemorrhagic pancreatitis (causes deposition of Mg in tissue)
3. Decreased intestinal absorption of Mg related to factors such as
  • Prolonged periods of total parenteral nutrition with inadequate Mg replacement
	Neuromuscular findings related to neuromuscular excitability may include
	• Alterations in mental status such as insomnia
	• Alterations in sensory and motor function such as nystagmus, dysphagia, vertigo, ataxia, muscle cramps and twitching, muscular spasms, tetany, and seizures
	• Hyperactive deep tendon reflexes
	• Positive Chvostek's sign
	• Positive Trousseau's sign
	Cardiac findings related to decreased activity of the Na^+-K^+-ATPase pump may include
	• ECG changes such as prolonged QT interval and ST segment depression

Table continued on following page

TABLE 13–5 Clinical Findings Associated with Electrolyte Imbalances *Continued*

History	Assessment Findings
• Malnutrition • Chronic alcoholism • Chronic diarrhea • Postsurgical fluid loss with ileal resection • Gastric drainage • Fistula drainage	• Tachycardia (increased spontaneous firing in the sinus node)

Hyponatremia. Hyponatremia is characterized by too little sodium for the amount of water present in the ECF. A dilutional imbalance may occur with a gain in water in excess of sodium. A depletional imbalance may occur with a loss of more sodium than water associated with an ECF volume depletion, inadequate replacement of sodium in an ECF volume depletion, or insufficient oral intake of sodium (see Table 13–5).

Hyponatremia decreases the osmolality of the ECF. The hypoosmolality causes water to move into the cell, resulting in IC swelling. Clinical findings primarily reflect neuromuscular manifestations associated with the decreased plasma osmolality and increased volume expansion in the brain cells (see Table 13–5). Additional findings may reflect an alteration in the ECF volume (see ECF Volume Deficit and ECF Volume Excess above).

Chloride (95–105 mEq/L)

Chloride is the primary EC anion. Chloride functions in tandem with sodium, which means that as the sodium concentration increases, the chloride concentration increases, and as the sodium concentration drops, the chloride concentration drops. Chloride assists in the regulation and distribution of fluid between body compartments, and in the regulation of acid-base balance. Chloride combines with hydrogen to produce the acidity in the stomach.

The kidney retains chloride with sodium in exchange for a potassium or hydrogen ion. To maintain acid-base balance, when the body fluids are acidic, the kidneys excrete chloride and sodium, and bicarbonate is reabsorbed. As well, chloride shifts in and out of the RBCs in exchange for bicarbonate.

Hyperchloremia. Hyperchloremia usually occurs with an excess of sodium or a deficit of bicarbonate. Hyperchloremia may also occur with dehydration. The clinical findings of hyperchloremia are similar to the clinical presentations of hypernatremia and metabolic acidosis (see Table 13–5).

Hypochloremia. Hypochloremia usually occurs with a deficit of sodium or an excess of bicarbonate. Hypochloremia may also occur with overhydration, the loss of chloride through the upper GI tract, or renal disease. The clinical findings of hypochloremia are similar to the clinical presentations of hyponatremia and metabolic alkalosis (see Table 13–5).

Potassium (3.5–5 mEq/L)

Potassium is primarily an IC cation. Responsible for many functions, potassium helps regulate the osmolality of the body's fluid compartments, is crucial to normal neuromuscular function including the conduction of impulses in nerves and muscles, and plays a role in acid-base balance.

The kidney regulates the balance of potassium in response to EC concentration. As sodium delivery to the renal tubule is increased, or retained in response to aldosterone, potassium is excreted, and vice versa. As well, cellular redistribution of potassium regulates the ECF concentration. In acidosis, hydrogen ions move into the cell in exchange for potassium ions, which increases the ECF concentration of potassium. In alkalosis, hydrogen ions move out of the cell and potassium ions move into the cell, decreasing the ECF concentration. Insulin also drives potassium into the cells with the movement of glucose.

Hyperkalemia. Hyperkalemia may occur with the decreased renal excretion of potassium, a shift of potassium from the ICF to the ECF, or increased oral or intravenous intake (rare unless decreased renal function). The clinical findings of hyperkalemia are related to the increased level of potassium in the ECF, which causes a decrease in resting potential of the cell membrane. The cell rapidly repolarizes and becomes irritable. If the hyperkalemia persists, the resting potential approaches the threshold potential, and the cell is unable to repolarize and respond to stimuli. The muscle most crucially affected is the heart (see Table 13–5).

Hypokalemia. Hypokalemia may occur with an excessive body loss of potassium, a shift of potassium from the ECF to the ICF, or decreased intake (rare as the kidney will minimize excretion with decreased intake). The clinical findings of hypokalemia are related to the decreased level of potassium, which causes the cell membrane to become hyperpolarized and less sensitive to excitation. Neuromuscular excitability is decreased, causing skeletal muscle weakness and decreased smooth muscle tone. Changes in the cardiac membrane excitability cause delayed ventricular repolarization and impaired cardiac contractility (see Table 13–5).

Calcium (8.2–10.2 mg/dl)

Calcium is primarily an IC cation. Responsible for many functions, calcium promotes normal skeletal and cardiac muscle contractility, maintains or decreases neuromuscular irritability, decreases capillary permeability, is the support matrix for bones, teeth, and nails, is an essential component of the clotting process, and plays a significant role in activation of the complement system.

The kidney regulates calcium in response to the parathyroid hormone (PTH). Low serum calcium concentrations increase the secretion of PTH, which stimulates the kidney to decrease renal excretion of calcium. With high concentrations of calcium, PTH stimulates the kidney to increase the excretion of calcium. In addition, with low concentrations of calcium, PTH stimulates the release of calcium from the bone. With high concentrations of calcium, calcitonin inhibits the release of calcium from the bone.

The concentration of calcium is also regulated by vitamin D. Vitamin D facilitates the increased absorption of calcium from the intestine and affects the response of bone calcium to PTH and calcitonin.

Hypercalcemia. Hypercalcemia may occur with increased calcium absorption from the GI tract or bone, or decreased calcium excretion. The clinical findings of hypercalcemia reflect the increased threshold potential of excitable cells, which results in decreased neuromuscular excitability or hypotonicity. Cardiac effects result from a shortened plateau phase of the action potential, delayed atrioventricular conduction, and increased contractility and peripheral vascular resistance (calcium has a positive inotropic effect on the cardiac muscle). Renal calculi may develop, related to the high concentration of calcium in the urine, and impaired renal function may develop secondary to obstruction of the renal tubules. Hypercalcemia may be accompanied by an osmotic diuresis and dehydration (see Table 13–5).

Hypocalcemia. Hypocalcemia may occur with a decreased level of PTH, abnormalities in vitamin D metabolism, pancreatitis, blood transfusions, hyperphosphatemia, or nutritional deficiencies. Clinical findings are related to a decrease in the threshold potential of excitable cells, which allows action potentials to be generated more easily and leads to an increase in neuromuscular irritability. Cardiac effects result from prolongation of the plateau phase of the cardiac action potential, impaired atrioventricular and intraventricular conduction, ventricular irritability, and decreased contractility and peripheral vascular resistance (see Table 13–5).

Phosphorus (2.5–4.5 mg/dl)

Phosphorus is a major IC anion. Most phosphorus is present in the blood as phosphate. Responsible for many functions, phosphate is a structural element of bone, is an important component of phospholipids, and plays a role in the metabolism of lipids, proteins, and carbohydrates. It is part of ATP and essential to oxidative phosphorylation, which is the main energy source of muscle tissue, and as a part of 2,3-diphosphoglycerate (2,3-DPG), it influences the oxygen carrying capacity of hemoglobin.

The kidney regulates phosphate balance by increasing renal excretion as the plasma concentration of phosphate increases. As well, PTH increases phosphate excretion from the kidneys and shifts phosphate from the bones as a homeostatic mechanism in relation to calcium levels.

Hyperphosphatemia. Hyperphosphatemia may occur with decreased renal excretion of phosphate, cell breakdown (movement of phosphate from the IC to the EC compartment), or increased intestinal absorption of phosphorous. Increased levels of phosphate lower serum calcium levels and cause clinical findings similar to the clinical presentation of hypocalcemia (see Table 13–5). Prolonged hyperphosphatemia causes increased amounts of phosphate and calcium to be deposited in the bones and soft tissues.

Hypophosphatemia. Hypophosphatemia may occur with increased renal excretion of phosphate, cellular redistribution of phosphorous (from the EC compartment to the IC compartment), or intestinal malabsorption. Clinical findings reflect decreased levels of 2,3-DPG and ATP, which may be harmful to the critically ill adult. Decreased levels of 2,3-DPG may result in the decreased transport and release of oxygen to the cells and lead to tissue hypoxia. Tissue hypoxia causes the release of lactic acid, which shifts the oxyhemoglobin curve to the left (see Figs. 13–3 and 13–4). Decreased levels of ATP alter the energy metabolism of cells, causing fragility of erythrocytes and RBCs, which may lead to hemolytic anemia and further compromise oxygen delivery. Leukocyte dysfunction increases the risk of infection, and platelet dysfunction affects blood clotting and increases the risk of hemorrhage. Nerve and muscle function may be affected, resulting in irritability and muscle weakness. Bone resorption may cause bone disease. Hypercalcemia and hypomagnesemia may be present (see Table 13–5).

Magnesium (1.5–2.5 mEq/L)

Magnesium is a prevalent IC cation. Responsible for many functions, magnesium is an important component of bone structure, a cofactor in enzymatic activity and necessary for the control of numerous metabolic processes, including oxidative phosphorylation, the production or maintenance of RNA, DNA, and ATP, and fat and protein metabolism. As well, magnesium has a direct effect on the neuromuscular junction (depresses the release of acetylcholine at neuromuscular junctions), which affects neuromuscular irritability and muscular contraction. In addition, magnesium affects calcium homeostasis. An antagonist of calcium, magnesium counterbalances the effect of calcium on bronchial and vascular smooth muscle contraction.

The kidney regulates magnesium balance by increasing renal excretion as the plasma level of magnesium rises and decreasing renal excretion of magnesium in the presence of low plasma levels. PTH, vitamin D, and thyrocalcitonin also affect renal regulation in conjunction with their role in calcium regulation.

Hypermagnesemia. Hypermagnesemia may occur with decreased renal excretion, liberation from cells (usually in the presence of renal dysfunction), or excessive intake. Clinical findings reflect a decreased release of acetylcholine at the neuromuscular junction, which causes depressed skeletal muscle contraction and nerve function, as well as cardiac effects related to decreased cardiac conduction, depression of membrane excitability, and peripheral vasodilation (see Table 13–5).

Hypomagnesemia. Hypomagnesemia may occur with increased renal excretion, cellular redistribution to the IC compartment, or decreased intake. Clinical findings primarily reflect central nervous system dysfunction related to excessive release of acetylcholine at the neuromuscular junction, and cardiac dysfunction related to a decrease in intracellular myocardial potassium related to a decrease in the activity of Na^+-K^--ATPase pump, which allows potassium to more readily escape from the cell (see Table 13–5).

Blood Urea Nitrogen (BUN) and Creatinine

The BUN may be used to evaluate the production and excretion of urea and as an indicator of glomerular function. The serum creatinine may be used to evaluate renal function and the effectiveness of glomerular filtration. However, because the creatinine is usually not affected by fluid or diet, the creatinine level is often considered a more sensitive indicator of renal dysfunction (see Table 13–6). In general, if there is a rise in both the BUN and creatinine, renal dysfunction is highly suspect.

TABLE 13–6 **BUN and Creatinine**

Description of Test and Reference Value	Clinical Significance
Blood Urea Nitrogen (BUN) (5–20 mg/dl)	
Urea is an end-product of protein and amino acid metabolism	Elevations in the BUN may be influenced by numerous nonrenal factors, including
Urea is primarily excreted from the body through glomerular filtration in the kidneys:	• Increased dietary protein intake
• More urea is resorbed with a low tubular flow of urine	• Increased protein catabolism
• Less urea is resorbed with a high tubular flow of urine	• Dehydration (should return to normal with fluid replacement)
	• GI hemorrhage (the BUN is usually elevated with an upper GI bleed as digested blood is absorbed, and the BUN is usually

Table continued on following page

TABLE 13–6 **BUN and Creatinine** *Continued*

Description of Test and Reference Value	Clinical Significance
	normal with a lower GI bleed as absorption of blood does not occur in the lower intestine) A decreased serum BUN may be associated with numerous nonrenal factors, including • Decreased protein intake (low-protein diet, malnutrition, and starvation) • Overhydration • Severe liver failure (decreased protein metabolism) Renal causes of an elevation in BUN include • Prerenal dysfunction (decreased renal perfusion associated with conditions such as heart failure and shock slows the glomerular filtration rate and limits renal function) • Intrarenal dysfunction (damage to the renal parenchyma associated with conditions such as acute tubular necrosis limits renal function) • Postrenal dysfunction (obstruction in the kidney or urinary tract leads to increased resorption of urea)
Creatinine **(0.7–1.3 mg/dl male;** **0.6–1.1 mg/dl female)** Creatinine is a by-product of muscle catabolism: The amount of creatinine produced is proportional to the amount of muscle mass (females	Increased levels of creatinine may be due to conditions causing prerenal, intrarenal, and postrenal failure (see BUN)

TABLE 13–6 BUN and Creatinine *Continued*

Description of Test and Reference Value	Clinical Significance

and the elderly may have slightly lower values)

Creatinine is primarily excreted from the body through glomerular filtration in the kidneys (creatinine is not usually resorbed)

- In early renal disease, the kidney is able to compensate and maintain relatively low serum creatinine levels by secreting greater amounts of creatinine from the renal tubules
- As renal disease progresses, the kidneys are unable to continue to compensate, and the creatinine level rises in proportion to the severity of the disease

Decreased levels of creatinine may be due to conditions that result in decreased muscle mass or muscle-wasting disorders such as paralysis, polymyositis, muscular dystrophy, hyperthyroidism, and long-term corticosteroid therapy, or advanced liver disease (less creatinine synthesis, storage, and production).

Creatinine Clearance (85–135 ml/min); females slightly less than males; males: 1–2 g/d; females: 0.8–1.8 g/d

Assists in determining the presence and progression of renal dysfunction by estimating the glomerular filtration rate:

- The total amount of creatinine excreted in a 12- or 24-hour urine collection is multiplied by the urine volume, and the result is divided by the plasma creatinine
- A creatinine clearance of less than 40 ml/min is highly indicative of moderate to severe renal dysfunction

Elevated levels of creatinine clearance may be due to disorders such as hypothyroidism

In addition to renal dysfunction, decreased levels of creatinine clearance may be due to disorders such as hyperthyroidism or muscular dystrophy

ENDOCRINE FUNCTION

Because the endocrine system inflences all body systems, several laboratory studies may be used to assist in the diagnosis of one endocrine disorder. Some laboratory studies may be used to assess glandular disorders by stimulating or suppressing hormone secretion, and others to confirm suspected glandular disorders (see Table 13–7).

TABLE 13–7 Common Laboratory Studies Used to Assist in the Diagnosis of Endocrine Disorders

Description of Test and Reference Value	Clinical Significance
Adrenocorticotropic Hormone (ACTH) (AM: 25–100 pg/ml; PM: 0–50 pg/ml) A plasma ACTH may be used to • Assist in the diagnosis of Addison's disease • Distinguish between primary and secondary adrenal insufficiency	Elevated levels of ACTH may be due to • Primary adrenal insufficiency (disease of the adrenal gland itself interferes with the feedback mechanism that regulates the hypothalamic-pituitary-adrenal hormonal responses) • Stress (severe physical or emotional stress increases the level of corticotropin-releasing hormone, which causes an increase in ACTH and leads to an increase in plasma cortisol levels) • Ectopic production of ACTH (ACTH-producing tumors) Decreased levels of ACTH may be due to hypopituitarism (a deficiency of ACTH causes secondary adrenal insufficiency)

TABLE 13–7 Common Laboratory Studies Used to Assist in the Diagnosis of Endocrine Disorders *Continued*

Description of Test and Reference Value	Clinical Significance
ACTH Stimulation Test **Plasma cortisol levels should increase to 18 μg/dl within 30–60 minutes following an IV bolus of 0.25 mg of synthetic ACTH (cosyntropin [Cortrosyn])** ACTH stimulation test is used to assist in the diagnosis of primary and secondary insufficiency	Elevated levels indicate a normal response Reduced values indicate an abnormal response and may be due to • Primary adrenal insufficiency (the diseased adrenal gland is unable to respond to the ACTH) • Secondary adrenal insufficiency (the adrenal gland is usually atrophied from ACTH deficiency and is unable to respond to the ACTH)
Aldosterone **(Supine: 3–10 ng/dl; upright: 5–30 ng/dl)** Aldosterone levels may be used to • Assist in the diagnosis of aldosteronism and hypertension • Distinguish between primary and secondary adrenal insufficiency	Elevated values may be due to • Primary aldosteronism associated with disorders such as adrenal adenoma • Secondary aldosteronism associated with disorders such as nephrotic syndrome, renin-producing renal tumors, and excessive diuretic therapy or laxative abuse

Table continued on following page

TABLE 13–7 Common Laboratory Studies Used to Assist in the Diagnosis of Endocrine Disorders *Continued*

Description of Test and Reference Value	Clinical Significance
	Decreased values may be due to Primary adrenocortical insufficiency (Addison's disease)
Cortisol (AM: 5–23 μg/dl; PM: 3–13 μg/dl) Cortisol levels may be used to assist in the diagnosis of • Cushing's syndrome • Cushing's disease • Primary adrenocortical insufficiency • Secondary adrenocortical insufficiency	Elevated values may be due to • Cushing's syndrome (adrenocortical hyperfunction resulting from a primary adrenal dysfunction) • Cushing's disease (adrenocortical hyperfunction resulting from a pituitary or hypothalamic disorder that causes an increase in the production of glucocorticoids) • Severe physical and emotional stress • Pregnancy Decreased values may be due to • Primary adrenocortical insufficiency • Secondary adrenocortical insufficiency
Catecholamines *Epinephrine (Supine: <50 pg/ml)* *Norepinephrine (Supine: 110–410 pg/ml)* Catecholamine levels may be used to assist in the diagnosis of • Adrenal medullary pheochromocytomas • Extraadrenal pheochromocytomas	Elevated values may be due to • Pheochromocytoma • Hyperthyroidism • Prolonged stress response (sympathetic nervous system stimulation)

TABLE 13-7 Common Laboratory Studies Used to Assist in the Diagnosis of Endocrine Disorders *Continued*

Description of Test and Reference Value	Clinical Significance
Vanillylmandelic Acid (VMA) *(Urine: 2–7 mg/24 h)* VMA is a by-product of catecholamines that may be used to assist in the diagnosis of pheochromocytoma	Elevated levels of VMA may be due to pheochromocytoma
Glucagon *(50–100 pg/ml)* Glucagon levels may be used to assist in the diagnosis of • Pancreatic tumors • Chronic pancreatitis	Elevated values may be due to • Acute pancreatitis • Diabetic ketoacidosis • Hypoglycemia (as blood glucose levels drop, plasma glucagon levels rise as glucagon is secreted to promote the breakdown of stored glycogen and maintain gluconeogenesis to meet the glucose needs of the tissue) • Stress (glucagon is secreted in response to sympathetic nervous stimulation to promote glycogenolysis and gluconeogenesis to meet the increased glucose needs of the tissue) Decreased values may be due to • Chronic pancreatitis • Hyperglycemia
Glucose, Blood *(60–110 mg/dl)* Blood glucose levels may be used to assist in the diagnosis of • Diabetes mellitus • Hypoglycemia	Elevated values may be due to a decrease in insulin production associated with disorders such as • Diabetes mellitus

Table continued on following page

TABLE 13–7   Common Laboratory Studies Used to Assist in the Diagnosis of Endocrine Disorders *Continued*

Description of Test and Reference Value	Clinical Significance
	• Diabetic ketoacidosis • Hyperglycemic, hyperosmolar, nonketotic syndrome Decreased values may be due to an increase in the amount of circulating insulin associated with disorders such as • Hypoglycemia • Excessive replacement of insulin
Serum Osmolality (285–319 mOsm/kg) Serum osmolality, a measure of the number of particles such as electrolytes, urea, and glucose dissolved in the plasma, may be used to • Assist in the evaluation of fluid and electrolyte imbalances • Assist in the differential diagnosis of ADH abnormalities	Elevated values may be due to • Dehydration • Diabetes insipidus (DI) • Hyperglycemia • Hypernatremia • Hyperkalemia • Hypercalcemia (Elevated values associated with hemoconcentration related to dehydration may be accompanied by physical findings such as thirst, dry mucous membranes, skin tenting over the sternum, and flat neck veins in the horizontal position) Decreased values may be due to • Fluid overload • Syndrome of inappropriate ADH • Primary adrenocortical insufficiency • Hyponatremia (Decreased values associated with hemodilution related to

**TABLE 13–7 Common Laboratory Studies Used to Assist in the
Diagnosis of Endocrine Disorders** *Continued*

Description of Test and Reference Value	Clinical Significance
	overhydration may be accompanied by physical findings such as full and bounding pulses, crackles, distended neck veins, or headache and irritability related to water intoxication)

**Urine Osmolality
(50–1200 mOsm/kg H$_2$O)**

Urine osmolality may be used to

- Assist in evaluating the kidney's ability to concentrate or dilute urine
- Assist in the differential diagnosis of ADH abnormalities

Elevated values may be due to

- Dehydration (the urine osmolality increases as the urine output decreases)
- SIADH
- Primary adrenocortical insufficiency
- Hyperglycemia
- Hypernatremia
- Azotemia

Decreased values may be due to

- Fluid overload (the urine osmolality decreases as the urine output increases)
- DI
- Hypocalcemia
- Hyponatremia
- Acute renal failure
- Glomerulonephritis
- Sickle cell anemia

**Vasopressin (ADH)
(If serum osmolality 285–319
mOsm/kg, ADH 1–12 pg/ml)**

Serum ADH levels may be used to assist in the diagnosis of

Elevated levels may be due to

- SIADH

Table continued on following page

TABLE 13-7 Common Laboratory Studies Used to Assist in the Diagnosis of Endocrine Disorders *Continued*

Description of Test and Reference Value	Clinical Significance
<ul><li>SIADH</li><li>DI</li></ul>	<ul><li>Severe physical or emotional stress</li></ul> Decreased levels may be due to DI
Water-Deprivation Test A water-deprivation test may be used to assist in the diagnosis of DI	Normally, as fluid is withheld, the serum osmolality increases, the urine output decreases, and the urine osmolality increases: <ul><li>In the water-deprivation test, the normal response to the fluid restriction and increased serum osmolality is an increase in ADH secretion</li><li>In DI, little or no increase in ADH secretion occurs, resulting in little or no change in urine output (the patient will continue to excrete dilute urine)</li></ul>
Vasopressin Test A vasopressin test may be used to differentiate neurogenic DI from nephrogenic DI	An exogenous form of ADH (usually aqueous vasopressin) is administered <ul><li>An increase in urine osmolality indicates neurogenic DI</li><li>Little or no response to the exogenous hormone indicates nephrogenic DI</li></ul>
Thyroxine (T_4) **(Total T_4 5–12 μg/dl)** T_4 levels may be used to <ul><li>Assist in the evaluation of thyroid function</li></ul>	Elevated values may be due to <ul><li>Hyperthyroidism</li><li>Thyrotoxicosis</li></ul>

TABLE 13–7   Common Laboratory Studies Used to Assist in the Diagnosis of Endocrine Disorders *Continued*

Description of Test and Reference Value	Clinical Significance
<ul><li>Confirm the diagnosis of hyper- or hypothyroidism</li><li>Evaluate antithyroid medication therapy in hyperthyroidism</li><li>Evaluate replacement therapy in hypothyroidism</li></ul>	<ul><li>Acute thyroiditis</li></ul>Decreased values may be due to<ul><li>Primary hypothyroidism</li><li>Secondary hypothyroidism</li></ul>
Triiodothyronine (T_3) Resin Uptake (T_3RU) **(25%–35% of total)** T_3 resin uptake assesses the binding capacity of blood proteins for the hormone T_3 and may be used to<ul><li>Estimate the free thyroxine index</li><li>Assist in the diagnosis of hyper- and hypothyroidism</li></ul>	Elevated levels may be due to hyperthyroidism Decreased levels may be due to hypothyroidism
Free Thyroxine Index (FTI) **(1.3–4.2)** The FTI (product of the T_4 level and the T_3RU) may be used to assist in the evaluation of thyroid function	Elevated values may be due to hyperthyroidism Decreased values may be due to hypothyroidism
Thyrotropin or Thyroid-Stimulating Hormone (TSH) **(0.4–8.9 U/ml)** Thyrotropin levels may be used to<ul><li>Assist in the diagnosis of hypothyroidism</li><li>Distinguish between primary and secondary hypothyroidism</li><li>Evaluate replacement therapy in</li></ul>	Elevated levels may be due to primary hypothyroidism Decreased values may be due to<ul><li>Hypothalamic-pituitary dysfunction</li><li>Hyperthyroidism</li><li>Thyroiditis</li><li>Excessive exogenous replacement therapy</li><li>Secondary hypothyroidism</li></ul>

HEMATOLOGIC FUNCTION

Disorders of the hematopoietic system may be evaluated through the study of the cells of the blood, including erythrocytes, platelets, clotting factors, and plasma proteins (see Table 13–8).

TABLE 13–8   **Common Laboratory Studies Used to Assist in the Diagnosis of Hematologic Disorders**

Description of Test and Reference Value	Clinical Significance

Red Blood Cell (RBC) Count (Male: 4.6–6.2 × 10^6/μl; female: 4.5 × 10^6/μl)
 	
The RBC count may be used to
• Determine the total number of red blood cells
• Assist in the diagnosis of poly-cythemia and anemia
	Elevated values may be due to poly-cythemia (an excessive production of erythrocytes) related to condi-tions such as
	• Hyperactivity of the bone mar-row cells
	• Increased production of erythro-poietin, as in renal failure
	• Dehydration (hemoconcentration)
	Decreased values may be due to
	• Anemia (an excessive loss of erythrocytes) related to condi-tions such as
	  – Hemolysis
	  – Bone marrow dysfunction
	  – Recent blood loss or hemor-rhage
	  – Lack of erythropoietin (de-creased production of red blood cells)
	• Hemodilution (fluid retention or excessive administration of flu-ids in volume resuscitation)

TABLE 13–8 Common Laboratory Studies Used to Assist in the Diagnosis of Hematologic Disorders *Continued*

Description of Test and Reference Value

Clinical Significance

Hemoglobin (Hgb)
(Male: 13.5–18 g/dl;
  female: 12–16 g/dl)

The hemoglobin level may be used to
- Assist in the determination of oxygen transport
  - The heme molecule combines with oxygen in the lungs for transport to the cells
  - Oxygen is released at the cell level, and the globulin molecule combines with carbon dioxide for the return trip to the lungs
- Assist in the evaluation of polycythemia and anemia

Elevated values may be due to
- Polycythemia
- Dehydration (hemoconcentration)

Decreased values may be due to
- Anemia
- Hemolysis of RBCs
- Recent blood loss or hemorrhage (value may not drop for several hours after the bleeding episode)
- Hemodilution (fluid retention or excessive fluid replacement during volume resuscitation)

Physical findings associated with anemia may include pallor, dizziness, tachycardia, weakness, and dyspnea at rest related to the loss of erythrocytes, which decreases the oxygen-carrying capacity

Physical findings associated with severe blood loss may include thirst, restlessness, tachycardia, and tachypnea related to loss of blood volume and hypovolemia

Hematocrit (Hct)
(Male: 40%–54%;
  female: 36%–46%)

The hematocrit level may be used to assist in the evaluation of polycythemia, anemia, hemolytic anemia, blood loss, and dehydration

Elevated values may be due to
- Polycythemia
- Dehydration (reduction in fluid volume causes hemoconcentra-

Table continued on following page

TABLE 13–8 Common Laboratory Studies Used to Assist in the Diagnosis of Hematologic Disorders *Continued*

Description of Test and Reference Value	Clinical Significance
	tion and an increase in blood viscosity) Decreased values may be due to • Anemia • Hemolytic anemia • Hemorrhage (value may not drop for several hours after the bleeding episode) • Hemodilution (fluid retention or excessive fluid administration during volume resuscitation)
Platelet Count (150,000–400,000/μl) The platelet count may be used to • Evaluate platelet production by the bone marrow • Assess the destruction or loss of platelets in the circulation • Assess the effects of chemotherapy and radiation on platelet production and destruction	Elevated values (thrombocytosis) may be due to • Polycythemia vera • Cancers such as multiple myeloma, lymphomas, and chronic myelocytic leukemia • Chronic renal disease • Splenectomy • Acute or chronic infection • Inflammatory disease • Posthemorrhage regeneration Thrombocytosis places the critically ill adult at risk for possible hemorrhage related to defects in the platelets and the inability to form a clot, as well as thrombosis related to platelet aggregation and trapping of erythrocytes in the microcirculation Decreased values (thrombocytopenia) may be due to

**TABLE 13-8 Common Laboratory Studies Used to Assist in the
Diagnosis of Hematologic Disorders** *Continued*

Description of Test and Reference Value	Clinical Significance
	<ul><li>Disseminated intravascular coagulation (DIC; excessive coagulation defects)</li><li>Cardiac valve replacement (mechanical damage to platelets)</li><li>Massive blood transfusions (dilutional thrombocytopenia)</li><li>Anemias, including aplastic, megaloblastic, and severe iron deficiency (deficient platelet production)</li><li>Autoimmune processes (destruction of platelets by IgG antibodies)</li><li>Idiopathic thrombocytopenia purpura (widespread immune-mediated platelet aggregation causes microvascular thrombosis)</li><li>Infection infiltrates, congestion, and malignancy (abnormal distribution or pooling of platelets)</li><li>Radiation therapy</li><li>Chemotherapy</li><li>Liver disease</li><li>Thyroid disease</li></ul>Thrombocytopenia places the critically ill adult at risk for spontaneous hemorrhage, particularly cerebral, related to the compromised ability to form a clot

Table continued on following page

TABLE 13–8 Common Laboratory Studies Used to Assist in the Diagnosis of Hematologic Disorders *Continued*

Description of Test and Reference Value	Clinical Significance
Platelet Aggregation (Normally occurs in 3–5 minutes) The platelet aggregation test may be used to • Evaluate the ability of the platelets to adhere to one another and form a plug • Assist in the detection of a congenital or acquired platelet bleeding disorder	Elevated values may be due to Raynaud's phenomenon Decreased values may be due to • Leukemia • Liver disease • Uremia • Hypothyroidism • Macroglobulinemia • Myeloproliferative disorder
Prothrombin Time (PT) (11–15 seconds) The PT may be used to • Evaluate the extrinsic coagulation system • Assist in measuring the coagulation ability of or deficiency of factors I (fibrinogen), II (prothrombin), V, VII, and X • Evaluate oral anticoagulant therapy • Screen for vitamin K deficiency (prothrombin is a vitamin K–dependent clotting factor synthesized and removed by the liver) • Assist in the diagnosis of liver failure and DIC	Elevated values may be due to • Liver disease • Vitamin K deficiency • Deficiency of factor V, VII, or X • Deficiency of fibrinogen • Deficiency of prothrombin • DIC • Excessive anticoagulant therapy

TABLE 13-8 Common Laboratory Studies Used to Assist in the Diagnosis of Hematologic Disorders *Continued*

Description of Test and Reference Value	Clinical Significance
Partial Thromboplastin Time (PTT) (60–70 seconds) Activated Partial Thromboplastin Time (aPTT) (25–35 seconds) The PTT and aPTT (more sensitive than the PTT) may be used to • Assist in the evaluation of the coagulation system • Assist in the identification of congenital and acquired deficiencies of the intrinsic and extrinsic pathways of the coagulation system and inhibitors of the coagulation system (detects deficiencies in all clotting factors except VII and XIII) • Evaluate the effects of heparin anticoagulant therapy	Elevated values may be due to • Liver failure • Vitamin K deficiency • DIC • Deficiency of one or more coagulation factors • Excessive administration of heparin Decreased values may be due to • Hypercoagulable states (very early stages of DIC) • Acute hemorrhage
Fibrinogen (Factor I) (200–400 mg/dl) The fibrinogen level may be used to assist in the diagnosis of bleeding disorders, including DIC (fibrinogen produces the fibrin strands necessary for clot formation)	Elevated values may be due to • Acute injury • Inflammation • Infection • Malignancy Decreased values may be due to • Severe liver disease • DIC • Recent trauma

Table continued on following page

TABLE 13–8 Common Laboratory Studies Used to Assist in the Diagnosis of Hematologic Disorders *Continued*	
Description of Test and Reference Value	**Clinical Significance**

Fibrin Split Products
(<10 μg/ml)

Fibrin split products may be used to
- Assist in the diagnosis of DIC
- Assist in the evaluation of disorders that produce clot formation and lysis of the clot

Elevated values may be due to
- DIC
- Myocardial infarction
- Pulmonary embolism
- Liver disease
- Infection
- Inflammation

D-Dimer Test
(Latex Beads: <250 ng/ml);
Enzyme-Linked Immunosorbent Assay (ELISA)
(No D-dimer fragments present)

The D-Dimer test may be used to
- Screen for DVT
- Assist in the diagnosis of DIC
- Assist in determining the presence of a clot in acute myocardial infarction and unstable angina
- Assist in the diagnosis of hypercoagulable conditions causing recurrent thrombosis

Elevated values (the presence of D-Dimer fragments, which are fragments of fibrin that are formed as a result of fibrin degradation and clot lysis) may be due to
- DIC
- Thrombotic diseases such as DVT, pulmonary embolism, and arterial thromboembolism
- Malignancy
- Surgery

IMMUNOLOGIC FUNCTION

Disorders of the immune system may be evaluated through the study of leukocytes (see Table 13–9).

TABLE 13-9 Common Laboratory Studies Used to Assist in the Diagnosis of Immunologic Disorders

Description of Test and Reference Value	Clinical Significance
White Blood Cell (WBC) Count (5,000–10,000/μl) WBC levels may be used to • Assist in the identification and severity of infection or inflammation • Assess the bone marrow's response to radiation therapy and chemotherapy	Elevated values (leukocytosis) may be due to • Bacterial infection • Tissue necrosis associated with disorders such as acute myocardial infarction, burns, and gangrene • Inflammation • Leukemia • Lymphomas Decreased values may be due to • Bone marrow depression • Exhaustive infection • Viral infections such as influenza
White Blood Cell Differential *Neutrophils (50%–70%)* Neutrophils respond to inflammatory tissue damage and infection (body's first line of defense)	Elevated values (neutrophilia) may be due to • Acute infections (localized or systemic) • Inflammatory disorders such as rheumatoid arthritis, pancreatitis, nephritis • Tissue damage, including acute myocardial infarction, burns, crush injuries, and extensive surgery Decreased values (neutropenia) may be due to • Viral infection

Table continued on following page

TABLE 13-9 Common Laboratory Studies Used to Assist in the Diagnosis of Immunologic Disorders *Continued*

Description of Test and Reference Value	Clinical Significance
	• Bone marrow depression • Anemia (aplastic and iron deficiency)
Eosinophils (1%–3%) Eosinophils respond to allergic and parasitic infections, as well as to some malignancies, infections, inflammations, and tissue necrosis	Elevated values (eosinophilia) may be due to • Allergic disorders • Parasitic infections • Cancer • Renal disease • Asthma • Emphysema • Phlebitis • Thrombophlebitis Decreased values (eosinopenia) may be due to stress related to disorders such as burns, shock, trauma, surgery, and adrenocortical hyperfunction
Basophils (0.4%–1%) Basophils are involved in systemic allergic reactions and atelectasis, as well as the healing process of inflammation (during an acute episode of inflammation, basophils release histamine, serotonin, and heparin into the circulation)	Elevated values (basophilia) may be due to • Inflammatory process • Hypersensitivity reactions to food, drugs, inhalants, or foreign protein injections • Healing phase of inflammation • Hemolytic anemia • Myeloid leukemia • Hodgkin's disease Decreased values (basopenia) may be due to

TABLE 13–9 Common Laboratory Studies Used to Assist in the Diagnosis of Immunologic Disorders *Continued*

Description of Test and Reference Value	Clinical Significance
	• Hyperthyroidism • Stress • Acute infection
Lymphocytes (25%–35%) Lymphocytes are involved in the response to infection as well as the immune response (B lymphocytes and T lymphocytes)	Elevated values (lymphocytosis) may be due to • Infections, including mononucleosis, viral hepatitis, viral pneumonia, cytomegalovirus infection, and acute HIV infection • Lymphocytic leukemia Decreased values (lymphopenia) may be due to • Renal failure • Immunological deficiency disorders associated with decreased T lymphocytes • Impaired lymphatic drainage
Monocytes (4%–6%) Monocytes are the body's second line of defense against infection and foreign substances (once in circulation, they become macrophages capable of phagocytosis, similar to neutrophils)	Elevated levels (monocytosis) may be due to • Infections (bacterial, viral, mycotic, rickettsial, and protozoan) • Leukemias • Collagen diseases Decreased levels (monocytopenia) may be due to • Bone marrow dysfunction • Aplastic anemia

14

Bedside Monitoring Techniques

RESPIRATORY MONITORING

Pulse Oximetry

Pulse oximetry is a noninvasive method of measuring SaO_2. A sensor is applied to any site that is a pulsating vascular bed (most commonly the finger). A photodetector determines the percentage of arterial oxygen saturation by measuring light absorption based on the percentages of hemoglobin and oxyhemoglobin in the blood. When the measured SaO_2 level is greater than 70%, the SaO_2 level recorded by the pulse oximeter shows a high degree of accuracy.

Continuous monitoring of SaO_2 levels in the critically ill adult may be used to

- Assist in the calculation of oxygen delivery (DO_2), oxygen consumption ($\dot{V}O_2$), and oxygen extraction parameters (see Table 14–1)
- Evaluate the critically ill adult's response to treatments and therapeutic interventions, including adjustments in FIO_2 levels and weaning from mechanical ventilation
- Guide adaptations in nursing interventions, including endotracheal suctioning and repositioning
- Detect hypoxemic episodes and increasing intrapulmonary shunts (see Chapter 13 for information relating to $\dot{Q}s/\dot{Q}t$)

TABLE 14–1 Parameters of Oxygen Delivery and Consumption

Parameter	Formula	Normal Range
Oxygen delivery (Do_2): The amount of oxygen delivered to the tissues each minute	$CI \times Hgb \times 13.4 \times Sao_2$	550–650 ml/min/m²
Oxygen consumption ($\dot{V}o_2$): The amount of oxygen used by the tissues per minute	$CI \times Hgb \times 13.4 \times (Sao_2 - S\bar{v}o_2)$	110–150 ml/min/m²
Oxygen extraction ratio (O_2ER): Compares the amount of oxygen consumed to the amount of oxygen delivered	$\dot{V}o_2/Do_2$	20%–30%

Clinical Findings Associated with Tissue Hypoxia

Clinical findings reflecting tissue hypoxia may include

- Physical findings such as
  - Anxiety, restlessness, and confusion related to cerebral ischemia (may lead to behavioral changes such as agitation, aggression, combativeness, and refusal to cooperate with treatments, which may compound the problem)
  - Dyspnea and decreased respiratory excursion related to hypoxic respiratory muscles that become fatigued and weak
  - Tachycardia related to the compensatory effort to increase oxygen delivery to the cells
  - Decreased urine output related to renal tubular ischemia
- Laboratory findings such as
  - An increase in the base deficit (see Chapter 13)
  - An elevated serum lactate level (see Chapter 13)
- Hemodynamic findings such as
  - A decrease in stroke volume related to myocardial ischemia and decreased ventricular compliance (see Hemodynamic Monitoring below)

– May or may not have hypotension (compensatory responses
   may maintain blood pressure)
– A decrease in the mean arterial pressure (see Hemodynamic
   Monitoring below)
– Increased pulmonary artery pressures related to pulmonary
   hypertension secondary to constricted pulmonary arteries (see
   Hemodynamic Monitoring below)

POINT TO REMEMBER

▶ Factors such as severe hypotension, severe anemia, blood pressure cuffs, vasoconstrictive drugs, shivering, movement, and
  lack of a pulse in the extremity may interfere with the accuracy
  of the reading.

Mixed Venous Oxygen Saturation

Mixed venous oxygen saturation ($S\bar{v}O_2$) is monitored invasively
with a special pulmonary artery catheter. Light-transmitting fiberop-
tics incorporated in the catheter emit light into the mixed venous blood
in the pulmonary artery. Red blood cells reflect light according to the
oxygen saturation of the hemoglobin.

DO_2 and $\dot{V}O_2$

As discussed in Chapter 13, hemoglobin binds with oxygen in the
lungs and is transported to the tissues (DO_2) with a normal arterial saturation close to 100%. At the tissue level, hemoglobin unloads about
25% of the oxygen (normal oxygen extraction rate) to meet the oxygen consumption ($\dot{V}O_2$) rate of the cells and returns to the heart approximately 75% saturated. The normal range of oxygen saturation of
venous blood is 60% to 80%.

Alterations in DO_2 and $\dot{V}O_2$

A variety of compensatory mechanisms function to maintain the
balance between oxygen DO_2 and $\dot{V}O_2$. For example, with physical exercise and increased muscle activity, the sympathetic nervous system
is stimulated, and DO_2 is increased to meet the increased $\dot{V}O_2$ rate of
the cells. If DO_2 is decreased, a compensatory increase in oxygen extraction functions to maintain cellular oxygenation needs and maintain
a constant $\dot{V}O_2$ rate. However, when DO_2 is critically decreased, oxygen extraction may reach its maximum level, and $\dot{V}O_2$ may be limited

to less than tissue demands. When $\dot{V}O_2$ fails to meet oxygen demands, cells revert to anaerobic metabolism.

Alterations in $S\bar{v}O_2$

Because changes in the oxygen extraction ratio (O_2ER) or the ratio between $\dot{V}O_2$ and DO_2 (see Table 14–1) may be reflected by variations in the $S\bar{v}O_2$ (as oxygen extraction increases, the $S\bar{v}O_2$ decreases, and as oxygen extraction decreases, the $S\bar{v}O_2$ increases) in the critically ill adult, continuous monitoring of the $S\bar{v}O_2$ may be used to track changes in the balance between DO_2 and $\dot{V}O_2$. For example:

- Conditions such as fever, shivering, anxiety, pain, infection, and increased work of breathing may increase the metabolic rate and $\dot{V}O_2$
- Compounding the problem, routine nursing care such as suctioning and position changes can significantly increase oxygen demand
- Because of compromised pulmonary and cardiovascular systems, many of these critically ill adults may be unable to increase DO_2 to meet increased oxygen demands
- When demand exceeds DO_2, or DO_2 is critically decreased, the tissues extract a greater percentage of oxygen to meet consumption needs, which may reduce the $S\bar{v}O_2$

Decreased $S\bar{v}O_2$ Value. A declining $S\bar{v}O_2$ may be an indication that the cellular demand for oxygen is exceeding the critically ill adult's ability to keep up with the supply. There may be an increase in $\dot{V}O_2$, or there may be a decrease in DO_2.

Elevated $S\bar{v}O_2$ Values. A rising $S\bar{v}O_2$ may reflect

- A decreased demand, indicating that the critically ill adult's condition is improving
- The development of a left-to-right ventricular shunt associated with a condition such as rupture of the interventricular septum
- An indication that the critically ill adult is experiencing decreased $\dot{V}O_2$ related to
  - A decrease in the metabolic rate associated with conditions such as hypothermia
  - Precapillary shunting such as seen in sepsis (the demand for oxygen may be high, but cellular disturbances in oxygen utilization may decrease consumption)

▶ $S\bar{v}O_2$ results should not be interpreted in isolation but rather trended and carefully evaluated with the clinical presentation of the patient.

▶ Measurements of other parameters, including the cardiac output (CO) or cardiac index (CI), the SaO_2, hemoglobin level, and the serum lactate level should be simultaneously examined to provide meaningful data about tissue oxygenation and assist in determining which factor in DO_2 and $\dot{V}O_2$ is abnormal.

Capnography

Exhaled CO_2 may be monitored with an infrared gas analyzer. The CO_2 gas analyzer may be attached to the exhalation tubing of the ventilator. The infrared light passes across the exhaled CO_2. The recorded value corresponds to the amount of light absorbed by the exhaled breath. The more light absorbed, the higher the reading and the higher the CO_2 level.

Changes in CO_2 elimination during a single exhalation are recorded in a waveform called a capnogram (see Fig. 14–1). As exhalation proceeds, there is a rapid rise in CO_2 levels followed by a plateau near the end of expiration, which remains until the onset of inspiration. The CO_2 is measured at the end of exhalation, because when gas exchange in the lungs is normal, the exhaled CO_2 (end-tidal CO_2, or $PETCO_2$) should approximate the arterial CO_2. The $PaCO_2$ is usually slightly higher than the $PETCO_2$. However, with normal pulmonary blood flow, the $PaCO_2$-$PETCO_2$ gradient should be less than 5 mm Hg.

In the critically ill adult, continuous monitoring of exhaled CO_2 may be used to

• Evaluate alveolar ventilation (in the presence of normal $\dot{V}/\dot{Q}$ relationships, alveolar and arterial CO_2 levels should be nearly equal)

• Assist in the evaluation of ventilator parameters and weaning changes (if the $PETCO_2$ increases, respiratory acidosis may be developing)

• Confirm endotracheal intubation (minimal amounts of CO_2 should be detected with esophageal placement)

• Assess the adequacy of cardiopulmonary resuscitation (a reduction in pulmonary blood flow is associated with inadequate clearance of CO_2 and lower $PETCO_2$ levels)

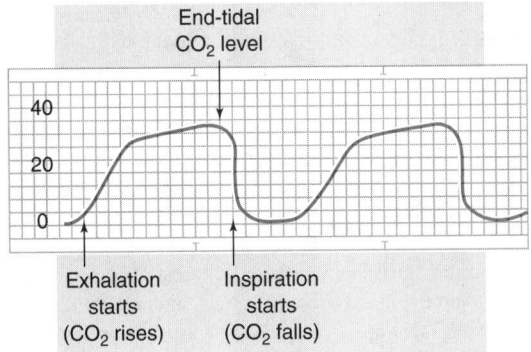

FIGURE 14–1

Capnograph tracing. On exhalation the capnograph tracing shows a rapid rise in carbon dioxide followed by a plateau. At the end of exhalation, the end-tidal carbon dioxide level is obtained. As inspiration begins, there is a dramatic decrease in carbon dioxide. (From Malarkey, L. M., & McMorrow, M. E. [1996]. *Nurse's manual of laboratory tests and diagnostic procedures* [p. 290]. Philadelphia: W. B. Saunders.)

Gastric Tonometry

The pH of the gastric mucosa is measured by inserting a nasogastric tube with a CO_2-permeable silicone balloon into the stomach. The balloon is filled with normal saline and left in contact with the gastric mucosa for 30 to 90 minutes to permit CO_2 to move into the balloon. When the CO_2 between the saline in the balloon and the gastric mucosa has had sufficient time to equalize, the saline is removed and sent to the laboratory with a blood gas sample. The saline PCO_2 is measured and used as the intramucosal PCO_2. The blood gas sample is used to determine the bicarbonate concentration, and then the Henderson-Hasselbalch equation is used to compute the intramucosal pH.

In the critically ill adult, gastric tonometry may be used to assist in determining the oxygenation status of the tissues. When DO_2 is compromised, splanchnic hypoperfusion occurs as blood is shunted away from the gastrointestinal tract to increase cardiac filling pressures and preserve the function of vital organs such as the heart and brain. An acidotic intramucosal pH (<7.32) may be an indication that the critically ill adult is at risk for cellular hypoxia and possible multiple organ dysfunction.

HEMODYNAMIC MONITORING

A fluid-filled, pressurized transducer system and catheters placed in the systemic arteries, superior vena cava, and pulmonary artery may be used to assist in the evaluation of the hemodynamic status of the critically ill adult. The waveforms and pressures obtained may provide valuable information about arterial blood pressure (BP), central venous pressure (CVP), right atrial pressure (RAP), pulmonary artery pressure (PAP), pulmonary capillary wedge pressure (PCWP), cardiac output (CO), cardiac index (CI), stroke volume index (SVI), pulmonary vascular resistance (PVR), systemic vascular resistance (SVR), right ventricular stroke work index, and left ventricular stroke work index (see Table 14–2), as well as parameters used in respiratory monitoring, including $S\overline{v}O_2$, DO_2, $\dot{V}O_2$, and O_2ER (see Table 14–1).

POINTS TO REMEMBER

▶ Variations in the waveforms and pressures obtained may be attributed to physiologic or technical factors as well as a variety of therapeutic interventions, including mechanical ventilation and positive end-expiratory pressure (PEEP).

▶ Because alterations in the intrathoracic pressure affect the measurement of intravascular pressures, these pressures should be measured at end-expiration.

▶ Transducers (and water manometers if used for central venous pressure) should be leveled to the phlebostatic axis (fourth intercostal space, midaxillary line) to avoid inaccurate pressure readings.

▶ Hemodynamic parameters should not be interpreted in isolation, but rather trended and carefully evaluated in conjunction with laboratory studies such as arterial blood gases and serum lactate levels.

▶ In addition hemodynamic parameters should be correlated with the critically ill adult's physical assessment findings:

   – For example, physical assessment findings such as distended neck veins and peripheral edema are noninvasive clinical observations that may indicate that blood is not moving forward from the right side of the heart to the left side of the heart as it should.

   – A correlating hemodynamic parameter may be an elevation in the right ventricular end-diastolic pressure or CVP (see Fig. 14–2).

TABLE 14-2 Hemodynamic Parameters

Parameter	Normal Range	Formula
Arterial blood pressure		
• Systolic (SP)	100–140 mm Hg	
• Diastolic (DP)	60–90 mm Hg	
• Mean (MAP)	70–105 mm Hg	$MAP = \dfrac{[(2)(DP)] + (SP)}{3}$
Central venous pressure (CVP)	4–7 cm H_2O	
Right atrial pressure (RAP)	–1–7 mm Hg	
Pulmonary artery pressure		
• Systolic (PAS)	15–25 mm Hg	
• Diastolic (PAD)	8–15 mm Hg	
• Mean (PAM)	10–20 mm Hg	$PAM = \dfrac{[(PAD)|(2)|] + PAS}{3}$
Pulmonary capillary wedge pressure (PCWP)	6–12 mm Hg	
Cardiac output (CO)	4–8 L/min	
Cardiac index (CI)	2.5–4.5 L/min/m²	CI = CO/BSA*
Stroke volume (SV)	60–130 ml/beat	
Stroke volume index (SVI)	40–50 ml/beat/m²	SVI = SV/BSA

*BSA = body surface area.

Table continued on following page

TABLE 14–2 Hemodynamic Parameters *Continued*

Parameter	Normal Range	Formula
Pulmonary vascular resistance (PVR)	150–250 dyne/s/cm^{-5}	$PVR = \dfrac{PAM - PCWP}{CO} \times 80$†
Pulmonary vascular resistance index (PVRI)	160–280 dyne/s/cm^{-5}/m^2	$PVRI = \dfrac{PAM - PCWP}{CI} \times 80$
Systemic vascular resistance (SVR)	800–1500 dyne/s/cm^{-5}	$SVR = \dfrac{MAP - RAP}{CO} \times 80$
Systemic vascular resistance index (SVRI)	1970–2390 dyne/s/cm^{-5}/m^2	$SVRI = \dfrac{MAP - RAP}{CI} \times 80$
Right ventricular stroke work index (RVSWI)	5–10 g/beat/m^2	$RVSWI = SVI \, (PAM - RAP)$‡ $\times 0.0136$§
Left ventricular stroke work index (LVSWI)	45–65 g/beat/m^2	$LVSWI = SVI \, (MAP - PCWP) \times 0.0136$

†80 = conversion factor.
‡CVP may be substituted for RAP.
§0.0136 = conversion factor.

Correlation of Hemodynamic Parameters and Physical Assessment Findings

Disorder	RA	PA	PCWP	LA	CO	BP	SVR	Physical assessment findings may include:
Left ventricular failure	→↑	PAD↑	↑	↑	→↓	→↓	↑	Tachycardia, crackles, S3, S4, cough productive of pink frothy sputum (see CF 5-1)
Right ventricular failure	↑	↑↓↑	→↓↑ PAD↑	→↓↑	→↓	→↓	↑	Tachycardia, distended neck veins, positive HJR, peripheral edema (see CF 5-2)
Mitral regurgitation	↑	↑	PAD↑	↑	→↓	→↓	↑	Giant V waves in PCWP, systolic murmur (see CF 5-1)
Pericardial tamponade	↑	↑	↑	↑	↓	↓	↑	Tachycardia, distended neck veins, pulsus paradoxus, muffled heart sounds, decreased ECG amplitude
Pulmonary embolism	→↑	→↓↑	→↑	→↑	→↓	→↑↓	↑	Crackles, wheezes, churning noise over right ventricle, pleural friction rub, increased intensity of S2 or fixed splitting of S2 (see CF 4-1)
Hypovolemic shock	↓	→↓↑	↓	↓	→↑↓	→↑↓	↑	Tachycardia, flat neck veins in the horizontal position, pale or cyanotic skin, cool and clammy skin (see CF 12-3)
Cardiogenic shock	↑	↑	↑	↑	↓	↓	↑	Tachycardia, distended neck veins, cool and clammy skin, S3, S4, crackles, peripheral edema (see CF 12-3)
Septic shock (early)	↓	↓	↓	↓	→↑	↓	↓	Tachycardia, warm and flushed skin, fever, edema, full and bounding pulses
Septic shock (advanced)	↓↑	↓	→↑	↓↑	↓	↓	↑	Tachycardia, cool and clammy skin, peripheral edema (see CF 12-3)
Anaphylactic shock	↓	↓	↓	↓	↓	↓	↓	Tachycardia, rash, swelling (see CF 12-3)
Neurogenic shock	↓	→↓	↓	↓	↓	↓	↓	Bradycardia, decreased bowel sounds, atonic bladder, impaired temperature regulation (see CF 6-7 and CF 12-3)

→ Normal   ↓ Decreased   ↑ Increased

RA=right atrial   PCWP=pulmonary capillary wedge pressure   BP=blood pressure
PA=pulmonary artery   LA=left atria   CO=cardiac output   SVR=systematic vascular resistance

FIGURE 14-2

Correlation of hemodynamic parameters and physical assessment findings.

▶ In the elderly, critically ill adult, alterations in hemodynamic parameters may be a combination of normal and pathologic changes (see Chapter 5, Function of the Cardiovascular System: Changes with Aging). Hemodynamic parameters should be cautiously evaluated with physical findings to avoid inaccurate interpretations.

Arterial Blood Pressure

Direct measurement of arterial blood pressure is the most reliable method of monitoring blood pressure in the hemodynamically unstable critically ill adult. Cuff measurements may show a high degree of error because vasoconstriction and low flow states may obliterate the Korotkoff sounds (see Table 5–1, Physical Examination: Blood Pressure for related information).

Waveform

Monitoring of intra-arterial blood pressure is achieved through cannulation of a systemic artery (usually the radial, brachial, or femoral). The normal arterial waveform should show a rounded peak reflecting systole, and a dicrotic notch reflecting closure of the aortic valve and the onset of diastole (see Fig. 14–3).

Variations in the waveform may reflect damping related to factors such as a catheter tip lodged against the vessel wall, air bubbles in the system, or systolic amplification. The catheter may have to be repositioned, or the system flushed, to improve the waveform and pressure reading. Using noncompliant tubing that is restricted in length from the catheter to the transducer may minimize systolic amplification of the pressure wave.

Mean Arterial Pressure

Blood pressure is the product of cardiac output and systemic vascular resistance. During systole, as blood is ejected from the ventricle into the aorta, pressure is exerted on the aortic and major arterial walls. This pressure is known as the systolic blood pressure. During diastole, passive recoil of the aorta and minimum pressure in the arterioles permits blood to flow into the peripheral arteries. The diameter of the arterioles contributes to the diastolic pressure and offers the greatest resistance to blood flow, or systemic vascular resistance (SVR). The mean arterial pressure (see Table 14–2) reflects the average pressure in the vascular system throughout the cardiac cycle. ·

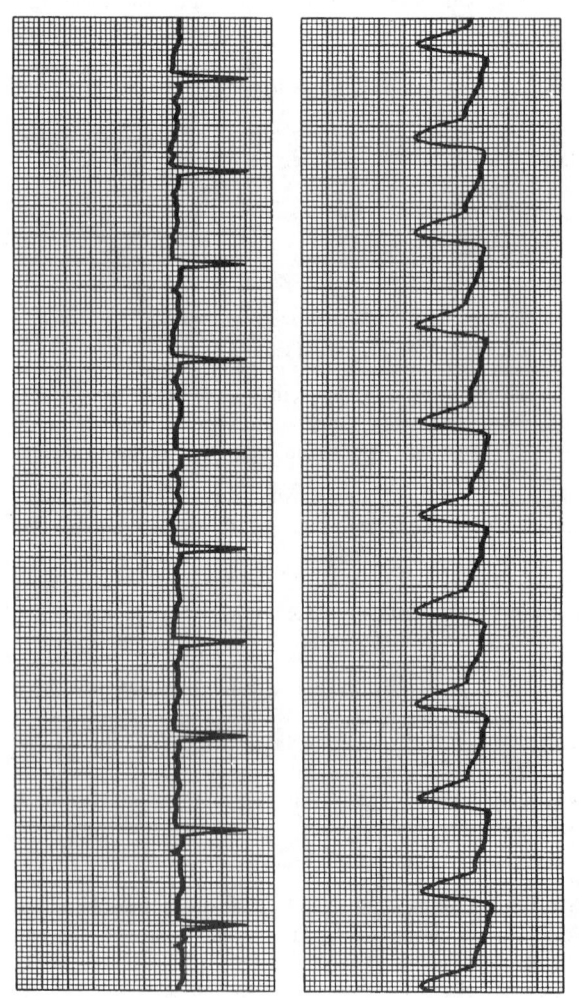

FIGURE 14-3

Intra-arterial pressure waveform with simultaneous electrocardiogram. (From Clochesy, J. M., Breu, C., Cardin, S., Whittaker, A. A., & Rudy, E. B. [Eds.]. [1996]. *Critical care nursing* [2nd ed., p. 20]. Philadelphia: W. B. Saunders.)

Alterations in Blood Pressure

Variations in numerous factors including heart rate, stroke volume, the elasticity and diameter of the arterial vessels, the sympathetic nervous system, and chemical mediators can influence the blood pressure.

Hypotension. In the critically ill adult, hypotensive values may be related to

- A decrease in cardiac output associated with hypovolemic or cardiogenic shock states
- A decrease in systemic vascular resistance associated with anaphylactic and septic shock states
- Disorders such as aortic stenosis

Physical Findings Associated with Hypotension. Physical findings associated with hypotension may include

- Confusion, restlessness, anxiety, increased respirations, tachycardia, cool extremities, peripheral cyanosis, capillary refill >2 seconds, sluggish bowel sounds, and decreased urine output

Clinical findings, including hypotension, vary with the shock state and may not be apparent in the initial stage of the shock syndrome (see Clinical Findings 12–3).

Hypertension. In the critically ill adult, hypertensive values may be related to

- High cardiac output states such as anemia, fever, and thyrotoxicosis
- Increased systemic vascular resistance associated with sympathetic nervous system stimulation
- Increased systemic vascular resistance associated with disorders such as arteriosclerosis and renal failure
- Disorders such as aortic insufficiency

Physical Findings Associated with Hypertension. Physical findings associated with hypertension may include headache, flushed skin, and full and bounding pulses.

POINTS TO REMEMBER

▶ Compensatory mechanisms, including sympathetic nervous system stimulation, may profoundly increase systemic vascular re-

sistance to maintain blood pressure during shock states (see Chapter 12).

▶ In hemodynamically unstable patients, the mean arterial pressure may give a more accurate reflection of arterial pressure and blood flow.

Central Venous Pressure

The central venous pressure (CVP) may be measured with a catheter inserted through the venous system into the right atrium and then attached to a water manometer and a conventional intravenous system, or with a flow-directed pulmonary artery catheter attached to a fluid-filled, pressurized, transducer monitoring system (see right atrial pressure).

Right Atrial Pressure

In the absence of a valvular obstruction between the right atrium and the right ventricle, the right atrial pressure (RAP) approximates the right ventricular end-diastolic pressure (RVEDP). RVEDP is reflected in the right atrial pressure because the open tricuspid valve permits atrial and ventricular pressures to equilibrate.

Waveform

Components of the RAP waveform (see Fig. 14–4) include the three positive waves, the A, C, and V waves. The A wave correlates with the PR interval on the ECG and reflects right atrial systole. The C wave correlates with the RT interval and reflects the bulging of the tricuspid valve into the right atrium with ventricular systole. The V wave correlates with the TP interval and reflects right atrial filling.

Abnormal wave forms include

- Absent A waves with atrial fibrillation
- Large A waves with increased resistance to right atrial emptying associated with disorders such as tricuspid stenosis, right ventricular hypertrophy, and a noncompliant right ventricle
- Giant A waves with contraction of the right atrium against a closed tricuspid valve, which may occur with dysrhythmias such as junctional rhythm, heart block, and ventricular irregularities
- Large V waves related to tricuspid regurgitation

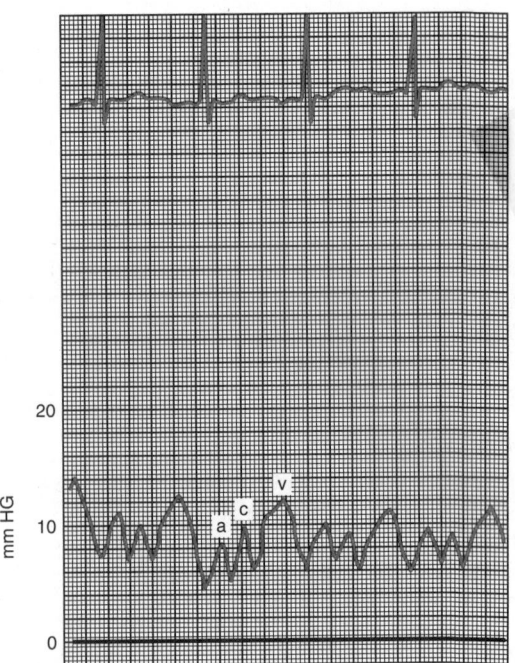

FIGURE 14–4
Right atrial pressure waveform with simultaneous ECG. (Adapted from Daily, E. K., & Schroeder, J. S. [1994]. *Techniques in bedside hemodynamic monitoring* [5th ed.]. St. Louis: Mosby.)

Alterations in RAP

The RAP varies with changes in the relationships between the amount of blood returning to the right atrium, blood volume distribution, and the function of the right ventricle.

Elevated RAP Values. In the critically ill adult, an elevated right atrial pressure may be caused by

- Volume overload associated with conditions such as the over-zealous administration of intravenous fluids and disorders such as renal failure

- An increase in venous return to the heart related to compensatory vasoconstriction and the redistribution of blood volume to maintain cardiac output (vasoconstrictive drug therapy may also increase venous return)
- Constriction of the pericardium related to constrictive disorders such as pericardial effusion and tamponade
- Right ventricular failure
  - Right ventricular failure is often systolic failure characterized by a decrease in contractility (see Chapter 5 for related information on systolic and diastolic heart failure, and Clinical Findings 5–2 for related information on right heart failure).
  - Impaired contractility leads to incomplete ventricular emptying (a decrease in the right ventricular ejection fraction), a decrease in the stroke volume, and an increase in the end-diastolic volume.
  - The decrease in contractility may be secondary to numerous disorders, including left ventricular failure (see Clinical Findings 5–1), right ventricular infarction (see Clinical Findings 5–3), ventricular septal defect, tricuspid or pulmonic valve disease (see Chapter 5), and pulmonary hypertension associated with disorders such as ARDS (see Clinical Findings 4–1), COPD (see Clinical Findings 4–8), and pulmonary embolism (see Clinical Findings 4–7).

Physical Findings Associated with an Elevated RAP. Physical findings associated with an increase in RAP may include

- Distended neck veins, peripheral edema, anasarca, positive hepatojugular reflex (HJR), hepatomegaly, and ascites related to an increase in the RAP and venous congestion.
- Other findings related to the etiology of the increase in the RAP may include murmurs, extra heart sounds such as an S_3 or an S_4, muffled heart sounds, crackles, wheezes, tachypnea, dyspnea, hypotension, and hypertension

Decreased RAP Values. In the critically ill adult, a decreased right atrial pressure is usually caused by a decrease in volume load or venous return to the heart associated with hypovolemia or vasodilation.

- Hypovolemia may be related to numerous disorders (see Section II) that may lead to hemorrhage, diuresis, prolonged vomiting or diarrhea, or a redistribution of blood volume from the vascular to the interstitial spaces.

- Vasodilation may be related to disorders such as the systemic inflammatory response syndrome, anaphylactic or neurogenic shock (see Chapter 12), and therapeutic interventions such as vasodilating drug therapy.

Physical Findings Associated with a Decrease in RAP. Physical findings associated with a decrease in RAP are generally related to the etiology of hypotension or vasodilation and may include flat neck veins in the horizontal position, restlessness, thirst, dry mucous membranes, increased respiratory rate, tachycardia (bradycardia with neurogenic shock), and hypotension.

POINTS TO REMEMBER

▶ The CVP or RAP is often used clinically as an indicator of right ventricular volume or preload (preload is defined as the amount of blood in the ventricle at the end of diastole, the ventricular filling pressure, or the distending force that stretches the ventricles just prior to contraction).

▶ However, with conditions such as myocardial ischemia or pericardial tamponade where ventricular compliance (the ability of the ventricle to distend and fill during diastole) is decreased, the CVP or RAP may not be an accurate reflection of end-diastolic volume (see Pulmonary Capillary Wedge Pressure below for further explanation).

Pulmonary Artery Pressure

The pulmonary artery pressure (RAP) is a product of right ventricular contraction and pulmonary vascular resistance (PVR).

Waveform

Components of the PAP waveform (see Fig. 14–5) include the peak systolic pressure (PAS), which represents right ventricular contraction and occurs after the QRS complex on the ECG, the dicrotic notch, which reflects closure of the pulmonic valve, and the diastolic pressure (PAD), which represents the PVR.

Alterations in the PAP

The pulmonary artery pressure may reflect changes in the volume of blood in the pulmonary vasculature as well as changes in pulmonary vascular resistance.

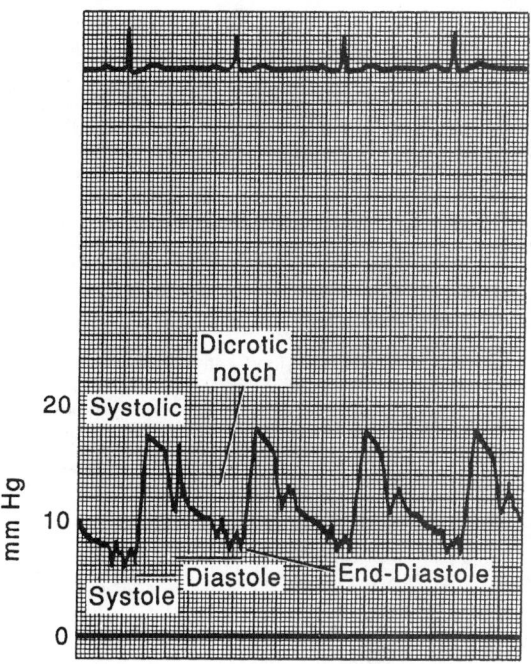

FIGURE 14–5
Pulmonary artery waveform with simultaneous ECG. (Adapted from Daily, E. K., & Schroeder, J. S. [1994]. *Techniques in bedside hemodynamic monitoring* [5th ed.]. St Louis: Mosby.)

Elevated PAP Values. In the critically ill adult, elevated pulmonary artery pressures may be caused by

- An increase in pulmonary blood volume related to hypervolemia
- An increase in pulmonary blood volume related to the backward effects of left ventricular failure and cardiogenic shock (see Chapters 5 and 12)
- The constrictive effects of disorders such as pericardial tamponade or constrictive pericarditis (see Chapter 5)
- An increase in pulmonary vascular resistance related to hypoxemia and disorders such as pulmonary embolism, ARDS, and COPD (see Chapter 4)

Physical Findings Associated with an Increase in PAP. Physical findings associated with an increase in pulmonary artery pressures may include

- Dyspnea, crackles, wheezes, and distended neck veins
- Other findings related to the etiology of the increase in pulmonary artery pressures may include murmurs, extra heart sounds such as S_3 and S_4, hypertension or hypotension, and tachycardia

Decreased PAP Values. In the critically ill adult, decreased pulmonary artery pressures may be caused by

- A decrease in pulmonary blood volume related to hypovolemia or vasodilation
- Right ventricular failure
- Pulmonary stenosis

Physical Findings Associated with a Decrease in PAP. Physical findings associated with a decrease in pulmonary artery pressures are generally related to the etiology.

POINTS TO REMEMBER

▶ In the absence of increased PVR and valvular disease or obstruction, the PAD pressure should correlate with the pulmonary capillary wedge pressure (PCWP).

▶ When the PVR is elevated, for example, in disorders such as ARDS and COPD, the PAD will be higher than the PCWP.

▶ A normal PAS pressure with an elevated PAD pressure may reflect disorders such as left ventricular failure and mitral regurgitation.

Pulmonary Capillary Wedge Pressure

The pulmonary capillary wedge pressure (PCWP) is measured with the balloon on the tip of the pulmonary artery catheter inflated. When the pulmonary artery catheter is properly positioned (below the level of the left atrium) and the balloon is inflated, in the absence of a valvular obstruction between the left atrium and the left ventricle, the PCWP should approximate the left atrial pressure and the left ventricular end-diastolic pressure (LVEDP). This is because, under these conditions, an open channel of blood exists from the left heart back to the pulmonary artery.

Waveform

Components of the PCWP waveform (see Fig. 14–6) include two positive waves, the A and the V wave. The A wave correlates with the QRS complex on the ECG and reflects left atrial contraction. The V wave follows the T wave on the ECG (occurs during the TP interval) and reflects bulging of the mitral valve during left ventricular systole and left atrial filling. Abnormal waveforms include

- Absent A waves with atrial fibrillation
- Large A waves with an increase in resistance to left atrial emptying associated with disorders such as mitral stenosis, left ventricular hypertrophy, and a noncompliant left ventricle

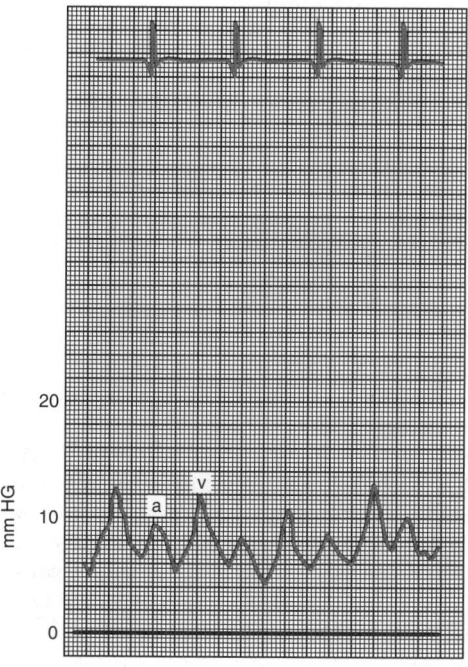

FIGURE 14–6
Pulmonary capillary wedge pressure waveform with simultaneous ECG. (Adapted from Daily, E. K., & Schroeder, J. S. [1994]. *Techniques in bedside hemodynamic monitoring* [5th ed.]. St Louis: Mosby.)

- Giant A waves may occur if the left atrium contracts against the closed mitral valve, which may occur with dysrhythmias such as junctional rhythm, heart block, and ventricular irregularities
- Large V waves related to mitral regurgitation

Alterations in the PCWP

The PCWP varies with changes in the relationships between volume load, blood volume distribution, and the function of the left ventricle.

Elevated PCWP Values. In the critically ill adult, an elevated PCWP may be caused by

- An increase in volume load related to hypervolemia
- Constriction of the pericardium related to constrictive disorders such as pericardial tamponade and constrictive pericarditis
- Left ventricular failure or cardiogenic shock
  - Left ventricular failure may occur during systole or during diastole (see Chapter 5 for related information on heart failure and Clinical Findings 5–1 for related information on left ventricular failure).
  - Systolic failure is characterized by a decrease in contractility, which leads to incomplete ventricular emptying (a decrease in the ejection fraction), a decrease in the stroke volume, and an increase in the end-diastolic volume.
  - The decrease in contractility may be secondary to numerous disorders, including acute myocardial infarction (see Clinical Findings 5–3), mitral and aortic valve disease, and increased systemic vascular resistance associated with disorders such as hypertension.
  - Diastolic failure is characterized by a decrease in compliance, which impairs diastolic filling and leads to a decrease in the end-diastolic volume and a decrease in the stroke volume.
  - The decrease in compliance may be secondary to a variety of disorders, including myocardial ischemia, ventricular hypertrophy, and pericardial tamponade, as well as therapeutic interventions such as positive pressure mechanical ventilation and PEEP.

Physical Findings Associated with an Increase in the PCWP. Physical findings associated with an increase in the PCWP vary with the clinical conditions. For example:

- With normal plasma oncotic pressure and pulmonary capillary permeability,
  - PCWP <16–18 mm Hg may be associated with dry lungs
  - PCWP >16–18 mm Hg: Fluid generally enters the tissue and findings such as tachypnea, dyspnea, cough, crackles, and wheezes may reflect pulmonary edema and congestion
  - PCWP >30 mm Hg is generally associated with acute pulmonary edema
- The critically ill adult with increased pulmonary capillary permeability associated with a disorder such as ARDS (see Clinical Findings 4–2) may develop severe pulmonary edema with a PCWP in the normal range.
- The critically ill adult with poor myocardial contractility may need a higher than normal PCWP to improve left ventricular function and provide an adequate cardiac output.

Additional physical findings may reflect the etiology of the increase in the PCWP and may include murmurs, extra heart sounds such as an S_3 and an S_4, muffled heart sounds, hypotension, and hypertension.

Decreased PCWP Values. A decreased PCWP may be caused by

- A decrease in volume load related to hypovolemia or vasodilation (see Right Atrial Pressure above)
- A decrease in volume load related to disorders such as right ventricular infarction, right ventricular failure, and pulmonary embolism

Physical Findings Associated with a Decrease in the PCWP. Physical findings associated with a decrease in the PCWP are generally related to the etiology of hypovolemia or vasodilation (see Right Atrial Pressure above).

POINTS TO REMEMBER

► The PCWP is often used clinically as an indicator of left ventricular volume or preload (preload is defined as the amount of blood in the ventricle at the end of diastole, the ventricular filling pressure, or the distending force which stretches the ventricle just prior to contraction).

▶ However, in the critically ill adult with decreased ventricular compliance (see discussion of diastolic failure), the PCWP may not accurately reflect the actual end-diastolic volume (as compliance decreases, the EDP increases and the PCWP may overestimate the actual left ventricular volume).

Cardiac Output

Cardiac output (CO) is the product of heart rate and stroke volume. The rate at which blood is ejected from the heart is measured with a thermistor at the distal tip of the pulmonary artery catheter and expressed in liters per minute. The cardiac index is calculated to standardize the CO to the size of the patient.

Alterations in Cardiac Output

Elevated CO Values. In the critially ill adult an elevated CO may be related to

- A hyperdynamic state associated with an increase in catecholamine release or hypermetabolism in disorders such as burns, multiple trauma, and thyrotoxicosis
- A compensatory response to increase oxygen delivery in disorders such as anemia
- An initial response to profound vasodilation in disorders such as the systemic inflammatory response syndrome
- Hypervolemia (excessive fluid resuscitation)

Physical Findings Associated with an Increase in CO. Physical findings associated with an elevated cardiac output may include full and bounding peripheral pulses, systolic murmurs, warm and flushed skin, and high urine output.

Decreased CO Values. In the critically ill adult, a decrease in cardiac output may be related to

- A loss of intravascular blood volume associated with conditions such as hypovolemia or vasodilation
- Decreased myocardial contractility
- Decreased ventricular compliance
- Increased systemic vascular resistance
- Alterations in cardiac rhythm (see Dysrhythmias)

Physical Findings Associated with a Decrease in CO. Physical findings associated with a decreased cardiac output may include anxiety, restlessness, dizziness, confusion, syncope, fatigue (muscle weakness), decreased urine output, cool and moist skin, capillary refill >2 seconds, and weak peripheral pulses.

Stroke Volume

Stroke volume (SV) is the amount of blood ejected by the ventricles with each contraction. The stroke volume index (SVI) is calculated to standardize the SV to the size of the patient.

Determinants of Stroke Volume

Determinants of stroke volume include preload, afterload, and contractility.

Preload. In the clinical setting the CVP or RAP (see discussion of RAP) is frequently used to reflect right ventricular preload and the PCWP (see discussion of PCWP) is frequently used to reflect left ventricular preload.

Afterload. Afterload, or the resistance the heart muscle must overcome to eject blood into the pulmonary artery or the aorta during contraction, is evaluated by calculating the pulmonary vascular resistance (PVR) for the right ventricle, and the systemic vascular resistance (SVR) for the left ventricle. The higher the resistance, the harder the heart muscle has to work. Increases in PVR and SVR may increase myocardial oxygen demands and precipitate myocardial ischemia or right or left ventricular failure respectively. The pulmonary vascular resistance index (PVRI) and the systemic vascular resistance index (SVRI) are calculated to adjust the measurements to body size.

Alterations in Afterload

Alterations in the PVR. PVR represents the total resistance to blood flow in the pulmonary circulation (pulmonary arteries and arterioles). The pulmonary circulation is more compliant than the systemic circulation; therefore the PVR is much less than the SVR.

Elevated PVR Values. An increased PVR may be related to

- Pulmonary vasoconstriction associated with disorders such as hypoxia, ARDS, COPD, and pulmonary embolism
- An increase in left atrial pressure associated with mitral valve disorders and other causes of left ventricular failure

Physical Findings Associated with an Increase in PVR. Physical findings associated with an increase in PVR may include

- Dyspnea and increased work of breathing related to intrapulmonary shunting and ventilation-perfusion mismatching
- Tachycardia related to hypoxemia (compensatory mechanism to increase oxygen delivery to the tissues)

Decreased PVR Values. A decreased PVR may be related to

- Vasodilation associated with disorders such as the systemic inflammatory response syndrome and the distributive shock states (see Chapter 12)
- Vasodilating drug therapy

Physical Findings Associated with a Decrease in PVR. Physical findings associated with a decrease in PVR are generally related to the etiology of the vasodilation.

Alterations in the SVR. SVR represents the total resistance to blood flow in the systemic circulation (systemic arteries and arterioles).

Elevated SVR Values. An increased SVR may be related to

- Compensatory vasoconstriction associated with disorders such as decreased cardiac output, hypovolemia, hypovolemic and cardiogenic shock, and hypothermia
- Vasopressor therapy

Physical Findings Associated with an Increase in SVR. Physical findings associated with an increase in SVR may include

- Hypertension
- Decreased peripheral pulse volumes, cool and clammy skin, pale or cyanotic extremities with capillary refill >2 seconds, possible mottling of the extremities and torso, decreased urine output, and sluggish bowel sounds reflective of the vasoconstrictive state

Decreased SVR Values. A decreased SVR may be related to

- Vasodilatation associated with disorders such as the systemic inflammatory response syndrome and the distributive shock states (see Chapter 12)
- Vasodilating drug therapy

Physical Findings Associated with a Decrease in SVR. Physical findings associated with a decrease in the SVR may include

- Hypotension
- Full and bounding pulses, warm and flushed skin, and findings related to the etiology of the vasodilation

Contractility

Contractility, or the ability of the heart muscle fibers to shorten and develop tension, cannot be measured directly, but inferences can be made from a number of derived parameters including cardiac index (see discussion of CO), stroke volume index (see discussion of SV), right ventricular stroke work index (RVSWI), and left ventricular stroke work index (LVSWI).

Right Ventricular Stroke Work Index. The right ventricular stroke work index is calculated to determine the amount of work needed to move the right ventricular stroke volume against the pulmonary vascular resistance (move blood from the right ventricle through the pulmonary circulation).

Left Ventricular Stroke Work Index. The left ventricular stroke work index is calculated to determine the amount of work needed to move the left ventricular stroke volume against the systemic vascular resistance (move blood from the left ventricle into the aorta).

DYSRHYTHMIAS

In the critically ill adult, alterations in cardiac rhythm may cause rapid, slow, or irregular heart rates. Variations in heart rates, such as tachycardia, may affect diastolic filling times and lead to weak or absent ventricular contractions that may not be perfused to the extremities.

Abnormalities in the heart rate (Table 14–3) may be felt when palpating the peripheral pulse. In the presence of an irregular rhythm, the pulse should be carefully palpated to evaluate the pattern of irregularity. Rapid, slow, and irregular rates should be cautiously evaluated with changes in other clinical parameters such as blood pressure, urine output, mental status, and skin signs (cool and clammy versus warm and dry) to assist in the evaluation of blood flow to the tissues.

TABLE 14-3 Dysrhythmias

Rhythm and Criteria	Clinical Significance; Physical Findings; Geriatric Considerations

Sinus Rhythms
Normal Sinus Rhythm (NSR)

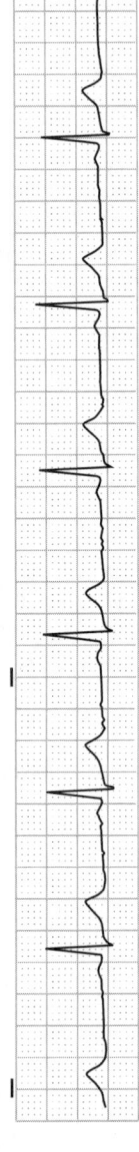

Rate: 60–100 bpm
Rhythm
Atrial rhythm (PP interval) regular
Ventricular rhythm (RR interval) regular
P wave: Upright in leads I, II, and aVF
PR interval: 0.12–0.20 seconds
QRS complex: 0.06–0.10 seconds

CLINICAL SIGNIFICANCE
In the presence of normal cardiac muscle contraction and relaxation, NSR should
   provide an optimal cardiac output

GERIATRIC CONSIDERATIONS
Slightly prolonged PR interval
Slightly prolonged QT interval without an increase in the QRS duration

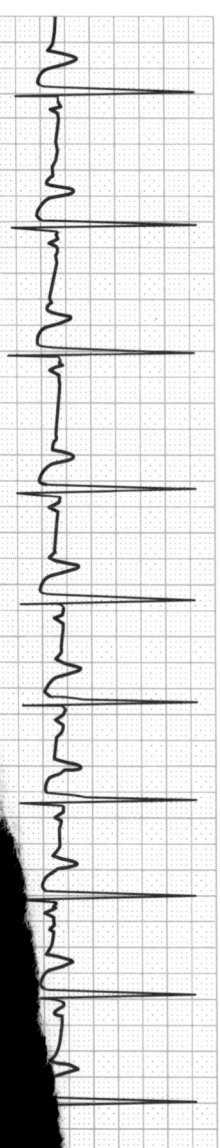

── Inspiration ──────── Expiration ──────

Rate: Same as NSR but may be <60 bpm or >100 bpm

Rhythm: PP and RR intervals are regularly irregular

P wave: Same as NSR

PR interval: Same as NSR

QRS complex: Same as NSR

CLINICAL SIGNIFICANCE

Sinus arrhythmia is a normal variation of NSR associated with respiration (the heart rate increases with inspiration and decreases with expiration)

Physiological explanation:

- The increased blood volume in the lungs on inspiration decreases the blood volume in the right heart chambers, and the sinus node responds to the decreased pressure by increasing the firing rate

- On expiration, the volume compliance of the pulmonary circulation is reduced Consequently, the blood volume in the right heart chambers increases, and the sinus node responds to the increasing pressures by decreasing the firing rate

Sinus arrhythmia is more common in the young adult

Note: All rhythm strips in this table from Paul, S., & Hebra, J. D. (1998). *The nurse's guide to cardiac rhythm interpretation: Implications for patient care.* Philadelphia: W. B. Saunders.

Table continued on following page

TABLE 14-3 Dysrhythmias *Continued*

Rhythm and Criteria	Clinical Significance; Physical Findings; Geriatric Considerations
	PHYSICAL FINDINGS In general, sinus arrythmia does not alter cardiac output unless there is underlying cardiac disease Slow rates may lead to • Complaints of dizziness • Fainting • Ectopic beats

Sinus Tachycardia

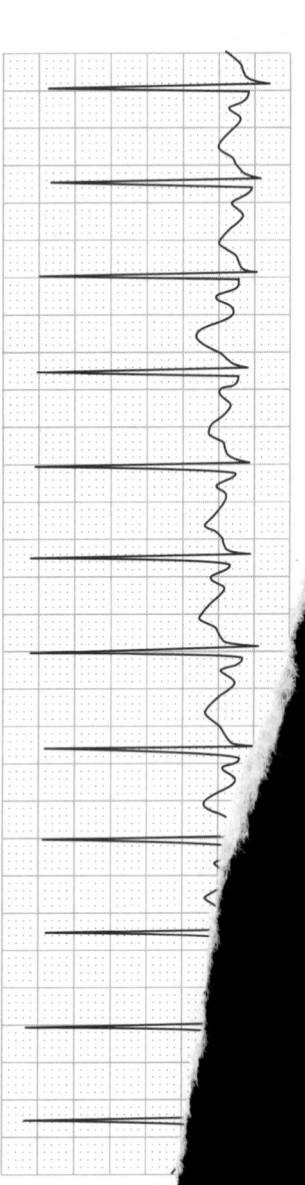

Rate: 100–150 bpm
Rhythm: Same as NSR
P wave: Same as NSR
PR interval: Same as NSR
QRS complex: Same as NSR

CLINICAL SIGNIFICANCE

Sinus tachycardia is generally a compensatory response to the body's demand for an increased cardiac output

In the critically ill adult, sinus tachycardia may be initiated by physical stress, emotional stress, and clinical conditions such as hypoxia, hypotension, fever (sepsis), and hypovolemia (sympathetic stimulation)

Sinus tachycardia is not usually harmful in the healthy adult; however, in the elderly adult, the adult with compromised cardiac function, and the critically ill adult, sinus tachycardia may increase myocardial workload and oxygen demand, and lead to myocardial ischemia and left ventricular failure (see Chapter 5)

Sinus tachycardia is a dangerous rhythm in the critically ill adult with angina or myocardial infarction because decreased filling of the coronary arteries may lead to increased myocardial ischemia and potentiate or extend myocardial injury and necrosis (see Chapter 5)

PHYSICAL FINDINGS

Indicators of deterioration in hemodynamic status may include

- Complaints of chest pain
- Restlessness, anxiety, and alterations in mental status, such as confusion or drowsiness
- Hypotension
- Cool and moist skin

Table continued on following page

TABLE 14-3 Dysrhythmias Continued

Rhythm and Criteria	Clinical Significance; Physical Findings; Geriatric Considerations
	GERIATRIC CONSIDERATIONS With aging, the heart becomes less responsive to sympathetic stimulation The mean maximum heart rate is decreased by about one beat per year to age 80 in deconditioned individuals Expected tachycardia may not develop with fever, early heart failure, or volume-depleting drugs Occult blood loss and anemia should be ruled out as causes of supraventricular tachycardia in the elderly

Sinus Bradycardia

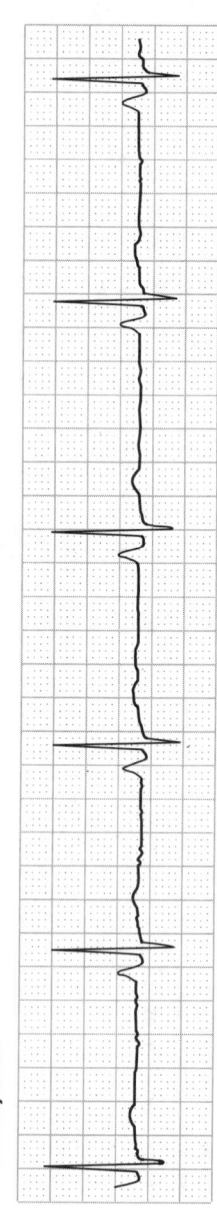

Rate: <60 bpm
Rhythm: Same as NSR
P wave: Same as NSR
PR interval: Same as NSR
QRS complex: Same as NSR

CLINICAL SIGNIFICANCE

Sinus bradycardia may be normal in the conditioned adult

In the critically ill adult, sinus bradycardia may be caused by disease of the sinus node, increased vagal stimulation, or drugs such as β-blockers

Slow heart rates may lead to decreased cardiac output, heart failure, ventricular dysrhythmias, and cardiac arrest

PHYSICAL FINDINGS

Indicators of deterioration in hemodynamic status may include

- Complaints of dizziness and chest pain
- Hypotension
- Premature junctional or ventricular beats
- Ventricular tachycardia
- Signs of heart failure (see Chapter 5)

Premature beats may be palpated as isolated extra beats

GERIATRIC CONSIDERATIONS

The incidence of bradydysrhythmias increases with aging (the sinus node pacemaker cells decrease with aging; also, the sinus node may become encased in fat, which can affect conduction)

- Many elderly are prescribed β-blocking drugs that may further potentiate bradycardia

Table continued on following page

TABLE 14-3 Dysrhythmias *Continued*

Rhythm and Criteria	Clinical Significance; Physical Findings; Geriatric Considerations
	• With aging, the heart is less responsive to sympathetic stimulation and compensation for decreased cardiac output

Sinus Pause

Sinus pause

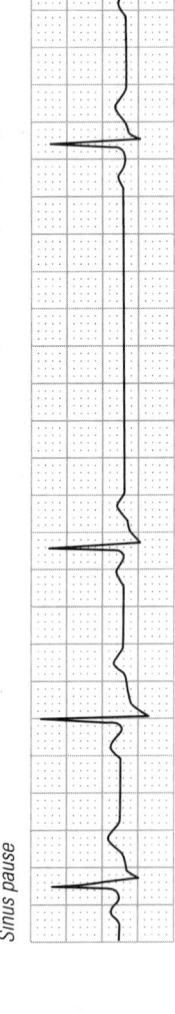

Sinus arrest

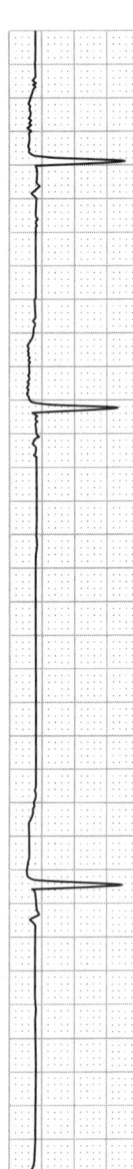

Sinoatrial block

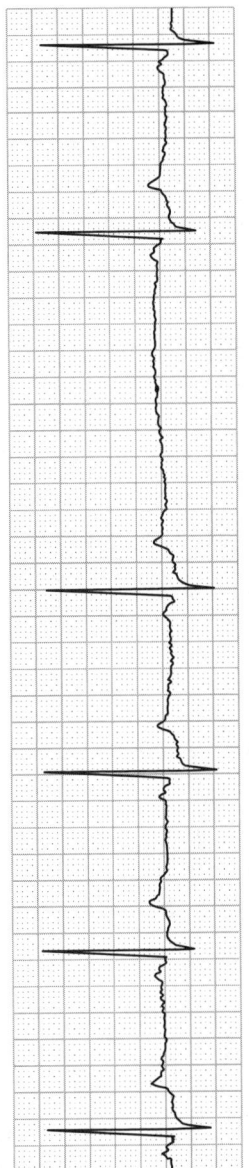

Rate: Usually slower than normal

Rhythm

- In **sinus pause** there is a momentary cessation of sinus rhythm
- In **sinus arrest** the intrinsic rhythm of the node is interrupted; there is a prolonged failure of the sinus node (>3 seconds) and the cycle of the dropped beat is not a multiple of the preceding PP interval
- **Sinoatrial block** resembles a sinus pause, but the intrinsic rhythm of the node is not interrupted (the du-

CLINICAL SIGNIFICANCE

Periods of sinus pause, sinus arrest, and sinoatrial block may be normal in the critically ill adult with increased vagal tone, or they may be related to

- Drug toxicity (for example: digitalis, lidocaine, quinidine, and atropine)
- Disease of the sinus node associated with aging, or metabolic disorders such as hypothyroidism, hyperthyroidism, hypokalemia, hypercarbia, and hypothermia
- Inflammatory disorders such as myocarditis or systemic lupus
- Ischemic heart disease such as acute myocardial infarction

If the periods of sinus pause, sinus arrest, and sinoatrial block are frequent or of a prolonged duration, the heart rate may decrease (the decrease in cardiac output may precipitate cardiogenic shock or cardiac arrest)

Table continued on following page

TABLE 14-3 Dysrhythmias *Continued*

Rhythm and Criteria	Clinical Significance; Physical Findings; Geriatric Considerations
ration of the sinus pause from P wave to P wave is double the PP interval of the preceding beat) *P wave:* Absent in failure of impulse formation and block intervals but is otherwise normal *PR interval:* Absent in failure of impulse formation and block complex but is otherwise normal *QRS complex:* Absent in failure of impulse formation and block complex but is otherwise normal	Tachydysrhythmias may interrupt periods of bradycardia (bradycardia-tachycardia syndrome) *PHYSICAL FINDINGS* Indicators of deterioration in hemodynamic status may include • Complaints of dizziness, lightheadedness, or chest pain • Restlessness or confusion • Hypotension The peripheral pulse will be nonpalpable during the periods of block *GERIATRIC CONSIDERATIONS* *Sinus node dysfunction,* often referred to as *Sick sinus syndrome* (SSS), is characterized by severe sinus bradycardia, sinus pauses, and sinus arrest related to intrinsic disease of the sinus node SSS is a common cause of symptomatic bradycardias and erratic rhythms in the elderly population

Atrial Rhythms
Premature Atrial Contraction (PAC)

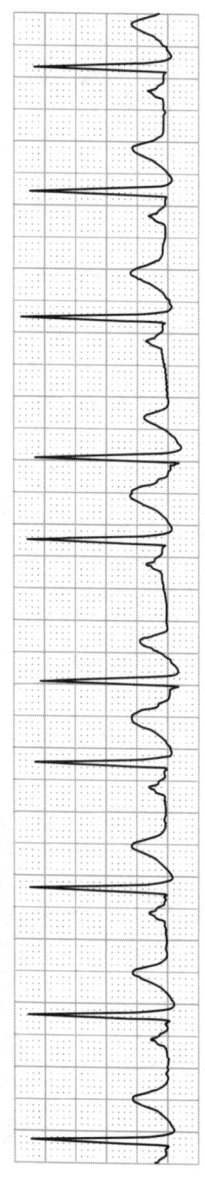

Rate: Underlying rate is usually normal

Rhythm: PP and RR intervals will be periodically irregular because of the early beat

P wave: Abnormal shape for the premature beat

PR interval: May be prolonged, normal, or shortened

QRS complex

Usually normal (narrow)

May be widened with abnormal conduction such as aberrancy

CLINICAL SIGNIFICANCE

A PAC is an electrical impulse from an irritable focus in the atrium

Causes may include excess caffeine, tobacco, alcohol, sympathomimetic drugs, hypoxia, heart failure, and digitalis intoxication

In the critically ill adult, frequent PACs may decrease ventricular filling and lead to a decrease in cardiac output

Frequent PACs may also lead to other dysrhythmias

PHYSICAL FINDINGS

The patient may complain of palpitations with frequent PACs

PACs may be palpated as an extra beat during a regular rhythm

Table continued on following page

TABLE 14-3 Dysrhythmias Continued

Rhythm and Criteria	Clinical Significance; Physical Findings; Geriatric Considerations

Atrial Tachycardia

Atrial tachycardia

Paroxysmal atrial tachycardia (PAT)

Paroxysmal supraventricular tachycardia (PSVT)

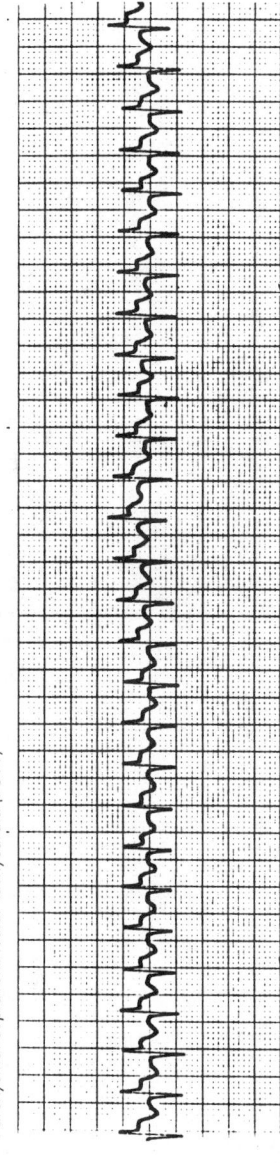

Rate: 150–250 bpm

Rhythm

In **atrial tachycardia** with a single focus of origin, the ventricular rhythm may be slightly irregular

In **multifocal atrial tachycardia** (MAT), the ventricular rhythm may be erratic

In **PAT** and **PSVT**, the atrial and ventricular rhythms are usually constant

One-to-one conduction

CLINICAL SIGNIFICANCE

In atrial tachycardia, a single focus or multiple atrial foci initiate a burst of three or more PACs (enhanced automaticity)

PAT refers to repeated episodes of atrial tachycardia with an abrupt onset and cessation (AV nodal reentrant tachycardia)

PSVT refers to repeated episodes of narrow QRS complex tachycardia with an abrupt onset and cessation, but without an identifiable P wave (AV nodal reentrant tachycardia)

Causes of atrial tachycardia may include disorders such as COPD, acute myocardial infarction, heart failure, pulmonary embolism, cardiomyopathy, and blunt

Table continued on following page

TABLE 14–3 Dysrhythmias *Continued*

Rhythm and Criteria	Clinical Significance; Physical Findings; Geriatric Considerations
P wave Abnormal shape In MAT the P wave may vary in shape from beat to beat In PAT and PSVT, the P wave is often difficult to identify *PR interval:* May be normal, prolonged, or shortened *QRS complex* Usually normal (narrow) May be widened with conduction abnormalities such as aberrancy	trauma; electrolyte imbalances such as hypomagnesemia and hypokalemia; and metabolic disturbances such as acidosis, alkalosis, and hypoxia In the critically ill adult, the rapid rate of these tachycardias may increase myocardial workload and oxygen demand, and decrease cardiac output (there may be decreased ventricular filling and decreased ventricular emptying) Myocardial hypoxia and decreased cardiac output may lead to disorders such as myocardial ischemia, left ventricular failure, and pulmonary edema PAT and PSVT are dangerous rhythms post–myocardial infarction, since myocardial ischemia may increase the area of myocardial injury and necrosis *PHYSICAL FINDINGS* Indicators of deteriorating hemodynamic status may include • Complaints of chest pain, palpitations, or weakness • Hypotension • Cool and moist skin • Signs of heart failure (see Chapter 5) or pulmonary edema (see Chapter 4) Pulsus alternans (alternating strong and weak pulses) may be palpable with left ventricular failure

Atrial Flutter

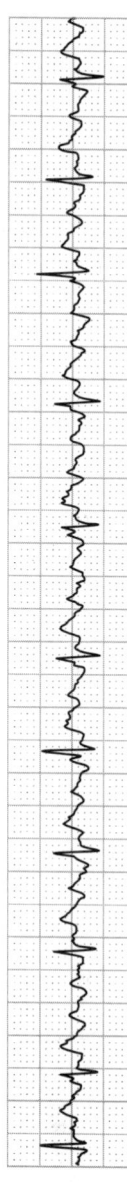

Rate

Atrial rate 250–350 bpm

Ventricular rate is slower (the atrial rate is usually a multiple of the ventricular rate: for example, 2:1, 4:1, etc.)

Rhythm

Atrial rhythm is regular

Ventricular rhythm is regular with constant AV conduction and irregular with variable conduction (the AV node blocks many of the F waves)

P wave: Sawtooth flutter (F) waves

PR interval: Absent

CLINICAL SIGNIFICANCE

Atrial flutter is often a transient dysrhythmia that converts to atrial fibrillation

The impulse originates in the atria and takes over from the sinus node

Causes include organic heart disease such as valvular disorders or cardiomyopathy, cardiac surgery, acute myocardial infarction, pulmonary disease, and thyrotoxicosis

In the critically ill adult with compromised cardiac function, increased workload on the ventricles may lead to an imbalance between oxygen supply and demand (demand exceeds supply) and potentiate myocardial ischemia

Rapid ventricular rates and loss of effective ventricular contraction may lead to decreased cardiac output, heart failure, and cardiogenic shock (decreased ventricular filling during diastole and decreased ventricular emptying during systole)

Table continued on following page

TABLE 14-3 Dysrhythmias *Continued*

Rhythm and Criteria	Clinical Significance; Physical Findings; Geriatric Considerations
QRS complex May be normal (narrow) May be widened with conduction abnormalities such as aberrancy	*PHYSICAL FINDINGS* Indicators of deteriorating hemodynamic status may include • Complaints of palpitations, chest pain, or shortness of breath • Restlessness and confusion • Hypotension • Cool and clammy extremities The pulse rate and rhythm may vary with the type of conduction (may be regular, regularly irregular, or irregularly irregular)

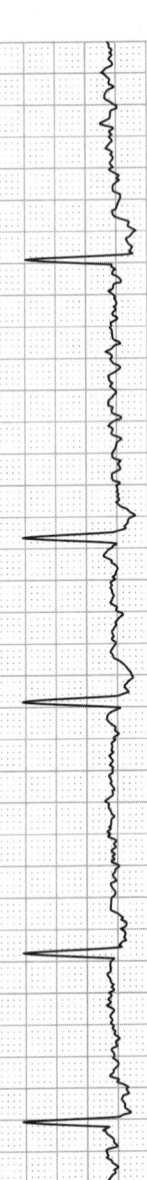

Atrial Fibrillation

Rate

Atrial rate >350 bpm

Ventricular rate may be slow or rapid (usually 160–180 bpm in the undigitalized patient)

Rhythm

Atrial rhythm irregular

Ventricular rhythm irregular (random AV node conduction)

P wave

Absent

Fine fibrillatory (F) waves

PR interval: Absent

QRS complex

May be normal (narrow)

May be widened with conduction abnormalities such as aberrancy

CLINICAL SIGNIFICANCE

Atrial fibrillation may be acute or chronic

Multiple areas of atrial foci result in rapid, uncoordinated atrial activity

Causes include cardiac surgery, acute myocardial infarction, digitalis toxicity, and organic heart disease such as valvular disorders

In the critically ill adult, ineffective atrial contraction (loss of atrial contribution to ventricular end-diastolic volume), decreased ventricular filling, and decreased ventricular emptying may contribute to decreased cardiac output

Decreased cardiac output may lead to myocardial ischemia or heart failure

PHYSICAL FINDINGS

Indicators of deteriorating hemodynamic status may include
- Complaints of palpitations, flutters, chest pain, and shortness of breath
- Restlessness and confusion
- Hypotension
- Signs of heart failure (see Clinical Findings 5–1 and 5–2) or pulmonary edema (see Clinical Findings 4–2)

Thrombi may form in the fibrillating atrium and lead to cerebral embolism (see Clinical Findings 6–5) or pulmonary embolism (see Clinical Findings 4–7)

The pulse rate will vary with the rate of conduction

Pulse deficit is common (the apical rate is faster than the peripheral pulse), because many of the contractions are too weak to perfuse to the extremities (the

Table continued on following page

TABLE 14-3 Dysrhythmias *Continued*

Rhythm and Criteria	Clinical Significance; Physical Findings; Geriatric Considerations
	heart rate should be obtained by auscultation rather than by palpation of a peripheral artery)
	The rhythm is usually irregularly irregular
	GERIATRIC CONSIDERATIONS
	Atrial fibrillation is a common dysrhythmia with aging due to changes in the SA node

Junctional Rhythms
Junctional Rhythm

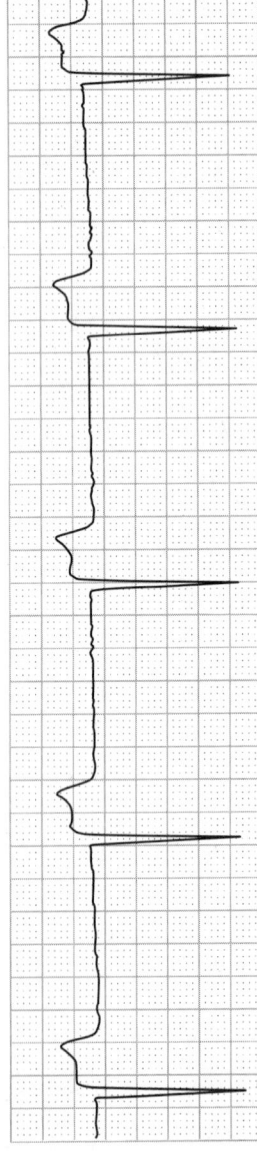

Rate: 40–60 bpm

Rhythm: Regular

P wave

May be before the QRS if the impulse depolarizes the atria before the ventricles

May be after the QRS if the impulse depolarizes the ventricles and then the atria

May be during the QRS if the impulse depolarizes the atria and the ventricles simultaneously

May be inverted in leads II, III, and aVF, and upright in aVR if the atria are activated by retrograde conduction from the AV junction

PR interval: If present, <0.12 seconds

QRS complex

May be normal (narrow)

May be widened with conduction abnormalities such as aberrancy

CLINICAL SIGNIFICANCE

Junctional rhythm is usually a slow, passive rhythm that escapes when the sinus node discharges slowly or fails to stimulate the atria

Causes include heart disease such as acute myocardial infarction, and drug toxicities, including digitalis, procainamide, quinidine, and other antiarrhythmic agents used to treat supraventricular tachycardias

Loss of atrial contribution to ventricular filling and the slow ventricular rate may contribute to a decreased cardiac output

The slow ventricular rate may potentiate life-threatening dysrhythmias such as ventricular tachycardia or fibrillation

PHYSICAL FINDINGS

Indicators of deteriorating hemodynamic status may include

- Complaints of chest pain
- Hypotension

Table continued on following page

TABLE 14–3 Dysrhythmias *Continued*

Rhythm and Criteria	Clinical Significance; Physical Findings; Geriatric Considerations

Premature Junctional Complex

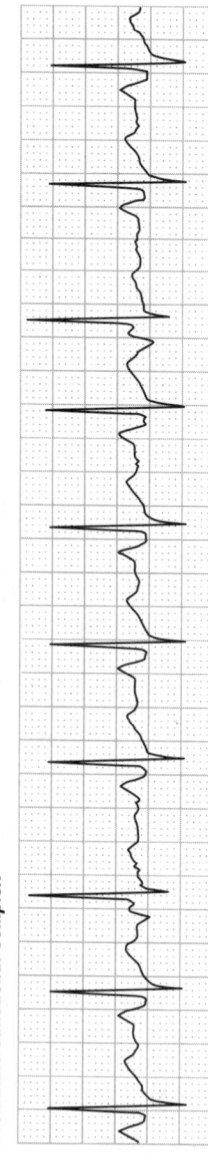

Rate: Underlying rate may be normal or slow

Rhythm: Periodically irregular because of the early beat

P wave: Same as junctional rhythm

PR interval: Same as junctional rhythm

QRS complex: Same as junctional rhythm

CLINICAL SIGNIFICANCE

A PJC is an impulse that arises prematurely in the AV junction

Retrograde atrial depolarization is usually present

Causes include acute myocardial infarction and drug toxicities (see Junctional Rhythm)

If frequent, PJCs may lead to decreased cardiac output or supraventricular tachycardia

PHYSICAL FINDINGS

A PJC may be palpated as an extra beat during a regular rhythm

Accelerated Junctional Rhythm or Nonparoxysmal Junctional Tachycardia

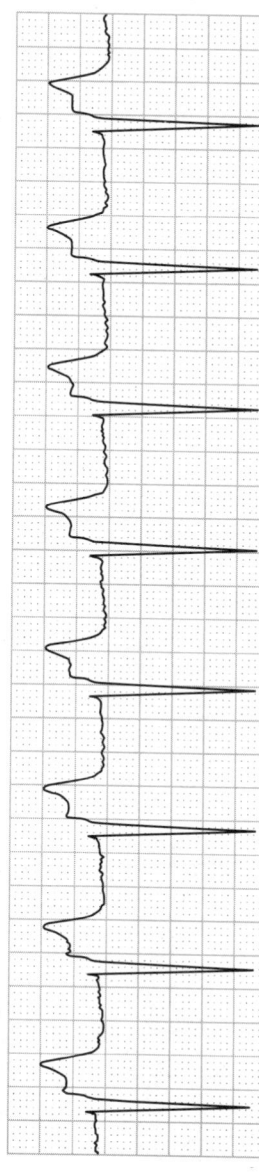

Rate: 60–130 bpm
Rhythm: Regular
P wave: Same as junctional rhythm
PR interval: Same as junctional rhythm
QRS complex: Same as junctional rhythm

CLINICAL SIGNIFICANCE

Usually results from enhanced automaticity of the AV junction associated with conditions such as inferior myocardial infarction, cardiac surgery, myocarditis, and digitalis toxicity

Decreased cardiac output (loss of atrial contribution) or heart failure (decreased ventricular emptying) may result depending on the rate and the underlying disease

PHYSICAL FINDINGS

Indicators of hemodynamic deterioration may include
* Complaints of chest pain

Table continued on following page

TABLE 14–3 Dysrhythmias *Continued*

Rhythm and Criteria	Clinical Significance; Physical Findings; Geriatric Considerations
	• Restlessness and confusion • Cool and moist extremities and signs of pulmonary edema (see Chapter 4)

Paroxysmal Junctional Tachycardia (PJT)

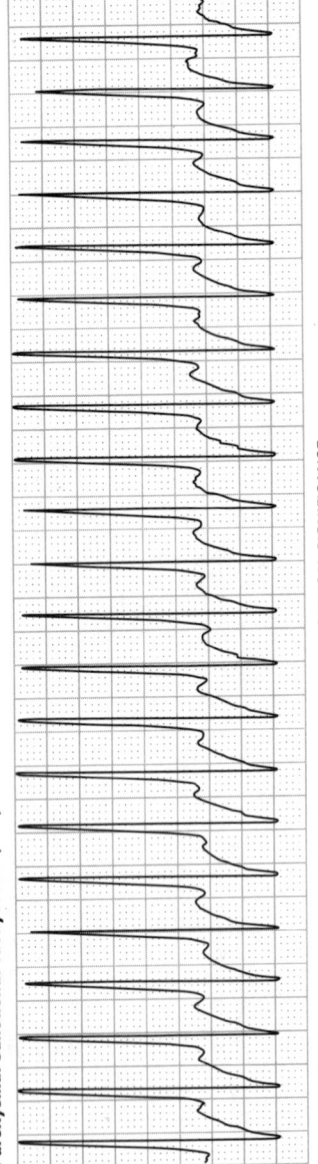

Rate: 140–250 bpm

Rhythm: Regular

P wave: Same as junctional rhythm

PR interval: Same as junctional rhythm

QRS complex: Same as junctional rhythm

CLINICAL SIGNIFICANCE

An irritable junctional focus takes over as pacemaker

PJT is initiated by a premature complex, starts and stops abruptly, and may progress to ventricular tachycardia, fibrillation, or cardiac arrest

Causes may include heart disease such as acute myocardial infarction, ischemia of the AV junction, rheumatic heart disease, hypertension, increased catecholamine secretion, and hyperthyroidism

Rapid heart rates may increase myocardial oxygen demand and decrease ventricular and coronary artery filling (shortened diastole), causing decreased cardiac output, myocardial ischemia, and left ventricular failure

PHYSICAL FINDINGS

Indicators of deteriorating hemodynamic status may include

- Complaints of chest pain
- Confusion
- Hypotension
- Cool and moist skin

Ventricular Rhythms
Premature Ventricular Complex (PVC)

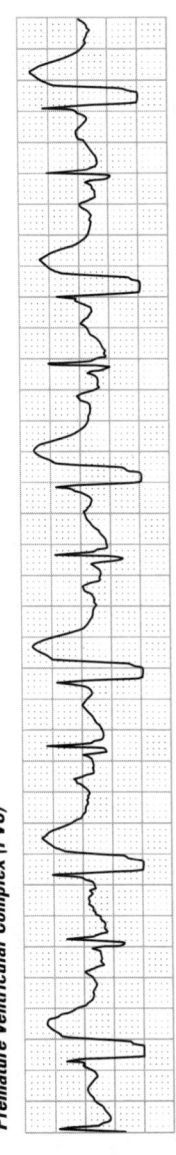

Table continued on following page

TABLE 14-3 Dysrhythmias *Continued*

Rhythm and Criteria	Clinical Significance; Physical Findings; Geriatric Considerations
Rate: Underlying rate may be normal, slow, or fast	*CLINICAL SIGNIFICANCE*
Rhythm: Irregular with premature beat	A PVC originates from an irritable focus in the ventricles
P wave: Usually not visible	Conduction is abnormal through the ventricles, resulting in a widened QRS
PR interval: Not measurable	Repolarization is also altered, resulting in ST and T wave changes in polarity opposite in direction to the QRS
QRS complex: Wide, bizarre complex with the ST segment and T wave opposite in polarity to the QRS	PVCs usually do not depolarize the atria and interrupt the firing of the SA node; therefore, there is a compensatory pause equal to two RR intervals following the PVC
	PVCs usually indicate myocardial irritability due to such factors as heart disease, electrolyte imbalances, hypoxia, acidosis, drug toxicities, poisonings, or slow heart rates
	PVCs may occur in isolation or >6/min
	PVCs may be unifocal, multifocal, bigeminal, trigeminal, or paired

Unifocal PVC

Multifocal PVC

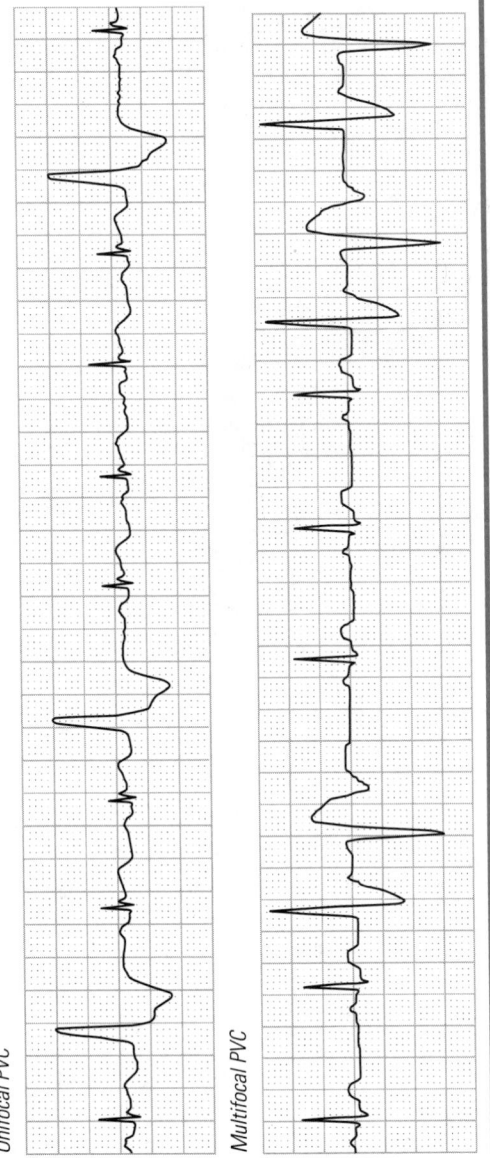

Table continued on following page

TABLE 14-3 Dysrhythmias Continued

Rhythm and Criteria	Clinical Significance; Physical Findings; Geriatric Considerations

Bigeminal PVC

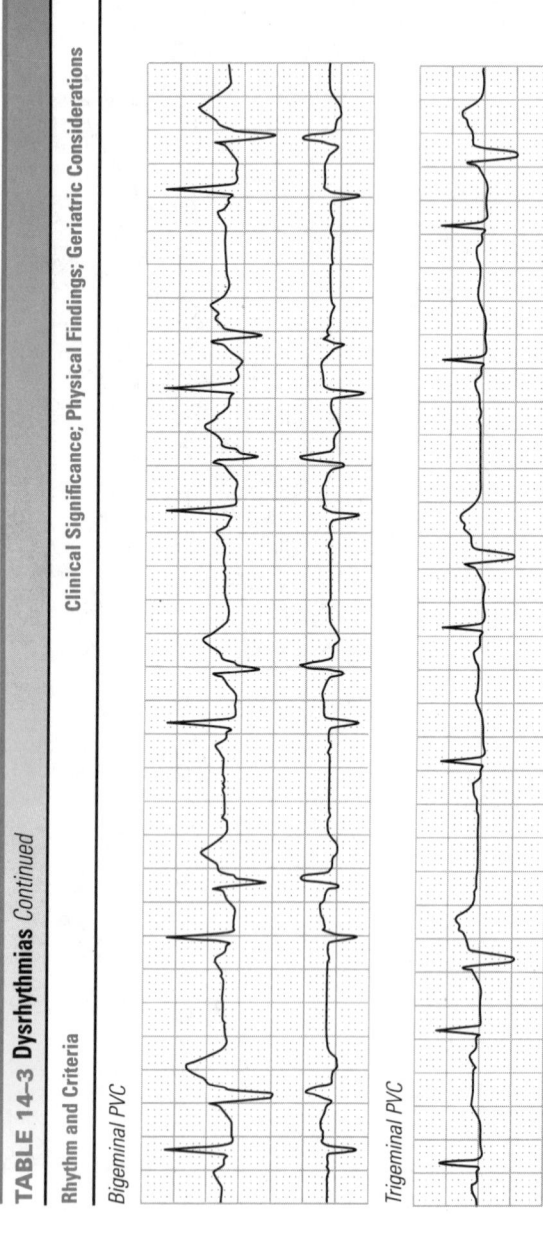

Trigeminal PVC

Paired PVC

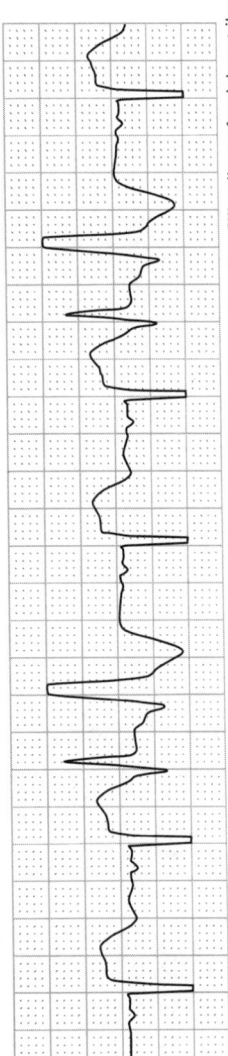

Frequent PVCs may interrupt cardiac filling (loss of atrial contribution and compensatory pause) and lead to a decreased cardiac output

Increasing frequency or types of PVCs may lead to ventricular tachycardia or fibrillation

If a PVC lands on the T wave of the preceding complex, ventricular tachycardia or fibrillation may occur (R on T phenomenon)

PHYSICAL FINDINGS

A PVC may be palpated as an extra beat in a regular rhythm

Table continued on following page

TABLE 14-3 Dysrhythmias Continued

Rhythm and Criteria	Clinical Significance; Physical Findings; Geriatric Considerations
	A bigeminal pulse may be felt as two beats in rapid succession, the first beat is the sinus beat and the second beat is the PVC The PVC may be weaker than the sinus beat and may be missed in palpating the peripheral pulse

Ventricular Tachycardia

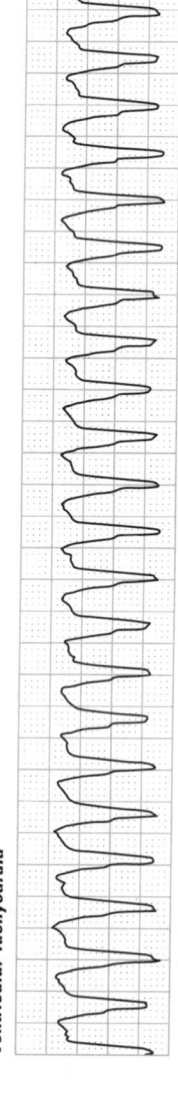

Rate: 100–200 bpm
Rhythm: Usually regular
P wave
Usually not seen
If present, is usually unrelated to the ventricular rhythm (AV dissociation)
PR interval: Usually not measurable
QRS complex: Same as PVC

CLINICAL SIGNIFICANCE

A ventricular focus initiates a burst of PVCs (three or more in succession)

Ventricular tachycardia usually indicates severe myocardial irritability secondary to myocardial infarction, heart failure, hypoxia, electrolyte imbalance, acidosis, or drug poisonings

Cardiac output decreases due to loss of appropriately timed atrial contraction, decreased cardiac filling, and decreased cardiac emptying

730

Increased myocardial workload and oxygen consumption may lead to increased myocardial ischemia, heart failure, cardiogenic shock, and ventricular fibrillation

Is considered a life-threatening dysrhythmia; often leads to cardiovascular collapse and cardiac arrest

Torsades de pointes is a special form of ventricular tachycardia associated with a prolonged QT interval

PHYSICAL FINDINGS

Indicators of deteriorating hemodynamic status may include

- Confusion
- Loss of consciousness
- Signs of cardiogenic shock (see Chapter 12)
- Cardiac arrest

Torsades de pointes

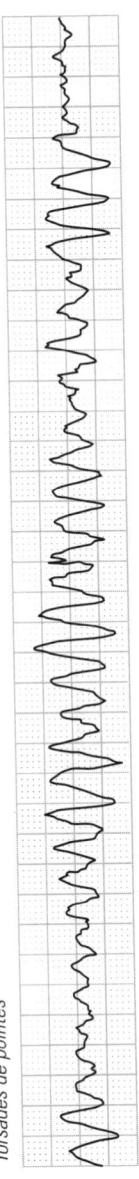

Table continued on following page

731

TABLE 14-3 Dysrhythmias *Continued*

Rhythm and Criteria	Clinical Significance; Physical Findings; Geriatric Considerations

Ventricular Fibrillation

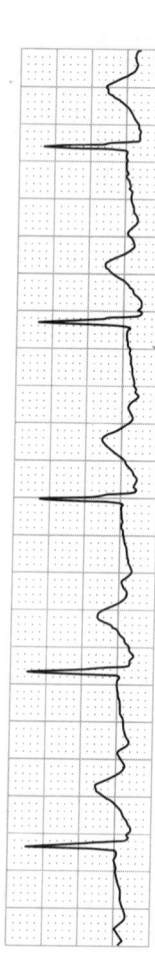

Rate: Unable to identify
Rhythm: Irregular
P wave: Absent
PR interval: Not measurable
QRS complex: Waveform varies in size and shape (irregular, bizarre deflection)

CLINICAL FINDINGS
Chaotic ventricular rhythm without organized ventricular depolarization or contraction
Etiology same as ventricular tachycardia
No effective contraction, therefore no cardiac output
Usually leads to sudden death

PHYSICAL FINDINGS
Peripheral pulses are not palpable

Atrioventricular Blocks
First-degree AV Block

Rate: Same as underlying rhythm (for example, NSR, sinus tachycardia, or sinus bradycardia)

Rhythm: Regular

P wave: Normal

PR interval
- >0.20 seconds
- Usually constant

QRS complex: Normal

CLINICAL SIGNIFICANCE

Delay in conduction of the impulse from the atria to the ventricles

Usually occurs at the AV node

May be associated with myocardial infarction or ischemia, digitalis toxicity, and cardiac surgery

Usually no adverse effects; however, it may progress to second-degree block

Type I, Second-degree AV Block, Mobitz I, or Wenckebach

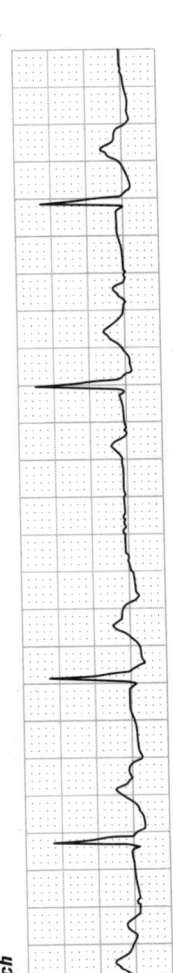

Rate
Atrial rate is usually unaffected
Ventricular rate is usually less than the atrial

Rhythm
Atrial regular
Ventricular irregular

CLINICAL SIGNIFICANCE

Sinus impulses are delayed at the AV node in progressively lengthening intervals until an impulse is completely blocked, and then the pattern repeats itself

Usually is a transient dysrhythmia associated with myocardial infarction or ischemia, increased parasympathetic stimulation, or drug therapy such as digitalis or calcium channel blockers

Table continued on following page

TABLE 14-3 Dysrhythmias Continued

Rhythm and Criteria	Clinical Significance; Physical Findings; Geriatric Considerations
Progressive shortening of the RR interval prior to the dropped beat *P wave* Normal Each P wave is followed by a QRS complex except for the dropped beat *PR interval:* Progressively lengthens until an impulse is completely blocked, and then the cycle repeats itself *QRS complex:* Normal	Usually benign, but cardiac output may decrease if there is excessive slowing of the ventricular rate *PHYSICAL FINDINGS* Indicators of deterioration in hemodynamic status may include • Complaints of lightheadedness, dizziness, chest pain, and dyspnea • Hypotension • Progression of block • The pulse rate and rhythm may be variable with the ventricular rate and rhythm (regularly irregular)

Type II, Second-degree AV Block or Mobitz II

Rate

Atrial unaffected

Ventricular rate less than the atrial rate (depends on the frequency of the block, for example, 2:1, 3:1, 4:1, etc.)

Rhythm

Atrial regular

Ventricular usually irregular but may be regular with a constant conduction ratio

P wave

Normal

Blocked P waves are not followed by a QRS complex

PR interval

May be normal or prolonged

Is constant for conducted beats

QRS complex

May be normal if the block is at the His bundle

May be widened if the block is at the bundle branch level

CLINICAL SIGNIFICANCE

The sinus impulse is blocked below the level of the AV node at the His bundle or bundle branches

Usually associated with disease or injury to the AV node, His bundle, or bundle branches

Cardiac output may be decreased with slow ventricular rates

PHYSICAL FINDINGS

Indicators of deteriorating hemodynamic status may include

- Complaints of light headedness, dizziness, chest pain, and dyspnea
- Confusion
- Hypotension
- PVCs
- Progression to complete heart block

Pulse rate and rhythm variable with ventricular rate and rhythm

GERIATRIC CONSIDERATIONS

His bundle loses cells with aging

Increase in fibrous and adipose deposits in cardiac tissue may further affect cardiac compliance and conduction

Table continued on following page

TABLE 14-3 Dysrhythmias Continued

Rhythm and Criteria	Clinical Significance; Physical Findings; Geriatric Considerations

Third-degree AV Block

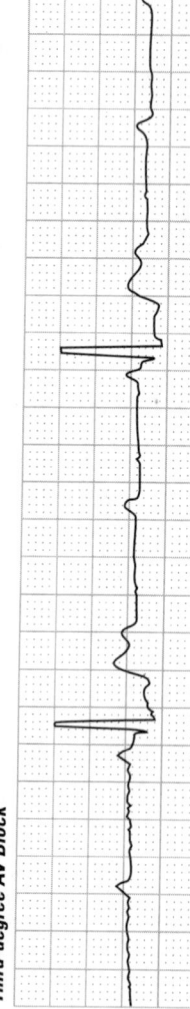

Rate

Atrial rate is unaffected

Ventricular rate is slower than the atrial rate (a junctional escape rhythm is 40–60 bpm; a ventricular escape rhythm is <40 bpm)

Rhythm

Atrial rhythm is usually regular

CLINICAL SIGNIFICANCE

Conduction through the atria and ventricle is absent

The block may occur at the AV node, the His bundle, or the bundle branch level

May be associated with ischemia or injury from acute myocardial infarction, drug toxicities, increased parasympathetic stimulation, and electrolyte imbalances

Slow rate may predispose to ventricular dysrhythmias

Cardiac output may decrease because of the slow ventricular rate and loss of synchronized contractions

Ventricular rhythm is usually regular

P wave
Normal
Not associated with a QRS complex

PR interval: Variable

QRS complex
May be narrow if the block is at the AV node
May be wide if the block is at the bundle branch level

Is a life-threatening dysrhythmia: may lead to hypotension, heart failure, cardiogenic shock, or ventricular standstill

INTRACRANIAL PRESSURE MONITORING

A catheter connected to a fluid-filled pressure system or a fiberoptic device is placed into an area in the cranium to continuously monitor intracranial pressure. In the critically ill adult, information obtained from the intracranial monitor may be used to

- Determine cerebral perfusion pressure and cerebral compliance
- Assess the individual's cerebral hemodynamic response to environmental stimuli
- Evaluate the effectiveness of therapeutic interventions
- Guide nursing interventions to avoid prolonged elevations in intracranial pressure

Intracranial Dynamics

Intracranial Pressure (ICP)

The contents of the skull include blood, cerebrospinal fluid (CSF), and brain tissue. The pressure these components exert within the skull constitutes the ICP. Various disorders can increase brain volume, blood volume, or CSF volume and potentiate an increase in the ICP.

- Brain volume may be increased by conditions such as an abscess, infection, tumor, hemorrhage, hematoma, or cerebral edema.
- Blood volume may be increased by factors such as an increased P_{CO_2}, a decreased P_{O_2}, hyperthermia, and impairment of venous drainage.
- CSF volume may be increased by disorders such as obstructive tumors and congenital abnormalities, and conditions such as a decrease in the reabsorption of CSF related to subarachnoid hemorrhage or meningitis.

Compliance

When the volume of one component in the skull increases, the volume of one or both of the other components will decrease to maintain an ICP value in the normal range of 0–15 mm Hg (Monro-Kellie doctrine). When compensatory mechanisms fail, compliance, or the ability to adapt to changes in volume, decreases, and intracranial pressure rises. With decreased compliance, small increases in volume may result in large increases in pressure and lead to decreased cerebral blood flow, cellular hypoxia, and possible brain herniation (see Chapter 6 and Clinical Findings 6–1 for related information).

Compliance levels vary with the individual. In the critically ill adult, compliance levels may be assessed by reading the ICP pulse waveform (see Fig. 14–7A). The pulse waveform has three or more peaks that correspond to the heartbeat:

- P_1, referred to as the percussion wave, reflects transmission of the arterial pressure from the choroid plexus. P_1 has a sharp peak and is generally consistent in amplitude.
- P_2, referred to as the tidal wave, is generated by venous pressure. P_2 is variable in shape and amplitude and ends on the dicrotic notch.
- P_3, referred to as the dicrotic wave, generally tapers down to the diastolic position (retrograde venous pulsations may add a few more peaks).

Intracerebral compliance is most directly reflected in the P_2 portion of the waveform. A P_2 elevation equal to or higher than P_1 is an indication of decreased compliance (see Figs 14–7B and C).

Cerebral Perfusion Pressure (CPP)

Cerebral perfusion pressure is a reflection of blood flow to the brain. It is the difference between the mean arterial pressure (MAP) and the ICP:

- CPP = MAP − ICP
- Normal range = 60 to 100 mm Hg

The brain has the ability to maintain blood flow to the tissue when the CPP is >60 mm Hg (autoregulation). When the CPP is <60 mm Hg (ICP is high or MAP is low), blood flow to the brain is decreased, and the cerebral tissue is deprived of oxygen and nutrients. Consistently low CPP may result in death of brain tissue. Cerebral ischemia may be reflected in the trend waveforms A, B, and C (see Fig. 14–8).

- A waves, referred to as plateau waves, are caused by rapid and sustained increases in ICP (>20 mm Hg) that may last 5 to 20 minutes. A waves reflect the presence of cerebral ischemia.
- B waves are sharp, rhythmic oscillations with a sawtooth appearance that may occur every 0.5 to 2 minutes with ICP elevations up to 50 mm Hg. B waves fluctuate with respiratory patterns and may be affected by arterial pressure. B waves occur

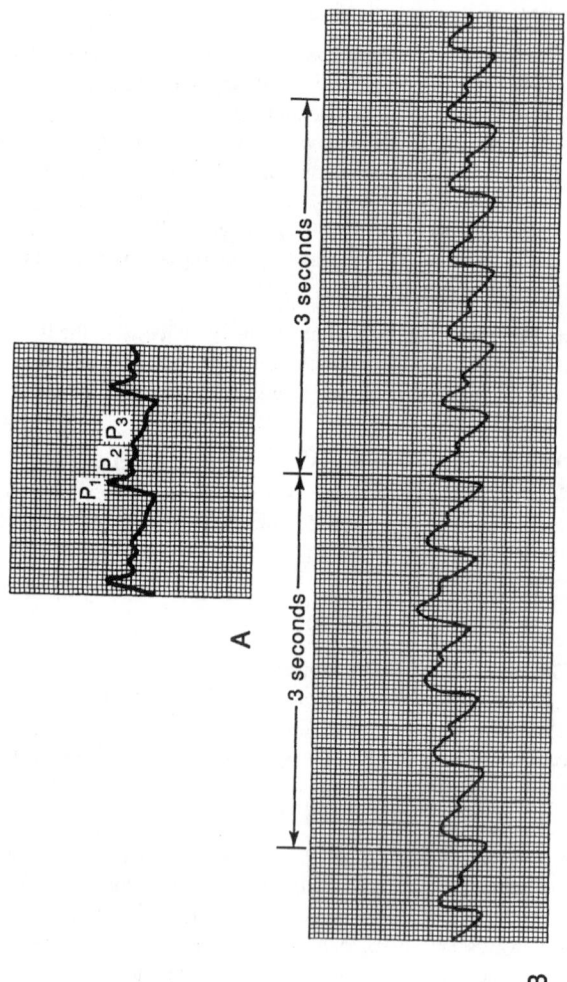

A

B

3 seconds

3 seconds

P₁ P₂ P₃

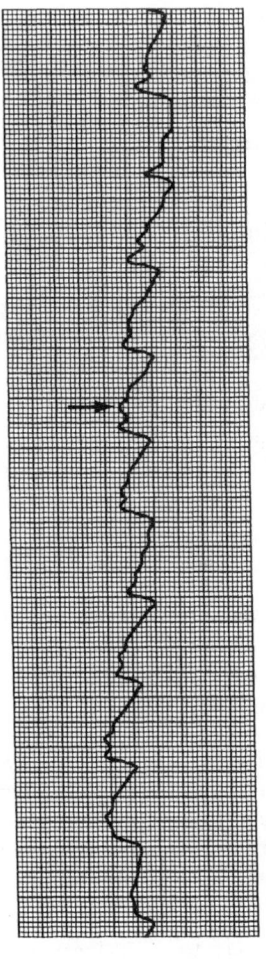

C

FIGURE 14–7

Normal intracranial pressure waveforms. **A,** ICP pulse wave with three main components: P_1, P_2, and P_3. The clarity of the three distinct waves will vary with the type of ICP monitoring device used and the calibration range of the bedside monitor. **B,** Waveform obtained from fluid-coupled intraventricular catheter. Calibration range is 0–50 mm Hg. **C,** ICP waveform obtained from ventriculostomy catheter. Arrow illustrates elevation of P_2 in relationship to P_1 due to increased ICP in a patient with ICP ranging from 20 to 40 mm Hg. (From Clochesy, J. M., Breu, C., Cardin, S., Whittaker, A. A., & Rudy, E. B. [Eds.]. [1996]. *Critical care nursing* [2nd ed., p. 302]. Philadelphia: W. B. Saunders.)

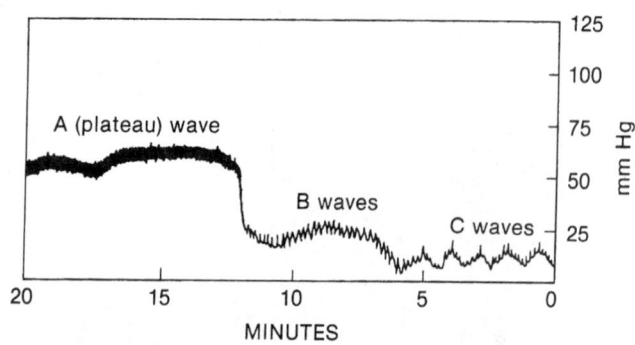

FIGURE 14–8

Abnormal ICP waves. Composite drawing of pressure waves that may be
recorded over time with a slow strip chart recorder, including A (plateau)
waves, B waves, and C waves. Note that this type of recording is used to
illustrate trends in ICP over time. (Redrawn from *Nursing the critically ill
adult,* 4th Edition, by Nancy Meyer Holloway. Copyright © 1993
Addison-Wesley Nursing, a division of Benjamin/Cummings Publishing
Company, Inc. Reprinted by permission.)

more frequently with increasing decompensation and may
progress to A waves.

- C waves are small, frequent waves that may occur every 4 to
  8 minutes with ICP elevations up to 20 mm Hg. C waves fluctuate with respiration and normal changes in arterial pressure and
  are not clinically significant.

Physical Findings Associated with an Increased ICP. Because the
accuracy of intracranial pressure monitoring may vary with the type
and location of the intracranial pressure monitor (see Table 14–4), the
ICP value should be evaluated in conjunction with the neuromuscular
assessment (see Tables 2–1 and 6–1). In general, physical findings reflecting an increase in the intracranial pressure may include

- Headache that increases in intensity and may be aggravated by
  straining or movement
- Vomiting (may be projectile)
- A change in the level of consciousness, including progressive alterations in orientation, speech, and arousal

TABLE 14-4 Types of ICP Monitoring Systems

Type of System	Advantages	Disadvantages
Intraventricular Technique A catheter is inserted into the lateral ventricle through a burr hole and then connected to a closed, fluid-filled pressure system and transducer	Direct and most accurate measurement of pressure Reliable waveform Able to drain and sample CSF Access for instillation of medication	Highest risk of infection (may permit CSF leakage) Catheter placement more difficult Occlusion of catheter by blood clots Can cause tissue damage or neurological deficits
Intraparenchymal Technique A fiberoptic, transducer-tipped catheter is inserted through a subarachnoid bolt and advanced into the white matter of the brain	Easy to insert Eliminates the flush system, which may reduce the risk of infection Accurate ICP values Sharp and distinct waveforms	Unable to sample or drain CSF Expensive Catheter breakage
Subarachnoid Technique A screw is inserted through the skull and dura into the subarachnoid space and generally attached to a closed, fluid-filled system and transducer (a fiberoptic device may also be used)	Easy to insert Ability to obtain pressures in patients with compressed and dislocated ventricles	Less reliability and accuracy of waveforms and pressures (the device is easily occluded by brain tissue) CSF leakage may occur
Subdural Technique A catheter is placed in the subdural space and then connected to a closed, fluid-filled system and transducer (a fiberoptic system may also be used)	Low risk of infection and hemorrhage (less invasive)	Accuracy and reliability of waveforms and pressures is poor (catheter lumen may become obstructed)

- Changes in the respiratory pattern (tachypnea may occur early and then progress to apnic periods)
- Abnormal pupil responses and eye movements, including conjugate and deviant eye movements, blurred or double vision, pupil dilation, inability of the pupil to react to light, and ipsilateral pupil changes
- Motor and sensory disturbances, including abnormal posturing, hemiplegia, hemiparesis, and seizures
- Changes in vital signs (late manifestation), which may include widening pulse pressure, bradycardia related to the increasing systolic pressure (baroreceptor response), then tachycardia as the ICP continues to rise and CPP is not maintained

References

Abels, L. (1986). *Critical care nursing: A physiologic approach.* St. Louis: C. V. Mosby.

Abrams, W. B., & Berkow, R. (1990). *The Merck manual of geriatrics.* Rahway, NJ: Merck, Sharp & Dohme Research Laboratories.

Adelman, R. D., Berger, J. T., & Macina, L. O. (1994). Critical care for the geriatric patient. *Clinics in Geriatric Medicine: Critical Illness in the Elderly, 10,* 19–30.

Ahrens, T. (1993). Respiratory monitoring in critical care. *AACN Clinical Issues in Critical Care Nursing, 4*(1), 56–65.

Alspach, J. G. (Ed.). (1991). *Core curriculum for critical care nursing* (4th ed.). Philadelphia: W. B. Saunders.

Alspach, J. G. (Ed.). (1998). *Core curriculum for critical care nursing* (5th ed.). Philadelphia: W. B. Saunders.

American Nurses' Association. (1991). *Standards of clinical nursing practice.* Washington, DC: Author.

Anderson, R. J., & Miller, S. W. (1988). Geriatric drug therapy. In E. T. Herfindal, D. R. Gourley, & L. L. Hart (Eds.), *Clinical pharmacy and therapeutics* (4th ed., pp. 996–1010). Baltimore: Williams & Wilkins.

Armstrong S. L. (1994). Cerebral vasospasm: Early detection and intervention. *Critical Care Nurse, 14*(4), 33–37.

Bates, B. (1987). *A guide to physical examination and history taking* (4th ed.). Philadelphia: J. B. Lippincott.

Bates, B. (1995). *A guide to physical examination and history taking* (6th ed.). Philadelphia: J. B. Lippincott.

Beattie, S., & Pike, C. (1996). Left ventricular diastolic dysfunction: A case report. *Critical Care Nurse, 16*(2), 37–50.

Bennett, A. F., & Sauer, H. C. (1991). Special considerations in cardiovascular assessment of the aged. *Nurse Practitioner Forum, 2*(1), 55–60.

Bradway, C. W. (1996). *Nursing care of geriatric emergencies.* New York: Springer.

Butts, D. E. (1987). Fluid and electrolyte disorders associated with diabetic ketoacidosis and hyperglycemic hyperosmolar nonketotic coma. *Nursing Clinics of North America, 22*(4), 827–836.

Byers, J. F., & Flynn, M. B. (1996). Acute burn injury: A trauma case report. *Critical Care Nurse, 16*(4), 55–65.

Carpenter, K. D. (1991). Oxygen transport in the blood. *Critical Care Nurse, 11*(9), 20–31.

Cassel, C. K., Riesenberg, D. E., Sorensen, L. B., & Walsh, J. R. (Eds.). (1990). *Geriatric medicine* (2nd ed.). New York: Springer-Verlag.

Chernecky, C. C., & Berger, B. J. (1997). *Laboratory tests and diagnostic procedures* (2nd ed.). Philadelphia: W. B. Saunders.

Clochesy, J. M., Breu, C., Cardin, S., Whittaker, A. A., & Rudy, E. B. (Eds.). (1996). *Critical care nursing* (2nd ed.). Philadelphia: W. B. Saunders.

Coburn, K. (1992). Traumatic brain injury: The silent epidemic. *AACN Clinical Issues in Critical Care Nursing, 3*(1), 9–18.

Coen, D. S. (1992). Spinal cord injury: Preventing secondary injuries. *AACN Clinical Issues in Critical Care Nursing, 3*(1), 44–54.

Copstead, L. C. (Ed.). (1995). *Perspectives on pathophysiology.* Philadelphia: W. B. Saunders.

Daily, E. K., & Schroeder, J. S. (1994). Techniques in bedside hemodynamic monitoring (5th ed.). St. Louis: Mosby.

Darovic, G. O. (1987). *Hemodynamic monitoring: Invasive and noninvasive clinical applications.* Philadelphia: W. B. Saunders.

Darovic, G. O. (1998). *Hemodynamic monitoring: Invasive and noninvasive clinical applications* (2nd ed.). Philadelphia: W. B. Saunders.

Dickson, S. L. (1995). Understanding the oxyhemoglobin dissociation curve. *Critical Care Nurse, 15*(5), 54–58.

Dworken, H. J. (1989). Gastrointestinal hemorrhage. In W. C. Shoemaker et al. (Eds.), *Textbook of critical care* (pp. 697–710). Philadelphia: W. B. Saunders.

Faldmo, L., & Kravitz, M. (1993). Management of acute burns and burn shock resuscitation. *AACN Clinical Issues in Critical Care Nursing, 4*(2), 351–366.

Fitzsimmons, L. (1994). Consequences of trauma: Systemic inflammation and multiple organ dysfunction. *Critical Care Nursing Quarterly, 17*(2), 74–90.

Forbes, C. D., & Jackson, W. F. (1997). *Color atlas and text of clinical medicine* (2nd ed.). London: Mosby-Wolfe.

Foreman, M. D., Gillies, D. A., & Wagner, D. (1989). Impaired cognition in the critically ill elderly patient: Clinical implications. *Critical Care Nursing Quarterly, 12*(1), 61–73.

Fulmer, T. T., & Walker, M. K. (Eds.). (1992). *Critical care nursing of the elderly.* New York: Springer.

Gardner, P. E. (1993). Pulmonary artery pressure monitoring. *AACN Clinical Issues in Critical Care Nursing, 4*(1), 98–119.

Germon, K. (1994). Intracranial pressure monitoring in the 1990s. *Critical Care Nursing Quarterly, 17*(1), 21–32.

Gordon, M., & Goodwin, C. W. (1997). Burn management: Initial assessment, management, and stabilization. *The Nursing Clinics of North America, 32*(2), 237–249.

Gorny, D. A. (1993). Arterial blood pressure measurement technique. *AACN Clinical Issues in Critical Care Nursing, 4*(1), 66–79.

Grossbach, I. (1994). The COPD patient in acute respiratory failure. *Critical Care Nurse, 14*(6), 32–40.

Guyton, A. C., & Hall, J. E. (1997). *Human physiology and mechanisms of disease* (6th ed.). Philadelphia: W. B. Saunders.

Guzzetta, C. E., Dossey, B. M., & Kenner, C. V. (1985). Nursing assessment and diagnosis. In C. V. Kenner, C. E. Guzzetta, & B. M. Dossey (Eds.), *Critical care nursing: Body, mind, spirit* (2nd ed., pp. 41–72). Boston: Little, Brown.

Halloran, T. H. (1990). Nursing responsibilities in endocrine emergencies. *Critical Care Nursing Quarterly, 13*(3), 74–81.

Hamner, J. (1995). Challenging diagnosis: Adult respiratory distress syndrome. *Critical Care Nurse, 15*(5), 46–51.

Hazinski, M. F., & Cummins, R. O. (Eds.). (1996). *Handbook of emergency cardiac care for health providers.* Dallas: American Heart Association.

Hazzard, W. R., Bierman, E. L., Blass, J. P., Ettinger, Jr., W. H., & Halter, J. B. (1994). *Principles of geriatric medicine and gerontology* (3rd ed.). New York: McGraw-Hill.

Hebra, J., & Kuhn, M. A. (1996). *Manual of critical care nursing.* Boston: Little, Brown.

Holloway, N. M. (1993). *The critically ill adult* (4th ed.). Menlo Park, CA: Addison Wesley Longman.

Houston, M. C. (1990). Pathophysiology of shock. *Critical Care Nursing Clinics of North America, 2*(2), 143–149.

Hoyt, N. J. (1990). Preventing septic shock: Infection control in the intensive care unit. *Critical Care Nursing Clinics of North America, 2*(2), 287–296.

Hudak, C., Gallo, B., & Lohr, T. (1986). *Critical care nursing: A holistic approach* (4th ed.). Philadelphia: J. B. Lippincott.

Hudak, C., Gallo, B., & Lohr, T. (1994). *Critical care nursing: A holistic approach* (6th ed.). Philadelphia: J. B. Lippincott.

Ignatavicius, D. D., Workman, M. L., & Mishler, M. A. (1995). *Medical-surgical nursing* (2nd ed.). Philadelphia: W. B. Saunders.

Jarosz, D. A., Yoram, K., Ellias, M. E., Farls, K. A., & Diamond, D. L. (1994). The tertiary nursing survey in the assessment of trauma patients: An important addendum to survival. *Critical Care Nurse, 14*(2), 98–103.

Jarvis, C. (1992). *Physical examination and health assessment.* Philadelphia: W. B. Saunders.

Jarvis, C. (1996). *Physical examination and health assessment* (2nd ed.). Philadelphia: W. B. Saunders.

Jessup, M., Lakatta, E. G., Leier, C. V., & Santinga, J. T. (1992). CHF in the elderly: Is it different? *Patient Care, 26*(14), 40–43, 46, 49, 52, 58–61.

Johnson, M. M., & Brown, M. A. (1986). Assessment. In D. A. Zschoche (Ed.), *Mosby's comprehensive review of critical care* (3rd ed., pp. 121–161). St. Louis: C. V. Mosby.

Joseph, D. H., & Larrivee, C. (1992). A decision-making algorithm for blood pressure measurements. *Dimensions of Critical Care Nursing, 11*(3), 145–150.

Kee, J. L. (1991). *Laboratory and diagnostic tests with nursing implications* (3rd ed.). Norwalk: Appleton & Lange.

Keith, J. S. (1985). Hepatic failure: Etiologies, manifestations, and management. *Critical Care Nurse, 5*(1), 60–86.

Kellum, J. A., & Decker, J. M. (1996). The immune system: Relation to sepsis and multiple organ failure. *AACN Clinical Issues in Critical Care Nursing, 7*(3), 339–350.

Kenner, C. V., Guzzetta, C. E., & Dossey, B. M. (Eds.). (1985). *Critical care nursing: Body, mind, spirit* (2nd ed.). Boston: Little, Brown.

Kenner, C. V., Guzzetta, C. E., & Dossey, B. M. (Eds.). (1991). *Critical care nursing: Body, mind, spirit* (3rd ed.). Boston: Little, Brown.

Kenney, R. A. (1989). *Physiology of aging: A synopsis.* Chicago: Year Book Medical Publishers.

Kernicki, J. G. (1993). Differentiating chest pain: Advanced assessment techniques. *Dimensions of Critical Care Nursing, 12*(2), 66–76.

Kinney, M. R., Packa, D. R., & Dunbar, S. B. (Eds.). (1988). *AACN's clinical reference for critical-care nursing* (2nd ed.). New York: McGraw Hill.

Kinney, M. R., Packa, D. R., & Dunbar, S. B. (Eds.). (1993). *AACN'S clinical reference for critical-care nursing* (3rd ed.). St. Louis: C. V. Mosby.

Kitt, S., Selfridge-Thomas, J., Proehl, J. A., & Kaiser, J. (1995). *Emergency nursing: A physiologic and clinical perspective* (2nd ed.). Philadelphia: W. B. Saunders.

Kravitz, M. (1988). Thermal injuries. In V. D. Cardona, P. D. Hurn, P. J. Bastnagel Mason, A. M. Scanlon, & S. W. Veise-Berry (Eds.). *Trauma nursing: From resuscitation through rehabilitation.* Philadelphia: W.B. Saunders.

Kuhn, M. A. (1994). Multiple trauma with respiratory distress. *Critical Care Nurse, 14*(2), 68–80.

Lakatta, E. G. (1990). The aging heart. In M. C. Geokas (moderator). The aging process. *Annals of Internal Medicine, 113,* 455–466.

Lakatta, E. G. (1993). Cardiovascular regulatory mechanisms in advanced age. *Physiological Reviews, 73,* 413–467.

Lasater-Erhard, M. (1995). The effect of patient position on arterial oxygen saturation. *Critical Care Nurse, 15*(5), 31–36.

Leibowitz, R. E., Tatarakis, J., & Delgado, J. (1995). HIV infection/AIDS and critical care. *Critical Care Nursing Clinics of North America, 7*(4), 651–658.

Long, L., & McAuley, J. W. (1996). Epilepsy: A review of seizure types, etiologies, diagnosis, treatment, and nursing implications. *Critical Care Nurse, 16*(4), 83–91.

Lueckenotte, A. G. (1996). *Gerontologic nursing.* St. Louis: Mosby.

Marino, P. L. (1998). *The ICU Book* (2nd ed.). Baltimore: Williams & Wilkins.

Malarkey, L. M., & McMorrow, M. E. (1996). *Nurse's manual of laboratory tests and diagnostic procedures.* Philadelphia: W. B. Saunders.

Matteson, M. A., McConnell, E. S., & Linton, A. D. (1997). *Gerontological nursing: Concepts and practice* (2nd ed.). Philadelphia: W. B. Saunders.

McMahon, K. (1995). Multiple organ failure: The final complication of critical illness. *Critical Care Nurse, 15*(6), 20–30.

Mezey, M. D., Rauckhorst, L. H., & Stokes. S. A. (1993). *Health assessment of the older individual.* New York: Springer.

Misasi, R. S., & Keyes, J. L. (1994). The pathophysiology of hypoxia. *Critical Care Nurse, 14*(4), 55–64.

Misasi, R. S., & Keyes, J. L. (1996). Matching and mismatching ventilation and perfusion in the lung. *Critical Care Nurse, 16*(3), 23–40.

Morrison, C. A. M. (1987). Brain herniation syndromes. *Critical Care Nurse, 7*(5), 34–38.

Murray, S. E. (1989). Patient assessment in the postanesthesia care unit: A critical care approach. *Journal of Post-Anaesthesia Nursing, 4*(4), 232–238.

Murray, S. E. (1990). *Utilization of physical assessment skills in acute care settings.* Unpublished Master's thesis, California State University, Long Beach.

Nikas, D. L. (1988). Pathophysiology and nursing interventions in acute spinal cord injury. *Trauma Quarterly, 4*(3), 23–44.

Noone, J. (1995). Acute pancreatitis: An Orem approach to nursing assessment and care. *Critical Care Nurse, 15*(4), 27–35.

Oppeneer, J. E., & Vervoren, T. M. (1983). *Gerontological pharmacology.* St. Louis: C. V. Mosby.

Paul, S. (1995). The pathophysiologic process of ventricular remodelling: From infarct to failure. *Critical Care Nursing Quarterly, 18*(1), 7–21.

Paul, S., & Hebra, J. D. (1998). *The nurse's guide to cardiac rhythm interpretation: Implications for patient care.* Philadelphia: W. B. Saunders.

Paul, S., & Lee, C. L. (1994). Trauma case review: Survival following impalement. *Critical Care Nurse, 14*(2), 55–59.

Phillips, R. E., & Feeney, M. K. (1990). *The cardiac rhythms: A systematic approach to interpretation* (3rd ed.). Philadelphia: W. B. Saunders.

Planchock, N. Y., & Slay, L. E. (1996). Pharmacokinetic and pharmacodynamic monitoring of the elderly in critical care. *Critical Care Nursing Clinics of North America, 8*, 79–89.

Porth, C. M. (1994). *Pathophysiology: Concepts of altered health states* (4th ed.). Philadelphia: J. B. Lippincott.

Price, S. A., & Wilson, L. M. (1982). *Pathophysiology: Clinical concepts of disease processes* (2nd ed.). New York: McGraw-Hill.

Price, S. A., & Wilson, L. M. (1992). *Pathophysiology: Clinical concepts of disease processes* (4th ed.). New York: McGraw-Hill.

Purcell, J. A., & Holder, C. K. (1989). Cardiomyopathy: Understanding the problem. *American Journal of Nursing, 89*(1), 57–74B.

Raffin, T. A. (1987). ARDS: Mechanisms and management. *Hospital Practice, 22,* 65–80.

Ramsey, J. D., & Tisdale, L. A. (1995). Use of ventricular stroke work index and ventricular function curves in assessing myocardial contractility. *Critical Care Nurse, 15*(1), 61–67.

Reasner, C. A. (1990). Adrenal insufficiency. *Critical Care Nursing Quarterly, 13*(3), 67–73.

Reilly, E., & Yucha, C. B. (1994). Multiple organ failure syndrome. *Critical Care Nurse, 14*(2), 25–31.

Rice, V. (1991). Shock, a clinical syndrome: An update. Part 1, An overview of shock. *Critical Care Nurse, 11*(4), 20–27.

Rice, V. (1991). Shock, a clinical syndrome: An update. Part 2, The stages of shock. *Critical Care Nurse, 11*(5), 74–82.

Rice, V. (1991). Shock, a clinical syndrome: An update. Part 4, Nursing care of the shock patient. *Critical Care Nurse, 11*(7), 28–38.

Richmond, T. S. (1993). Intracranial pressure monitoring. *AACN Clinical Issues in Critical Care Nursing, 4*(1), 148–160.

Roberts, S. L. (1996). *Critical care nursing: Assessment and intervention.* Stamford: Appleton & Lange.

Rusnak, R. A. (1989). Adrenal and pituitary emergencies. *The Emergency Medicine Clinics of North America, 7*(4), 903–915.

Rusy, K. L. (1996). Rebleeding and vasospasm after subarachnoid hemorrhage: A critical care challenge. *Critical Care Nurse, 16*(1), 41–48.

Sabo, C. E., & Michael, C. E. (1989). Diabetic ketoacidosis: Pathophysiology, nursing diagnosis, and nursing interventions. *Focus on Critical Care, 16*(1), 21–28.

Sanford, S., & Disch, J. (1989). *Standards for nursing care of the critically ill* (2nd ed.). San Mateo, CA: Appleton & Lange.

Sansevero, A. C., & Ruddy, Y. (1996). Managing aortic dissections: A critical care challenge. *Critical Care Nurse, 16*(5), 44–50.

Schira, M. G. (1987). Steroid dependent states and adrenal insufficiency: Fluid and electrolyte disturbances. *Nursing Clinics of North America, 22*(4), 837–841.

Schwertz, D. W., & Buschmann, M. T. (1989). Pharmacogeriatrics. *Critical Care Nursing Quarterly, 12*(1), 26–37.

Seidel, H. M., Ball, J. W., Dains, J. E., & Benedict, G. W. (1991). *Mosby's guide to physical examination* (2nd ed.). St. Louis: Mosby.

Seidel, H. M., Ball, J. W., Dains, J. E., & Benedict, G. W. (1994). *Mosby's guide to physical examination* (3rd ed.). St. Louis: Mosby.

Sheehy, S. B. (1984). Primary trauma survey and immediate intervention with the use of the mnemonic ABC. *Journal of Emergency Nursing, 10*(4), 220–221.

Sheehy, S. B., & Jimmerson, C. L. (1994). *Manual of clinical trauma care* (2nd ed.). St. Louis: C. V. Mosby.

Sheehy, S. B., & Lombardi, J. E. (1995). *Manual of emergency care* (4th ed.). St. Louis: C. V. Mosby.

Shekleton, M. E., & Litwak, K. (1991). *Critical care nursing of the surgical patient.* Philadelphia: W. B. Saunders.

Shoemaker, W. C. (1996). Temporal physiologic patterns of shock and circulatory dysfunction based on descriptions by invasive and noninvasive monitoring. *New Horizons, 4,* 300–318.

Sinclair, A. J., & Woodhouse, K. W. (Eds.). (1995). *Acute medical illness in old age.* London: Chapman & Hall Medical.

Sinski, A., & Corbo, J. (1994). Surfactant replacement in adults and children with ARDS: An effective therapy? *Critical Care Nurse, 14*(6), 54–59.

Sommers, M. S. (1994). Alcohol and trauma: The critical link. *Critical Care Nurse 14*(2), 82–93.

Staller, A. G. (1987). Systemic effects of severe head trauma. *Critical Care Nursing Quarterly, 10*(1), 58–68.

Stroud, M., Swindell, B., & Bernard, G. R. (1990). Cellular and humoral mediators of sepsis syndrome. *Critical Care Nursing Clinics of North America, 2*(2), 151–159.

Summers, G. (1990). The clinical and hemodynamic presentation of the shock patient. *Critical Care Nursing Clinics of North America, 2*(2), 161–165.

Swartz, M. H. (1989). *Textbook of physical diagnosis.* Philadelphia: W. B. Saunders.

Swartz, M. H. (1994). *Textbook of physical diagnosis* (2nd ed.). Philadelphia: W. B. Saunders.

Swonger, A. K. & Burbank, P. M. (1995). *Drug therapy and the elderly.* Boston: Jones and Bartlett.

Task Force on Pain in the Elderly of the International Association for the Study of Pain. (1996). *Pain in the elderly.* (B. R. Ferrell & B. A. Ferrell, Eds.). Seattle: IASP Press.

Thierer, J., Perhus, S., McCracken, M. L., Reynolds, M. A., Holmes, A. M., Turton, B., Berkowitz, D. S., & Disch, J. M. (Eds.). (1981). *Standards for nursing care of the critically ill.* Reston, VA: Reston.

Tietz, N. W. (Ed.). (1995). *Clinical guide to laboratory tests* (3rd ed.). Philadelphia: W. B. Saunders.

Timiras, P. S. (Ed.). (1988). *Physiological basis of geriatrics.* New York: Macmillan.

Timiras, P. S. (Ed.). (1994). *Physiological basis of aging and geriatrics* (2nd ed.). Boca Raton: CRC Press.

Turner, D. M., & Turner, L. A. (1995). Right ventricular myocardial infarction: Detection, treatment, and nursing implications. *Critical Care Nurse, 15*(1), 22–27.

Turner, J. G., & Williamson, K. M. (1986). AIDS. *Focus On Critical Care, 13*(4), 41–50.

Urban, N. (1986). Integrating hemodynamic parameters with clinical decision-making. *Critical Care Nurse, 6*(2), 48–61.

Urban, N. (1993). Integrating the hemodynamic profile with clinical assessment. *AACN Clinical Issues in Critical Care Nursing, 4*(1), 161–179.

Vazquez, M., Lazear, S. E., & Larson, E. L. (1992). *Critical care nursing* (2nd ed.). Philadelphia: W. B. Saunders.

Wachtel, T. L. (1994). Critical care concepts in the management of abdominal trauma. *Critical Care Nursing Quarterly, 17*(2), 34–50.

Walleck, C. A. (1992). Preventing secondary brain injury. *AACN Clinical Issues in Critical Care Nursing, 3*(1), 19–30.

Waxman, K. (1996). Ischemia, reperfusion, and inflammation. *New Horizons, 4,* 153–160.

White, K. M. (1993). Using continuous $S\overline{v}O_2$ to assess oxygen supply/demand balance in the critically ill patient. *AACN Clinical Issues in Critical Care Nursing, 4*(1), 134–147.

Wiener, S. L. (1993). *Differential diagnosis of acute pain: By body region.* New York: McGraw-Hill.

Woods, S. L., & Osquthorpe, S. (1993). Cardiac output determination. *AACN Clinical Issues in Critical Care Nursing, 4*(1), 81–97.

Workman, M. L., Ellerhorst-Ryan, J. & Hargrave-Koertge. V. (1993). *Nursing care of the immunocompromised patient.* Philadelphia: W. B. Saunders.

Bibliography

Agana-Defensor, R., & Proch, M. (1992). Pheochromocytoma: A clinical review. *AACN Clinical Issues in Critical Care Nursing, 13*(2), 309–318.

Angerio, A. D., & Kot, P. A. (1994). Pathophysiology of pulmonary edema. (1994). *Critical Care Nursing Quarterly, 17*(3), 21–26.

Batcheller, J. (1992). Disorders of antidiuretic hormone secretion. *AACN Clinical Issues in Critical Care Nursing, 13*(2), 370–378.

Bridges, E. J., & Middleton, R. (1997). Direct arterial vs. oscillometric monitoring of blood pressure: Stop comparing and pick one: A decision-making algorithm. *Critical Care Nurse, 17*(3), 58–72.

Carrougher, G. J. (1993). Inhalation injury. *AACN Clinical Issues in Critical Care Nursing, 4*(2), 365–377.

Cheney, P. (1994). Early management and physiologic changes in crush syndrome. *Critical Care Nursing Quarterly, 17*(2), 62–73.

Gumowski, J., & Loughran, M. (1996). Diseases of the adrenal gland. *The Nursing Clinics of North America, 31*(4), 747–768.

Fein, A. M., & Adelman, R. D. (Eds.). (1994). Critical illness in the elderly. *Clinics in Geriatric Medicine 10*, 1–229.

Johannsen, J. M. (1993). Update: Guidelines for treating hypertension. *American Journal of Nursing, 93*(3), 42–49.

Kowalak, M. M., & Criddle, L. M. (1997). Laryngotracheal disruption. *Critical Care Nurse, 17*(3), 87–93.

Lee, L. M., & Gumowski, J. (1992). Adrenocortical insufficiency: A medical emergency. *AACN Clinical Issues in Critical Care Nursing, 13*(2), 319–330.

Loriaux, T. C. (1996). Endocrine assessment: Red flags for those on the front lines. *The Nursing Clinics of North America, 31*(4), 695–713.

Pousada, L. (Ed.). (1993). Geriatric emergency care. *Clinics in Geriatric Medicine 9*, 491–681.

Prociuk, J. L. (1995). Management of cerebral oxygen supply-demand balance in blunt head injury. *Critical Care Nurse, 15*(4), 38–45.

Rusterholtz, A. (1996). Interpretation of diagnostic laboratory tests in selected endocrine disorders. *The Nursing Clinics of North America, 31*(4), 715–724.

Sauve, D. O., & Kessler, C. A. (1992). Hyperglycemic emergencies. *AACN Clinical Issues in Critical Care Nursing, 13*(2), 350–360.

Secor, V. H. (1994). The inflammatory/immune response in critical illness: Role of the systemic inflammatory response syndrome. *Critical Care Nursing Clinics of North America, 6*(2), 251–264.

Sikes, P. J. (1992). Endocrine responses to the stress of critical illness. *AACN Clinical Issues in Critical Care Nursing, 13*(2), 379–391.

Sommers, M. S. (1995). Missed injuries: A case of trauma hide and seek. *AACN Clinical Issues in Critical Care Nursing, 6*(2), 187–195.

Spittle, L. (1992). Diagnoses in opposition: Thyroid storm and myxedema coma. *AACN Clinical Issues in Critical Care Nursing, 13*(2), 300–308.

Tasota, F. J., Fisher, E. M., Coulson, C. F., & Hoffman, L. A. (1998). Protecting ICU patients from nosocomial infections: Practical measures for favorable outcomes. *Critical Care Nurse, 18*(1), 54–65.

Teplitz, L. (1993). Hypertensive crisis: Review and update. *Critical Care Nurse, 13*(6), 20–35.

Thompson, C. L. (1995). Critical care-acquired pneumonia. *Critical Care Nursing Clinics, 7*(4), 695–702.

Urden, L. D., Lough, M. E., & Stacy, K. M. (1996). *Priorities in critical care nursing* (2nd ed.). St. Louis: C. V. Mosby.

Von Rueden, K. T., & Harris, J. R. (1995). Pulmonary dysfunction related to immobility in the trauma patient. *AACN Clinical Issues in Critical Care Nursing, 6*(2), 212–228.

Winfree, J., & Barillo, D. J. (1997). Nonthermal injuries. *The Nursing Clinics of North America, 32*(2), 275–296.

Wirtz, K. M., La Favor, K. M., & Ang, R. (1996). Managing chronic spinal cord injury: Issues in critical care. *Critical Care Nurse, 16*(4), 24–35.

Index

Note: Page numbers in *italics* refer to illustrations; page numbers followed by t refer to tables.